Evaluation of the Lovell Federal Health Care Center Merger

Findings, Conclusions, and Recommendations

AF621727

Committee on Evaluation of the Lovell Federal Health Care Center Merger

Board on the Health of Select Populations

INSTITUTE OF MEDICINE
OF THE NATIONAL ACADEMIES

THE NATIONAL ACADEMIES PRESS
Washington, D.C.
www.nap.edu

THE NATIONAL ACADEMIES PRESS 500 Fifth Street, NW Washington, DC 20001

NOTICE: The project that is the subject of this report was approved by the Governing Board of the National Research Council, whose members are drawn from the councils of the National Academy of Sciences, the National Academy of Engineering, and the Institute of Medicine. The members of the committee responsible for the report were chosen for their special competences and with regard for appropriate balance.

This study was supported by Contract/Grant No. HT0011-10-C-0002 between the National Academy of Sciences and the Department of Defense. Any opinions, findings, conclusions, or recommendations expressed in this publication are those of the author(s) and do not necessarily reflect the views of the organizations or agencies that provided support for the project.

International Standard Book Number-13: 978-0-309-26279-8
International Standard Book Number-10: 0-309-26279-8

Additional copies of this report are available for sale from the National Academies Press, 500 Fifth Street, NW, Keck 360, Washington, DC 20001; (800) 624-6242 or (202) 334-3313; http://www.nap.edu.

For more information about the Institute of Medicine, visit the IOM home page at: **www.iom.edu.**

Copyright 2012 by the National Academy of Sciences. All rights reserved.

Printed in the United States of America

The serpent has been a symbol of long life, healing, and knowledge among almost all cultures and religions since the beginning of recorded history. The serpent adopted as a logotype by the Institute of Medicine is a relief carving from ancient Greece, now held by the Staatliche Museen in Berlin.

Suggested citation: IOM (Institute of Medicine). 2012. *Evaluation of the Lovell Federal Health Care Center merger: Findings, conclusions, and recommendations.* Washington, DC: The National Academies Press.

"Knowing is not enough; we must apply.
Willing is not enough; we must do."

—Goethe

INSTITUTE OF MEDICINE
OF THE NATIONAL ACADEMIES

Advising the Nation. Improving Health.

THE NATIONAL ACADEMIES

Advisers to the Nation on Science, Engineering, and Medicine

The **National Academy of Sciences** is a private, nonprofit, self-perpetuating society of distinguished scholars engaged in scientific and engineering research, dedicated to the furtherance of science and technology and to their use for the general welfare. Upon the authority of the charter granted to it by the Congress in 1863, the Academy has a mandate that requires it to advise the federal government on scientific and technical matters. Dr. Ralph J. Cicerone is president of the National Academy of Sciences.

The **National Academy of Engineering** was established in 1964, under the charter of the National Academy of Sciences, as a parallel organization of outstanding engineers. It is autonomous in its administration and in the selection of its members, sharing with the National Academy of Sciences the responsibility for advising the federal government. The National Academy of Engineering also sponsors engineering programs aimed at meeting national needs, encourages education and research, and recognizes the superior achievements of engineers. Dr. Charles M. Vest is president of the National Academy of Engineering.

The **Institute of Medicine** was established in 1970 by the National Academy of Sciences to secure the services of eminent members of appropriate professions in the examination of policy matters pertaining to the health of the public. The Institute acts under the responsibility given to the National Academy of Sciences by its congressional charter to be an adviser to the federal government and, upon its own initiative, to identify issues of medical care, research, and education. Dr. Harvey V. Fineberg is president of the Institute of Medicine.

The **National Research Council** was organized by the National Academy of Sciences in 1916 to associate the broad community of science and technology with the Academy's purposes of furthering knowledge and advising the federal government. Functioning in accordance with general policies determined by the Academy, the Council has become the principal operating agency of both the National Academy of Sciences and the National Academy of Engineering in providing services to the government, the public, and the scientific and engineering communities. The Council is administered jointly by both Academies and the Institute of Medicine. Dr. Ralph J. Cicerone and Dr. Charles M. Vest are chair and vice chair, respectively, of the National Research Council.

www.national-academies.org

COMMITTEE ON EVALUATION OF THE LOVELL FEDERAL HEALTH CARE CENTER MERGER

MICHAEL M. E. JOHNS (*Co-Chair*), Chancellor, Emory University, Atlanta, GA
STEPHEN M. SHORTELL (*Co-Chair*), Dean of the School of Public Health, Blue Cross of California Distinguished Professor of Health Policy & Management, and Professor of Organization Behavior, School of Public Health and Haas School of Business, University of California, Berkeley
NANCY R. ADAMS, Senior Partner, Martin, Blanck & Associates, Falls Church, VA
GEORGE K. ANDERSON, Executive Director, Association of Military Surgeons of the United States, Bethesda, MD
PETER B. ANGOOD, Chief Executive Officer, American College of Physician Executives, Tampa, FL
LAWTON R. (ROBERT) BURNS, Chair of the Health Care Management Department, James Joo-Jin Kim Professor, and Professor of Health Care Management, Wharton School, University of Pennsylvania, Philadelphia
EMMANUEL G. CASSIMATIS, President and Chief Executive Officer, Educational Commission for Foreign Medical Graduates, Philadelphia, PA
TIMOTHY C. FLYNN, Senior Associate Dean for Clinical Affairs, College of Medicine, and Chief Medical Officer, Shands Hospital, University of Florida, Gainesville
LARRY M. MANHEIM, Research Professor in the Institute for Healthcare Studies and the Department of Physical Medicine and Rehabilitation, Northwestern University Feinberg School of Medicine, Chicago, IL
JOHN E. MAUPIN, JR., President and Chief Executive Officer, Morehouse School of Medicine, Atlanta, GA
KAREN L. MILLER, Senior Vice Chancellor for Academic and Student Affairs, University of Kansas Medical Center, Kansas City
FRANCES M. MURPHY, President, Sigma Health Consulting, LLC, Silver Spring, MD
J. MARC OVERHAGE, Chief Medical Informatics Officer, Siemens Health Services, Malvern, PA
SUSANNE TROPEZ-SIMS, Associate Dean of Clinical Affiliations and Professor of Pediatrics, Meharry Medical College, Nashville, TN
CAROLYN (CINDY) WATTS, Professor and Chair of the Department of Health Administration, Virginia Commonwealth University, Richmond

Consultants

DAVID K. BARNES, Advanced Policy Solutions, Bethesda, MD
THOMAS A. D'AUNNO, Executive Vice Dean, Mailman School of Public Health, Columbia University, New York, NY

IOM Study Staff

MICHAEL McGEARY, Study Director
SUSAN R. McCUTCHEN, Senior Program Associate
LaVITA SULLIVAN, Senior Program Assistant
FREDERICK (RICK) ERDTMANN, Director, Board on the Health of Select Populations

Reviewers

This report has been reviewed in draft form by individuals chosen for their diverse perspectives and technical expertise, in accordance with procedures approved by the National Research Council's Report Review Committee. The purpose of this independent review is to provide candid and critical comments that will assist the institution in making its published report as sound as possible and to ensure that the report meets institutional standards for objectivity, evidence, and responsiveness to the study charge. The review comments and draft manuscript remain confidential to protect the integrity of the deliberative process. We wish to thank the following individuals for their review of this report:

Elizabeth H. Bradley, Yale School of Public Health
Timothy G. Buchman, Emory University School of Medicine
Jon B. Christianson, University of Minnesota School of Public Health
Audrey C. Drake, Department of Veterans Affairs (Deputy Chief Nursing Officer Emeritus)
Nancy E. Dunlap, University of Alabama at Birmingham
Richard G. Frank, Harvard Medical School
Kyle L. Grazier, University of Michigan School of Public Health
James E. Hastings, Department of Veterans Affairs Pacific Islands Health Care System
Richard E. Oliver, University of Missouri School of Health Professions
Jonathan B. Perlin, Hospital Corporation of America

Lawrence M. Riddles, American College of Physician Executives
Paul H. Rockey, Accreditation Council for Graduate Medical Education
Hector P. Rodriguez, University of California, Los Angeles, School of Public Health
James M. Walker, Geisinger Health System

Although the reviewers listed above have provided many constructive comments and suggestions, they were not asked to endorse the conclusions or recommendations, nor did they see the final draft of the report before its release. The review of this report was overseen by **Charles E. Phelps,** University of Rochester, and **David R. Challoner,** University of Florida. Appointed by the National Research Council and the Institute of Medicine, they were responsible for making certain that an independent examination of this report was carried out in accordance with institutional procedures and that all review comments were carefully considered. Responsibility for the final content of this report rests entirely with the authoring committee and the institution.

Preface

An important experiment in federal health care delivery is taking place in North Chicago, Illinois. In 2010, the Navy and the Department of Veterans Affairs (VA) consolidated their medical centers, which had operated 1.5 miles apart from each other for many years, into a joint health care center named the Captain James A. Lovell Federal Health Care Center (FHCC) after the well-known astronaut who lives near the facility. In a time of severe fiscal constraints and heightened concern about smoothing the transition of injured military servicemembers from active duty to veteran status, the possibility of providing better care at less cost by combining military and VA medical centers in the same health care market has great appeal. The outcomes of the Lovell FHCC experiment, therefore, are of significant interest to federal policy makers.

The 1995 Defense Base Consolidation and Realignment Commission decided to consolidate Navy recruit training, then in three locations, at the Naval Station Great Lakes, located near the city of North Chicago. This decision gave more urgency to the need to replace the old and obsolete Navy hospital with a new hospital, an action the Navy had planned for 2007. In 1999, a VA task force proposed converting the North Chicago VA medical center from a hospital to an outpatient facility, which was strongly opposed by veterans, community leaders, and their representatives in Congress. The solution reached by the VA/Department of Defense (DoD) Health Executive Council (HEC) was to have the Navy use the VA hospital for inpatient and emergency services rather than to build a new Navy hospital. The new arrangement was expected to reduce costs for the Navy and the VA while increasing the patient workload enough to justify keeping the VA hospital open. The Navy began to use the North Chicago VA medical center for acute inpatient mental health services in 2003 and for all inpatient medical, surgical, and pediatric services in 2006.

In 2002, the HEC directed the Navy to build an outpatient facility next to the North Chicago VA medical center, so that all care for veterans and Navy servicemembers and other DoD beneficiaries could be provided in one location. This model had been pioneered in Albuquerque, New Mexico, where the VA medical center provides inpatient services to DoD beneficiaries, who receive their outpatient care at the Air Force ambulatory care center next to it. Similarly, veterans in Hawaii and south-central Alaska receive outpatient services from VA ambulatory care facilities built beside the Army and Air Force hospitals in Honolulu and Anchorage, respectively, where they go to receive inpatient services. These cooperative arrangements, in addition to several other similar, extensive VA/DoD health care sharing arrangements in various locations around the United States, are called "joint ventures." In joint ventures, the VA medical center and the military medical center agree to reimburse each other for services received.

In 2005, the HEC made the momentous decision to go beyond the joint venture model and create the first "integrated" FHCC in North Chicago, which was characterized by a combined medical staff organized in a single set of clinical departments under one chief medical executive, a single set of administrative units, and a single chain of command under one FHCC chief executive. The date set for full integration was October 1, 2010, barely 5 years in the future.

The decision was based on the idea that a single organization should be able to provide better care for patients at lower cost for taxpayers than would a joint venture. The care should be better because it would be more comprehensive and coordinated, and the financial costs should be reduced because of economies of scale, reduced duplication, and other efficiencies. Local Navy and VA leaders fully embraced the concept of the Lovell FHCC, especially the idea of having one staff and one system wherever possible rather than having two side by side. The systems in question included quality assurance, patient medical records, provider accreditation, budgeting and accounting, personnel management, purchasing, and physical plant management.

A long and complicated process ensued, which included accommodating the separate but overlapping missions of the DoD and the VA health systems; reconciling the different policies and procedures, performance measures, and organizational cultures of the Navy and the VA; and overcoming several statutory limitations on interdepartmental integration, such as strictures on transferring property and personnel. Chapter 3 in this report reviews this implementation process, identifies the main issues that had to be resolved between the Navy and the VA, and documents how they were resolved—sometimes fully, sometimes partially, and sometimes not at all.

Some areas of incomplete or nonintegration, such as having to operate the provider accreditation systems of both departments, have resulted in continued duplication and thus are reducing potential efficiencies. Others affect patient care. Most critically, the VA and the DoD electronic health record (EHR) systems are not compatible, and few of the software programs created to make them interoperable—that is, to make it possible to enter one EHR system (or an interface) and view and enter information in both EHR systems simultaneously so that care can be optimized—were operational when the Lovell FHCC opened. To ensure, at a minimum, that patient safety is not compromised by harmful drug interactions or allergies, the Lovell FHCC had to develop costly manual pharmacy workarounds. When DoD patients are seen by VA specialty, inpatient, and emergency medicine providers, manual workarounds are necessary to enter the clinical information recorded in the VA EHR system into the DoD EHR system. We should note that this problem has been recognized and was part of the reason that in early 2011 the DoD and VA secretaries committed their departments to developing a joint EHR system, beginning with the single pharmacy system that is greatly needed at the Lovell FHCC.

In Chapter 4, our committee assesses the results of the integration experiment, to the extent they can be ascertained after less than 2 years of operation. Clearly, the leaders of the North Chicago FHCC initiative have succeeded, through tremendous effort, in creating a single organization serving both beneficiary populations. However, the degree of integration of clinical and administrative services varies across the organization, mostly because of external constraints. Nonetheless, the more important questions are whether the creation of the FHCC in North Chicago has been worthwhile and if it is a good model for merging the VA and the DoD health care delivery systems in other locations where they have facilities in close proximity.

The Lovell FHCC has not been in operation long enough to determine the benefits accrued and to assess whether it has been cost effective. Appendix B contains an evaluation framework that would be useful for the DoD and the VA to adopt so that at the end of the 5-year demonstration period for the Lovell FHCC these organizations will be able to decide whether the merger is worthwhile and whether it can be replicated elsewhere. In the meantime, our report recommends some ways that the departments could facilitate integration by resolving differences in department policies, procedures, and systems at the national level.

We would like to thank many people who helped with this study. Most are listed in the Acknowledgments section of the report; others contributed by agreeing to give confidential interviews, which were extremely helpful.

We are particularly grateful to Janice Halkovich of the Lovell FHCC for arranging interviews and access to data and for helping to schedule presentations at the committee's two meetings in North Chicago. We would also like to thank the hardworking members of the committee who attended the meetings, read extensive materials between meetings, and helped draft the report and review its several iterations. Their experience and expertise were critical to this evaluation and in formulating the committee's consensus conclusions and recommendations. Finally, we would like to thank the Institute of Medicine staff—Michael McGeary, Susan R. McCutchen, and LaVita Sullivan—who diligently collected the enormous amount of information that forms the basis of this report and organized our meetings to facilitate productive discussions.

Michael M. E. Johns, and
Stephen M. Shortell, *Co-Chairs*
Committee on Evaluation of the
Lovell Federal Health Care Center Merger

Acknowledgments

Many individuals and organizations contributed to the study. In particular, the committee and staff would like to thank the individuals listed below who took the time to provide information about, and their views of, the implementation, operation, and impacts of the Captain James A. Lovell Federal Health Care Center (Lovell FHCC). The committee would also like to thank the approximately 50 individuals who agreed to be interviewed on a confidential basis, who cannot be listed here but who provided important input into the study.

Mark Albrecht, Lovell FHCC
Mary Ann Allred, Lovell FHCC
CDR Martin Anerino, Lovell FHCC
Norman Arnswald, Veteran/Lovell FHCC Customer
CAPT Dale Barrette, Lovell FHCC
CAPT David J. Beardsley, Lovell FHCC
CAPT Steven G. Bethke, Recruit Training Command, Naval Station Great Lakes
Thomas Bresciano, Lovell FHCC
Jill K. Center, Government Accountability Office (GAO)
Kenneth L. Cox, Office of the Assistant Secretary of Defense for Health Affairs, Department of Defense (DoD)
Joseph X. DiMario, Rosalind Franklin University of Medicine and Science
CDR Bridgette Faber, Lovell FHCC
Imran Faizi, Lovell FHCC

Debra M. Filippi, DoD/Department of Veterans Affairs (VA) Interagency Program Office
Lenny Floom, Veteran/Lovell FHCC Customer
LCDR Aaron Frank, Lovell FHCC
Leanne Fredrickson, Lovell FHCC
Sarah Fouse, Lovell FHCC
CMC Ross Gilliatt, Lovell FHCC
Janice Halkovich, Lovell FHCC
Tariq Hassan, Lovell FHCC
CAPT Rich Hayden, Lovell FHCC
COL Claude Hines, Jr., Military Health System, DoD
Patrick Hull, Lovell FHCC
Andre Greedan, Lovell FHCC
Ronald Kaplan, Rosalind Franklin University of Medicine and Science
Laura Kelly, VA Northern California Health Care System
CMDR Ruth Kline, Lovell FHCC
CDR Eileen Knoble, Lovell FHCC
CAPT Norman Lee, Lovell FHCC
Frank Maldonado, Lovell FHCC
Karen T. Malebranche, Office of Interagency Health Affairs, VA
John G. Manczko, Lovell FHCC
Tiffany McFadden, Lovell FHCC
Barbara Meadows, Lovell FHCC
Gloria E. Meredith, Rosalind Franklin University of Medicine and Science
James Miller, Lovell FHCC
Paul Morgan, Lovell FHCC
CAPT Maryalice Morro, Navy Medicine East, Bureau of Medicine and Surgery, U.S. Navy
Clifford Moudy, Lovell FHCC
Jeffrey A. Murawsky, Veterans Integrated Service Network 12, VA
Robert Opsut, Office of the Assistant Secretary of Defense for Health Affairs, DoD
CAPT Kevin Otte, Lovell FHCC
CAPT James Oxford, Lovell FHCC
Kelvin Parks, Lovell FHCC
Nancy L. Parsley, Rosalind Franklin University of Medicine and Science
Michael Peck, Lake County Veterans Assistance Commission
LCDR Donna Poulin, Lovell FHCC
Robert Charles Powell, Constituent, Illinois 10th Congressional District

Wendy Rheault, Rosalind Franklin University of Medicine and Science
Russell Robertson, Rosalind Franklin University of Medicine and Science
Mary Schindler, Lovell FHCC
Marianne Semrad, Lovell FHCC
Robert Sorensen, Lovell FHCC
Patrick L. Sullivan, Lovell FHCC
Gregory X. Swanson, TRICARE North Region
Keith Tietmeyer, Office of Information and Technology, VA
Estan Villarreal, Veteran/Lovell FHCC Customer
Piyush Vyas, Lovell FHCC
K. Michael Welch, Rosalind Franklin University of Medicine and Science
E. Jane Whipple, GAO
Lt. Col. Doreen Wilder, David Grant U.S. Air Force Medical Center
Malissa G. Winograd, GAO
Edwin Zarling, Lovell FHCC

Contents

Tables, Figures, and Boxes

TABLES

FIGURES

BOXES

Abbreviations and Acronyms

200H	Naval Hospital Great Lakes (also referred to as NHGL)
ACC	ambulatory care center
AHLTA	Armed Forces Health Longitudinal Technology Application
ANACI	Access National Agency Check with Inquiries
APC	ambulatory payment classification
APN	advanced practice nurse
ARC	Allocation Resource Center
BAH	Booz-Allen & Hamilton (former name for Booz Allen Hamilton)
BHIE	Bi-directional Health Information Exchange
BRAC	Base Realignment and Closure
BUMED	Bureau of Medicine and Surgery
CAC	common access card
CAP	community-acquired pneumonia
CARES	Capital Asset Realignment for Enhanced Services
CCQAS	Centralized Credentials and Quality Assurance System
CHAMPUS	Civilian Health and Medical Program of the Uniformed Services
CHDR	Clinical Data Repository/Health Data Repository
CMOP	Consolidated Mail Order Pharmacy
CMS	Centers for Medicare & Medicaid Services
CNA	Center for Naval Analyses

CO	commanding officer
CPRS	Computerized Patient Record System
CR	continuing resolution
CTG	clinical task group
DMHRSi	Defense Medical Human Resources Systems-internet
DMLSS	Defense Medical Logistics Standard Support
DoD	Department of Defense
DOS	disk operating system
DSS	Decision Support System
DWV	dental weighted value
EA	executive agreement
eDR	enhanced document referral
ED	emergency department
EDM	executive decision memorandum
EHR	electronic health record
ESA	executive sharing agreement
FHCC	federal health care center
FHCF	federal health care facility
FLITE	Financial and Logistics Integrated Technology Enterprise program
FMS	Financial Management System
FTE	full-time equivalent
FY	fiscal year
GAO	Government Accountability Office (since 2004) or General Accounting Office (prior to 2004)
GIP	Generic Inventory Package
GLAC	Great Lakes Acquisition Center
HEC	Health Executive Council
HEDIS	Healthcare Effectiveness Data and Information Set
HR	human resources
ICTB	Inter-facility Credentialing Transfer Brief
ICU	intensive care unit
IDC	independent duty corpsman
IDES	Integrated Disability Evaluation System
iEHR	integrated electronic health record
IM	information management
IM/IT	information management/information technology

IOM	Institute of Medicine
IPO	Interagency Program Office
IT	information technology
JEC	Joint Executive Council
JFURSWG	Joint Facility Utilization Resource Sharing Working Group
JIF	Joint Incentive Fund
JMFDF	Joint Medical Facility Demonstration Fund
LTG	leadership task group
MAXIMO	Department of Veterans Affairs asset management commercial, web-based software program
MHS	Military Health System
MOA	memorandum of agreement
MRI	magnetic resonance imaging
MSPT	mission specific pass-through
MS-RWP	Medicare severity relative weighted product
MTF	military treatment facility
NACI	National Agency Check with Inquiries
NCOD	National Center for Organizational Development
NCVAMC	North Chicago Veterans Affairs Medical Center
NDAA	National Defense Authorization Act
NFEC	Naval Facilities Engineering Command
NHCGL	Naval Health Clinic Great Lakes
NHCU	nursing home care unit
NHGL	Naval Hospital Great Lakes (also referred to as 200H)
NME	Navy Medicine East
NMLC	Naval Medical Logistics Command
NRMC	Naval Regional Medical Center
NSGL	Naval Station Great Lakes
OHA	Office of Health Affairs
OMB	Office of Management and Budget
OPM	Office of Personnel Management
ORYX	Joint Commission's performance measure
PA	physician's assistant
PACS	picture archiving and communication system
PIV	personal identity verification
PSC	personal services contract

RTC	Recruit Training Command
RTC Recap	Recruit Training Command Recapitalization Program
RVU	relative value unit
RWP	relative weighted product
SAC	Stakeholder Advisory Committee
SCIP	Surgical Care Improvement Project
TFL	TRICARE for Life
TRICARE	military health care insurance system
TSC	Training Support Center
USS	United States ship
VA	Department of Veterans Affairs
VAMC	Department of Veterans Affairs medical center
VHA	Veterans Health Administration
VISN	Veterans Integrated Service Network
VistA	Veterans Health Information Systems and Technology Architecture

Summary

The Captain James A. Lovell Federal Health Care Center (FHCC) in North Chicago, Illinois, is an effort by the Departments of Veterans Affairs (VA) and Defense (DoD) to create a national model for joint delivery of health care that is more accessible and less expensive than operating two federal medical centers serving overlapping beneficiaries in the same area. The creation of the Lovell FHCC also permits the VA to continue and even to expand inpatient services in North Chicago—where the North Chicago Veterans Affairs Medical Center (NCVAMC) had been threatened with closure—because of the additional workload provided by Navy beneficiaries after the Naval Hospital Great Lakes (NHGL) was closed.

North Chicago is the site of Naval Station Great Lakes, which houses the Recruit Training Command (RTC) and the Training Support Center (TSC). The RTC runs the Navy's boot camp for all new enlisted recruits, and the TSC runs the "A" schools, which are advanced training programs for enlisted sailors. Each year, approximately 35,000 recruits and 16,000 A-school students spend several months at Great Lakes. NHGL's catchment area also includes approximately 67,000 military retirees and family members. The NCVAMC was built on former Navy land, and its catchment area contains approximately 78,000 military veterans. When planning for the Lovell FHCC began in the early 2000s, NCVAMC recorded approximately 215,000 outpatient visits and 600 acute inpatient admissions per year. At the NHGL, there were approximately 600,000 medical outpatient visits, 187,000 dental outpatient visits, and 2,600 acute inpatient admissions per year.

The VA and the DoD had operated separate medical centers 1.5 miles apart in North Chicago since 1926. By the late 1990s, each was underused because of the shift of most patient care to outpatient settings. In addition, the naval hospital had become obsolete and needed to be replaced. When the NCVAMC's inpatient operations were recommended for closure in 1999, local veterans organized to keep it open. The Illinois congressional delegation, aware that the Navy was planning to build a replacement hospital, urged the DoD and the VA to combine their services in a state-of-the-art federal health care center. Senator Richard Durbin later explained that

> the aim of the delegation was to keep the North Chicago VA Medical Center open, improve options for medical care for the Navy, improve training options for VA and Navy medical personnel, reduce costs, and improve access to health care for veterans and Department of Defense beneficiaries. (Durbin, 2003)

In 2002, the assistant secretary of defense for health affairs and the VA under secretary for health—as co-chairs of the Health Executive Council (HEC)—agreed on a plan to share facilities and services in North Chicago. In a multistep process, the Navy would close its hospital and use the NCVAMC to provide emergency and inpatient care to its beneficiaries and build a shared ambulatory care center adjacent to the NCVAMC. The VA would renovate and upgrade the NCVAMC's inpatient medical and surgical facilities and emergency department and allow Navy surgeons to practice in the VA hospital building. According to William Winkenwerder, Jr., the assistant secretary of defense for health affairs,

> With this agreement, the Navy gains a modern ambulatory care center at a cost less than building a new hospital. VA beneficiaries gain increased access to surgical care closer to their homes and families. And the overall operating expenses of both departments should be reduced. (VA, 2002)

In 2003, the Navy closed its inpatient psychiatry ward and began sending patients to the NCVAMC for acute inpatient psychiatry care. In 2004, the Navy moved its blood processing center to vacant space in the NCVAMC, in return for providing a share of the blood products to the VA. The departments also agreed to move the rest of the NHGL's inpatient and emergency care and Navy surgeons to the NCVAMC in 2006, after the VA had completed a $13 million renovation of the NCVAMC's inpatient medical and surgical facilities and emergency room. In June 2006, Navy inpatients began to be treated at the NCVAMC, and the NHGL became the Naval Health Clinic Great Lakes (NHCGL).

In 2005, the assistant secretary of defense for health affairs and the VA under secretary for health agreed to develop a federal health care facility that would integrate clinical and administrative services under a single line of authority. The decision to adopt a single chain of command was unprecedented. The VA and the DoD had each built an ambulatory care center next to the other's hospital in Honolulu and Albuquerque and were even sharing a "federal" hospital built for that purpose by the DoD in Las Vegas; however, in each case, the organizations operated alongside each other and billed each other for the services provided to the other's beneficiaries. The Lovell FHCC was going to be, and still is, unique in having a single overall command structure, integrated staff, and unified budget. The intent was to create an organizational structure in which health care services could be better coordinated with patient needs, which would presumably improve the range of, the access to, and the quality of the services. The FHCC was expected to be a showplace for new software that would enable providers to enter either the DoD or the VA electronic health record (EHR), or a common interface, and see and enter information in both EHRs in real time, a capability called interoperability. It was also expected to increase efficiency—by enabling FHCC managers to match resources to needs in ways that would be impeded by having to coordinate separate bureaucracies and budgets—and to produce cost savings by eliminating duplication.

The 2005 decision to have an integrated federal health care facility also included approval for construction by the Navy of a 201,000-square-foot ambulatory care center (ACC) connected to the VA hospital building and expanded parking facilities and renovation of 45,000 square feet in the hospital building for outpatient clinics. The timeline for the completion of the ACC in 2010 gave the planners 5 years to prepare for the switch to a single organization.

IMPLEMENTATION

The HEC formed six task groups to develop the detailed operational plans for an integrated health care center.[1] Each task group was co-chaired by the VA and the DoD and included local, regional, and central office representatives of each department. They met monthly, except for the leadership task group, which met weekly and coordinated the overall effort.

[1] The six were the leadership, clinical, information management/information technology, administration, human resources, and finance/budget task groups. A seventh task group, for communications, was formed later.

The Vision

The local leaders of the leadership task group—the director of the NCVAMC[2] and the current commander of the NHGL/NHCGL,[3] as well as key members of their staffs—had a consistent vision of the way the Lovell FHCC should function to achieve its mission of providing seamless health care to all patients, regardless of their status as VA or DoD beneficiaries or as providers. The vision was to have, to the fullest extent possible, one set of organizational units and systems rather than two (VA and DoD) side by side within the FHCC. For example, the local leadership pushed for single systems for finance (e.g., purchasing, logistics and inventory, payroll, assets), personnel and human resources management, facilities management, appointment scheduling, medical records and other information management systems, credentialing, workload measurement, performance measures, and inspector general inspections. They wanted a single operating fund and budget so that the FHCC staff did not have to determine which department's funds were being used for what purpose in daily operations. They envisioned a combined medical staff organized into single departments and clinics under one chief medical officer and operating under a single set of bylaws and one standard of care for all patients.

Constraints on Integration

The FHCC planners did not anticipate being able to fully achieve their vision because they were aware at the outset of several critical constraints that would hinder achieving full integration. For example, while one personnel system could be put into place to accommodate the Navy and the VA civilians, this was not possible for uniformed personnel. The departments agreed at the time of the 2005 decision that the FHCC director would be from the VA and the deputy director from the Navy, but pay, promotion, and disciplinary authority over military personnel could not be assumed by the VA director. It was not practical to integrate the clinical operations of branch clinics on the naval base serving enlisted recruits and students, although they were included as part of the FHCC. The law governing DoD/VA health care sharing limits it to excess capacity on the part of one department or the other, which limits the number of clinics that can schedule

[2] Patrick Sullivan has been the director of the North Chicago Veterans Affairs Medical Center since 2003 and was the associate director for the previous 6 years.

[3] There have been three commanders since 2003: Captains Michael Anderson (2003–2006), Thomas McGue (2006–2010), and David Beardsley (2010–present). A new commander will be appointed in 2012. Both McGue and Beardsley were posted to North Chicago to work with their predecessors for months before taking command in an effort to preserve continuity of leadership.

appointments without regard to the departmental affiliation of the provider or patient.

A critical constraint was the existence of two EHR systems that had to be maintained separately although the ability to communicate patient information between them was limited. Using both systems was necessary because the Navy personnel would be using DoD's EHRs in other locations throughout their career and veterans might use other VA medical centers if they moved or were traveling. The departments agreed to develop novel software for entering, viewing, and revising information in both EHR systems simultaneously, but they constrained the development process at the outset by stipulating that neither of them could be changed. They also left little time for the software development—less than 2 years.

Another critical constraint was the need for local leaders and staff to continue to serve their current patients without reducing access or quality while the planning and implementation of the FHCC was taking place. Most of the planning and implementation work was done by existing staff in addition to their regular work, which limited the degree of change that could be considered. Time for education and training of staff in preparation for new FHCC policies and procedures was also limited.

The biggest constraint was—and is—the existence of the three departments involved—the DoD, the Navy, and the VA. The VA and the DoD have different missions and are separately accountable for their performances to the president of the United States and Congress. Each has its own priorities and goals and associated business processes. Although the Department of the Navy is part of the DoD, it has a certain amount of discretion in how it carries out its business, which can be more specific or strict than DoD's policies and procedures (and different from the Army's or the Air Force's policies and procedures).

Ultimately, no matter how seamlessly it conducts its daily business, the Lovell FHCC has to report to the Navy and to the DoD on how well it performs as a military treatment facility (MTF) and to the VA on how well it performs as a VA medical center (VAMC). This set of dual standards and reporting requirements is an extra burden for the FHCC compared with what is required for an MTF or a VAMC. It also limits the feasibility and cost effectiveness of integrating functions. For example, the VA and the DoD have different standards for timeliness of routine medical appointments, that is, within 14 and 7 days, respectively, which must be tracked and the performance reported. This is part of the reason the FHCC has separate call centers and primary care clinics for VA and DoD beneficiaries, using the Veterans Health Information Systems and Technology Architecture (VistA) and the Armed Forces Health Longitudinal Technology Application (AHLTA), respectively. Even when the departments have agreed on a single system, for example, for workload accounting or purchasing supplies, there must be an additional process performed after the fact to account for and to report the activities in different formats to the parent departments.

Resolving Obstacles to Integration

The task groups began by identifying all policies, regulations, and statutes specific to each department's administrative operations that would have to be modified or waived to allow for the integration of health care services and the development of recommendations for resolving differences that would affect the implementation of FHCC operations. Some of the main areas of difficulty were identified:

- Choosing a governance model
- Choosing whether to designate the facility as a DoD medical facility, a VA medical facility, a network provider, or a hybrid
- Determining the budgeting and reimbursement methodology
- Determining who would own and maintain the property, especially the ACC
- Deciding on the logistics system to put into place
- Choosing (with two different EHR systems) either AHLTA (DoD) or VistA (VA), operating both side by side, or developing interoperability solutions
- Choosing (with two civilian personnel systems) between Title 5 (DoD) or Title 38 (VA), or using both
- Determining how to privilege independent duty hospital corpsmen and hospital corpsmen
- Handling adverse events involving military personnel

The approach taken to resolve most of these issues and many others involved a three-step process. The first step was for the appropriate task group to draft an executive decision memorandum (EDM). The second step was to seek approval of the EDM up each level of the respective departmental chains. The third step was approval of the EDM by the co-chairs of the HEC.

Developing the EDMs was generally a lengthy process involving numerous revisions. They were circulated locally first, and then at the regional and national levels, which generally involved multiple offices within the VA, the Navy, and the DoD. The Office of Management and Budget and the Executive Office of the President reviewed matters involving legislation or funding. Most aspects of the Lovell FHCC operations required higher-level approval, usually changes in the standard procedures or program policies of one department or the other or of both. The task groups spent a great deal of time trying to identify who needed to be consulted and arranging to bring them to the table to make decisions. Most of the EDMs were not signed until July 2008, 3 years after the start of the process.

The obstacles to integration addressed by the EDMs and by other means were resolved to varying degrees, depending on the obstacle. (The resolution to the problem of incompatible information management/information technology [IM/IT] systems was handled differently—at the national level—and is summarized below.) In some cases, a solution allowing integrated operations was reached. For example, the departments agreed to use the VA administrative systems for most financial matters—for example, accounting, purchasing, inventory. The Navy civilians were integrated into the VA personnel system. Accounting for the applicable VA and DoD expenses is performed after the fact through a reconciliation process that is seamless to FHCC staff.

In other cases, integration proved to be impossible. For example, the departments could not agree on a single clinical credentialing system although both were designed to meet the same Joint Commission requirements. The law enforcement and protection function could not be integrated because the Navy's masters-at-arms could not be deployed off the Navy base due to the Posse Comitatus Act, which generally prohibits the use of the military for domestic law enforcement. A small number of Navy IM/IT civilians were not transferred because only DoD employees can access certain computer systems. The VA does not have authority for personal services contracts (PSCs), so the Navy retained the responsibility for maintaining nearly 300 PSCs used to staff the branch clinics on the Navy base.

Other solutions involved exemptions. The major example is the funding of the branch clinics on the Navy base that exclusively serves recruits, students, and active duty staff. They are part of the Lovell FHCC's budget, but the funds are passed directly through to them rather than accounted for as part of the reconciliation process. Similarly, the nursing home and long-term care programs for veterans are funded by the VA as direct pass-throughs.

In most cases, the solutions were compromises. For example, the Navy relented on its requirement of a secret clearance for access to patient records in the DoD EHR system. However, it required a more intensive security clearance investigation than the VA's—the Access National Agency Check with Inquiries (ANACI) versus the National Agency Check with Inquiries—although VA personnel were allowed a grace period of 1 year to undergo the ANACI investigation. Also, it was impossible to agree on a single computer access card, so military personnel use the DoD common access card and VA personnel use the VA personal identity verification card, each programmed to access the other's system.

The security clearance example illustrates the extensive time and effort expended in developing and coordinating the integration process. The DoD/VA memorandum of understanding was not signed until after October 1,

2010, when the Lovell FHCC became official. This, along with undelivered IM/IT interoperability solutions, was a factor in delaying the move of the Navy outpatient clinics until after the middle of December 2012.

Ultimately, legislative authority had to be obtained to resolve some matters. The Lovell FHCC planners were directed to resolve differences within existing law as much as possible, but four issues could not be resolved without legislation[4]:

1. Allowing DoD beneficiaries to use the Lovell FHCC as they had the NHCGL, that is, without paying deductibles and copayments. Legislation was needed to designate the FHCC as an MTF so that copayments for TRICARE beneficiaries could be waived.
2. Enabling the Lovell FHCC to manage the facilities on the west campus as a unit. This required legislation authorizing the transfer of the ACC to the VA.
3. Enabling the Lovell FHCC to administer a uniform human resources program for civilian employees. Legislative authority was required to transfer civilians from the DoD personnel system (Title 5) to the VA personnel system (Title 38).
4. Permitting the Lovell FHCC to budget and spend funds for an integrated operation. This required legislation authorizing the establishment of a Department of the Treasury (Treasury) fund to allow pooling of DoD and VA funds.

Legislation containing the needed authorities was introduced as an amendment to the National Defense Authorization Act (NDAA) for fiscal year (FY) 2009 but was not adopted until late 2009 as part of the NDAA for FY 2010, which created an extra year of uncertainty. The legislation was more limited in some ways than had been hoped. The Lovell FHCC was designated as an MTF only for purposes of eligibility and cannot take advantage of the other benefits of being an MTF. The FHCC could not take full advantage of efficiencies to reduce costs because the personnel transfer came with provisos that no one would lose his or her job or have his or her pay reduced. In addition, the legislation only applies to the FHCC as a 5-year demonstration project and cannot be used to establish other federal health care centers.

[4] A separate bill was required in 2009 to name the North Chicago Federal Health Care Center after retired Navy Captain James A. Lovell, commander of *Apollo 13*, who lives in the North Chicago area.

Limited Interoperability of Electronic Health Record Systems

In keeping with the Lovell FHCC vision, the clinical task group recommended having one patient record system, or at least a single-user interface between the DoD and the VA EHR systems, for entering and retrieving patient clinical information. The IM/IT task group was able to accomplish little, given the size of the task and the resources required. The lack of progress became urgent by 2008, given the lead time needed to develop software interoperability solutions for single entry into both systems. At this point, the VA and DoD enterprise (i.e., national) IT offices were directed to identify and develop the minimum set of capabilities needed to make the FHCC functional by October 1, 2010. It took time to identify the minimum capabilities (early 2009), develop the technical requirements, obtain the funding (more than $100 million from the Joint Incentive Fund) and award the contracts (late 2009 for the VA and early 2010 for the DoD because its budget was under a continuing resolution).

The first capabilities—single registration and single medical sign-on—were not delivered until December 2010. Orders portability for radiology was delivered in June 2011 and for laboratory in March 2012. The final two capabilities, orders portability for pharmacy and for consults, were not delivered as of the date of this report and are not expected until 2014 at the earliest.

The lack of interoperability requires time-consuming manual workarounds by clinical and support staff to keep both the DoD and the VA EHR systems current. For pharmacy services, it is necessary to have five pharmacists devoted full time to manually check for drug interactions and allergies. This hinders the Lovell FHCC's ability to efficiently provide safe and seamless care to DoD beneficiaries as they move from place to place within the FHCC.

RESULTS

The Lovell FHCC is unique among health care joint ventures in having a single command structure. FHCC proponents expected this structure to result in more integrated clinical and administrative operations. In turn, the integration was anticipated to lead to better care being provided at less cost to area DoD and VA beneficiaries than would have occurred if the separate VA and Navy medical centers had been maintained. According to the executive agreement (EA) among the VA, the DoD, and the Navy, the FHCC was expected to result in more accessible, higher-quality, and less costly health care; meet military readiness standards; maintain high patient and provider satisfaction; and increase research and training opportunities.

These outcomes are analyzed in detail in Chapter 4. In brief, as of June

2012, when information gathering for this report was completed, the shift from separate commands to a single, more integrated organizational structure on October 1, 2010, has not had a significant effect on trends in most available outcome measures in either the positive or the negative direction.

Unfortunately, data on changes in efficiency and cost savings are not readily available. However, given that no one could lose his or her job or receive less pay, and that the Lovell FHCC is receiving the same funding in its first 2 years as it did the year before it was launched, adjusted for inflation, one would not expect major cost reductions. There might be efficiencies—doing more with the same amount of funding—but this would be hampered by the limited degree of integration within the clinical and administrative departments. In addition, the need to operate two EHR systems manually is widely acknowledged to be significantly reducing clinical efficiency. FHCC planners expected a temporary loss of clinical efficiency (i.e., number of patient encounters per provider) of 10 to 15 percent because of the learning curve in using the new interoperability solutions, but interviewees indicated that the loss has been closer to 20 percent and was continuing.

CONCLUSIONS

The Institute of Medicine was asked to form a committee to evaluate the merger of a Navy MTF and a VAMC in North Chicago into a federal health care center in terms of its benefit to the DoD and the VA compared with maintaining separate VA and DoD facilities. Specifically, the sponsor asked the committee to undertake—but not be limited to—six tasks (see Box S-1).

In addition to addressing each of the tasks outlined by the sponsor, the committee developed six recommendations regarding the Lovell FHCC.

STUDY TASKS

Task 1: Assessment Criteria

Task 1 asks for criteria for assessing the "success" of the FHCC demonstration in the short term and the longer term. The committee recommends below (Recommendation 3) that the DoD and the VA conduct a comprehensive evaluation of the Lovell FHCC demonstration designed to provide the basis for determining at the end of the 5-year demonstration period whether the FHCC model has been a success and whether it should be adopted in other locations where the VA and the DoD share health care markets. Appendix B contains the framework for such an evaluation that could be adopted by the VA and the DoD. The framework considers short-

BOX S-1
Substantive Study Tasks*

1. Establish criteria for near-term and longer-term assessment of the success of facility integration that can be used in follow-on assessments. Determine if success criteria would be different if the partner DoD health care facility was supporting operational units instead of basic/advanced training units, such as the Navy Health Center Great Lakes.
2. Evaluate whether performance benchmarks that DoD and VA have established in their executive agreement have been achieved.
3. Examine the lessons learned from similar mergers elsewhere in the federal and private health sectors that may be applicable to DoD/VA mergers.
4. Evaluate the most pressing concerns of the stakeholders and recommend ways to mitigate or eliminate these concerns.
5. Evaluate the specific impact of the merger on the level and quality of training received by active duty medical personnel and VA providers.

---

* The sixth task was to prepare a written report with findings, conclusions, and recommendations for the DoD and the VA that will be available to the general public.

term outcomes to be those observed in the first year or two and long-term outcomes to be those that emerge after 3 to 5 years.

The EA for the Lovell FHCC identifies the desired outcomes. They are (compared with operating separate VA and DoD health care centers in the same health care market): more accessible health care, higher-quality health care (e.g., more preventive services and continuity and coordination of care), cost savings or cost avoidance, increased market share among eligible beneficiaries, greater patient satisfaction, greater provider satisfaction, improved clinical proficiency of active duty providers, improved training programs, and better research opportunities. The outcome criteria of most importance are *financial*, such as the net reduction in costs per episode of care or procedures; *clinical*, such as the numbers of preventable drug-drug interactions and allergic reactions to drugs; *patient-focused*, such as time to third appointment and standardized patient satisfaction survey results; and in the case of the Lovell FHCC, *military operational readiness-focused*, such as the percentage of recruits unable to graduate on time for medical reasons. The evaluation framework in Appendix B suggests some intermediate-term outcomes, such as higher patient volume and quality of care measures. Other metrics take longer to collect and analyze and are listed as long-term outcomes, such as cost per patient, increased market share, and health status of patients.

The committee was also asked to consider the differences in assessment criteria for FHCCs serving training units (such as the RTC at Great Lakes) and those serving operational units. Operational units are more varied, with more complex, mission-related medical issues than training units are, and they require medical personnel with knowledge of military medicine and who respect the unique cultural identity of servicemembers in operational units. Administrative business functions would be similar for medical units serving training and operational units. Despite the differences between training and operational units, however, the criteria for success in an operational versus a training unit would be similar, although the benchmarks might be set at different levels.

Task 2: Performance Benchmarks

The departments specified 15 "integration benchmarks" intended to measure the degree of integration success. As of June 2012, most scores had stayed the same as they were at baseline. Two measures scored a one or a two in June 2012 and therefore have not achieved a successful score: (1) the DoD component of evidence-based health care and (2) IM/IT implementation. The failure to achieve evidence-based health care goals is attributed to vacancies in the active duty provider workforce due to rotation and deployment. The delay in implementation of joint IM/IT capabilities is critical to services integration at the Lovell FHCC and is unlikely to improve further until parts of the new EHR system being developed jointly by the DoD and the VA become available, beginning with a joint pharmacy program scheduled to be operational in 2014.

Task 3: Lessons Learned from Other Federal and Private-Sector Health Care Mergers

The committee addressed the third task by commissioning a comprehensive overview of the private-sector health care merger literature and analyzing the lessons learned reported by the nine VA/DoD joint venture sites. The review of the private-sector merger literature appears in Appendix D, "Collaboration Among Health Care Organizations: A Review of Outcomes and Best Practices for Effective Performance," and is summarized in Chapter 5. The lessons learned from the VA/DoD joint ventures reported at the annual joint venture conferences are also summarized in Chapter 5, and short profiles of the individual joint ventures and the lessons learned they have reported are in Appendix C, "Department of Veterans Affairs/Department of Defense Joint Ventures: Brief Histories and Lessons Learned."

Task 4: Stakeholder Concerns

The committee was not able to conduct a statistically valid survey of the most important stakeholders, the patients. However, the committee heard from stakeholders, including several veteran and retired military enrollees at the Lovell FHCC, at its third meeting, held in North Chicago.

The commanding officer of the RTC, who receives daily reports on recruits being seen at the west campus emergency room or admitted to the hospital, said that the FHCC was performing as well as the Naval Hospital/Health Clinic Great Lakes had been, for example, in the percentage of recruits unable to go to their next assignment for medical reasons.

The president of the affiliated medical school, the Rosalind Franklin University of Medicine and Science, had a positive view of the effect of the Lovell FHCC merger on medical education and training and on research opportunities because the merger has created a larger and more varied clinical staff and patient mix.

The veterans testified that they were satisfied with the care they were receiving at the Lovell FHCC but had two major concerns, namely, the time it takes to fill prescriptions was much longer than before the merger (although the wait times had shortened significantly more recently) and the safety of locating the mental health clinic on the third floor of the ACC next to a railing over an open three-story atrium.

Task 5: Staff Training

The committee did not find that staff training was affected by the merger except in one area, which was of special concern to the Navy when agreeing to merge clinical operations with the VA in the FHCC. The concern was whether independent duty corpsmen (IDCs) and active duty advanced practice nurses (APNs) would be able to practice their skills in the merged FHCC, especially in the inpatient setting. As described in Chapter 3, special training of VA staff on the duties of corpsmen was provided, and several compromises were reached to allow APNs and IDCs to maintain needed clinical proficiencies at the Lovell FHCC.

RECOMMENDATIONS

Develop Uniform Policies, Procedures, and Business Practices for Federal Health Care Centers

Findings

The implementation of the Lovell FHCC highlights the difficulty of achieving unified policies and procedures when each parent department has its own planning, operating, and reporting procedures for the same health care center functions.

Recently, the VA and the DoD agreed to develop a unified approach at the enterprise level in some cases rather than to try to facilitate local solutions. Prime examples of joint enterprise-level solutions include the efforts to develop a joint EHR system (the integrated EHR, or iEHR) and the joint disability examination process for wounded, ill, or injured servicemembers (the Integrated Disability Evaluation System, or IDES). These agreements resulted from top-down directives from the DoD and VA secretaries, who are personally monitoring progress through regular meetings.

Conclusions

Additional opportunities remain to develop enterprise-level solutions to differing departmental requirements and business practices. This would enable more cost-effective joint health care delivery collaborations, whether they are DoD/VA joint ventures or FHCCs. An example of an opportunity to work out a common approach would be a unified process for credentialing health care providers. Other opportunities include uniform cost accounting, civilian workforce policies, performance and quality measures, access to care standards, drug formularies, and mail-order drug refill programs. The more that common policies and processes are adopted, the more integrated FHCCs can be, which in turn should increase opportunities to achieve more accessible and cost-effective patient care.

> **RECOMMENDATION 1. Before establishing additional federal health care centers, the Department of Veterans Affairs and the Department of Defense should agree on a governance plan and common policies and procedures for joint health care delivery functions.**

Achieving additional enterprise-level agreement on single policies and processes is a critical first step in planning additional future FHCCs and would also assist the Lovell FHCC in reaching its full potential.

Complete Development of a Jointly Usable Electronic Health Record System Before Establishing Additional Federal Health Care Centers

Findings

The IM/IT goal for the Lovell FHCC is to "safely interface VA and DoD legacy systems to support an integrated DoD/VA facility with multiple care locations" (Filippi, 2011). The Lovell FHCC expected the software capabilities that its clinicians and other subject matter experts had identified in early 2009 as the minimum needed for integrated use of the VA and the DoD EHR systems to be in place when the FHCC opened on October 1, 2010, but they were significantly delayed. These included single registration and single sign-on (implemented in December 2010), orders portability for radiology (implemented in June 2010), and orders portability for laboratory (implemented in March 2011). Two capabilities are still not ready for implementation, namely, orders portability for pharmacy and for consults, and are not expected to be ready for several years.

Conclusions

The lack of EHR interoperability, despite the development of work-arounds (such as hiring five pharmacists to manually check both EHR systems for possible drug allergies and interactions), significantly reduced the efficiency of health care delivery for at least the first year of Lovell FHCC operations. The lack of single-entry access to both EHR systems has hindered the ability of the Lovell FHCC to deliver higher-quality or more efficient, cost-effective health care and to provide better research opportunities. The ability to seamlessly deliver electronic health information from the veteran, military beneficiary, and health care provider perspectives should be the hallmark of an FHCC.

RECOMMENDATION 2. Additional federal health care centers should not be implemented until an interoperable or joint Department of Defense/Department of Veterans Affairs electronic health record system becomes available.

The DoD and VA secretaries have committed their departments to developing such a system together—a new joint EHR system (the iEHR)—rather than upgrading their current (now legacy) EHR systems and trying to develop interoperability solutions. The iEHR will be developed in phases with some modules, such as pharmacy, scheduled to be completed in 2014; the final modules are due for completion in 2017. It would be helpful for the iEHR to have the capabilities identified by the FHCC clinical task group as the initial set of core IT capabilities required by the Lovell FHCC earlier rather than later in the development process if establishing additional FHCCs is a priority.

Develop Criteria for Selecting Future Federal Health Care Center Sites

Findings

The VA and the DoD have developed criteria for identifying "joint market areas" for increased health care sharing. These are health care markets with large DoD and VA beneficiary populations where shared facilities and services would provide access to services or infrastructure not available in one or the other organization; improve efficiency through economies of scale; reduce duplication of services, infrastructure, or both; and mitigate the impact of deployment on access.

The VA and the DoD have adopted a definition of joint ventures. They are local alliances or partnerships formed to facilitate comprehensive cooperation, shared risk, and mutual benefit, and they are expected to last at least 5 years. To qualify as a joint venture, the departments look for regular ongoing interactions in at least several of the following areas: staffing, clinical workload, business processes, management, information technology, logistics, education and training, and research capabilities.

The VA and the DoD have not defined FHCCs and do not have criteria for choosing their locations. The Lovell FHCC is considered to be unique and is no longer a joint venture.

Conclusions

To a large extent, the criteria should address the juncture at which FHCC lower operating costs or greater effectiveness are shown to outweigh the associated significant implementation costs (i.e., a single organizational structure and integrated administrative and clinical processes) enough for the FHCC structure to be regarded as preferable to a joint venture sharing arrangement and its comparative cost effectiveness. At this time (June 2012), the costs of implementing the Lovell FHCC have been substantial, while efficiencies and cost savings that might be expected have had a limited time to transpire.

The VA and the DoD should base a decision to establish another FHCC on evidence that it would provide higher performance in quality, access, or cost effectiveness compared with other arrangements, including a joint venture agreement. An important source of evidence on the costs and benefits will be the comprehensive evaluation of the Lovell FHCC recommended below.

RECOMMENDATION 3. The Department of Veterans Affairs and the Department of Defense should develop criteria for selecting future federal health care center (FHCC) sites. The criteria should address the costs and benefits of establishing a fully integrated organization compared with the costs and benefits of other collaborative arrangements, such as joint ventures, taking into account local health care market trends, institutional capabilities and readiness, unique local circumstances, and departmental limiting factors. Only when firm criteria based on cost savings and the expectation of enhanced health care service delivery are met should the concept of a future FHCC be considered.

Analyze and Promulgate Lessons Learned from the Lovell Federal Health Care Center Experience

Findings

The leadership of the Lovell FHCC encountered numerous issues that had to be resolved to achieve an integrated organization and uniform policies and procedures. Many of the issues resulted from conflicting policies and procedures of the VA, the DoD, and the Navy. Some were the result of statutory requirements and the lack of statutory authority.

Many of the issues have been resolved by adopting the policy or procedure of one department with the agreement of the other department. In some cases, agreement on a single policy or procedure could not be reached and workarounds had to be developed to meet the requirements of the two departments. Some issues could not be resolved because of irreconcilable policy differences, such as an integrated police force including active duty masters-at-arms on the west campus. Ultimately, four critically necessary actions had to be authorized by legislation: (1) the authority to transfer civilian employees from one department to the other; (2) the authority to transfer the ambulatory care center and other Navy-built facilities and related personal property and equipment from the DoD to the VA; (3) the authority for the DoD to transfer funds to a joint Treasury account under the VA; and (4) the authority for DoD beneficiaries to be treated by the Lovell FHCC as they would be at an MTF. However, the legislation authorized these only as part of a 5-year demonstration in North Chicago.

Every difference between VA and DoD policies and procedures had to be addressed at multiple regional- and headquarters-level decision points. This often took months, and sometimes years, to resolve through numerous drafts and meetings. The extra burden of this process was very heavy, especially at the local level where planning the integration was an extra duty for most staff members.

Conclusions

The implementation of the Lovell FHCC provides a road map to issues that will be encountered in any future attempts to establish FHCCs and offers many examples of ways to overcome or bypass those impediments. It would be extremely beneficial for planners of future FHCCs, and in many cases for existing and future joint ventures, to adopt solutions developed and already approved by the VA and the DoD without having to undertake the long negotiation process that the FHCC had to go through. An important, groundbreaking contribution would be made by the FHCC staff if they developed joint DoD/VA guidance materials, including a best-practices document or guidebook to disseminate local solutions or "fixes" arrived at to solve problems that arose in the implementation of the merger.

RECOMMENDATION 4. The Department of Veterans Affairs and the Department of Defense should systematically compile and analyze the lessons learned from the Captain James A. Lovell Federal Health Care Center merger experience, including both what and what not to do, and disseminate them through onsite consultation, webinars, technical assistance, and other means to other federal health care center sites considering joint ventures and related collaborative arrangements.

Conduct a Comprehensive Evaluation of the Lovell Federal Health Care Center Demonstration

Findings

The Lovell FHCC has been in operation for less than 2 years and is still implementing parts of the integration plan. It is too early to tell how successful the overall integration effort has been or will be when the demonstration period ends in 2015. That there have been substantial one-time costs is clear, but whether these have led or will lead to lasting efficiencies or can be adopted by future FHCCs to avoid unnecessary costs is not yet known.

The Lovell FHCC is tracking certain performance indicators designed to inform about the relative degree of success or failure, for example, if the facility is providing poor, less, or more expensive care; hurting operational readiness; reducing patient satisfaction and staff morale; or providing fewer education and research opportunities. However, the VA and the DoD have not adopted a comprehensive evaluation plan to judge objectively the success of the Lovell FHCC at the end of the 5-year demonstration period and to help them to decide whether the Lovell FHCC would be applicable in other locations.

Conclusions

Without a formal evaluation plan, the success of the integration effort will be more difficult to determine after the 5-year demonstration period than it should be because not all the data needed for an evaluation are being collected prospectively.

RECOMMENDATION 5. In considering the Captain James A. Lovell Federal Health Care Center merger and future collaborative arrangements, the Department of Veterans Affairs and the Department of Defense should develop a comprehensive evaluation framework with defined and measurable criteria for assessing performance that take into account local and national contexts, organizational capabilities and readiness, implementation plans, intermediate outcomes, and likely long-term impact.

Expand the Knowledge Base on Federal Health Care Collaborations

Findings

The DoD and the VA have not systematically analyzed the experience of the Lovell FHCC and the lessons that may be learned from it in considering if and where to establish additional integrated health care centers modeled after the Lovell FHCC merger.

Conclusions

The Lovell FHCC offers a number of lessons learned about what works well—and what does not—that would be useful to future FHCC decision makers and planners. The mergers of private-sector health care organizations do not provide adequate models for integration of federal health care organizations because they are narrowly based on increasing market share and revenue and usually do not involve clinical integration, only administrative consolidation. Published studies demonstrate substantial variation in performance after collaborative ventures. Nonetheless, lessons learned and pertinent data would be useful for both the Lovell FHCC and future endeavors (Appendix D contains a paper commissioned by the committee on the experiences of VA/DoD joint ventures and private-sector health care mergers).

RECOMMENDATION 6. The Department of Veterans Affairs (VA) and the Department of Defense (DoD) should fund studies to address the key findings and questions raised by the experiences of the Captain

James A. Lovell Federal Health Care Center merger and other VA/DoD collaborative arrangements. These studies should address the implementation issues involved in establishing collaborative arrangements, including leadership, governance, communication, organizational culture, coordination, incentives, and related factors associated with improved access, quality, slowing of the increase in the cost of care, and military readiness.

REFERENCES

Durbin, R. 2003. Remarks on the Senate floor on an amendment to the Departments of Veterans Affairs and Housing and Urban Development and Independent Agencies Appropriations Act, 2004, relating to VA-Navy sharing of facilities at the North Chicago VA Medical Center. *Congressional Record* 149(Pt. 21):S14511. http://www.gpo.gov/fdsys/pkg/CREC-2003-11-12/pdf/CREC-2003-11-12-pt1-PgS14506.pdf (accessed July 25, 2012).

Filippi, D. 2011. *James A. Lovell Federal Health Care Center IT informational brief.* Presentation by the director of the DoD/VA Interagency Program Office to the Institute of Medicine Committee on Evaluation of the Lovell Federal Health Care Center Merger at its first meeting, Washington, DC, February 25.

VA (Department of Veterans Affairs). 2002. *VA and DoD agree on health care in North Chicago*. VA press release, October 18.

1

Introduction

On October 1, 2010, the Captain James A. Lovell Federal Health Care Center (FHCC) came into being in North Chicago, Illinois. The Lovell FHCC is the joint effort of the Department of Defense (DoD) and the Department of Veterans Affairs (VA) to provide health care to DoD and VA beneficiaries in northern Illinois and southern Wisconsin through a consolidated delivery system intended to be more accessible and of higher quality for patients and more cost effective for taxpayers than would operating separate VA and DoD health care systems.

North Chicago is the home of the Naval Station Great Lakes, which is currently responsible for the initial (boot camp) training and much of the advanced training of the enlisted personnel of the Navy. Historically, the U.S. Navy provided health care to active duty servicemembers and their dependents through its own facilities (the Naval Hospital Great Lakes), while the VA provided health care to military veterans in its own medical center located less than two miles from the naval hospital (the North Chicago VA Medical Center). As in other locations around the United States where DoD and VA health care facilities are located near each other, there was both local and national interest in sharing equipment, facilities, and staff to reduce costs, while providing patients with a broader range of services and more coordinated care. Over time, VA and DoD health care facilities have developed a large number of sharing and exchange relationships ranging from the simple, such as sharing the cost and staffing of magnetic resonance imaging equipment, to the complex, such as collocating and sharing the use of the outpatient center of one department and the hospital of the other department. Examples of these joint activities are discussed later in this report.

The Lovell FHCC differs from other DoD/VA health care collaborations in several significant aspects. It is intended to be a single organization—a federal health care center rather than a military treatment facility or a VA medical center—that features a single chain of command, a consolidated funding source, and, to the extent possible, health care service delivery that is seamless for the patient, regardless of whether he or she is a VA or a DoD beneficiary. The hope is that the design of the FHCC will overcome some of the barriers to cost reduction and integrated service delivery remaining in even the most functional joint ventures and other sharing and exchange arrangements between DoD and VA health care facilities.

The Lovell FHCC was planned to be a 5-year demonstration of what can and cannot be accomplished with an integrated organization, but pressure to establish additional federal health care centers is strong and increasing. It is driven partly by the desire for a seamless transition of the wounded and injured from the wars in Iraq and Afghanistan who can no longer serve from active duty to veteran status. It is also driven by the desire to reduce the costs of health care for active duty and retired servicemembers and their dependents and for military veterans, a desire that will only increase as the United States struggles to reduce the federal budget deficit.

In 2010, the acting assistant secretary of defense for health affairs asked the Institute of Medicine (IOM) to undertake and report on an evaluation of the Lovell FHCC by December 29, 2012. The formal DoD statement of task is found in Box 1-1.

In response, the IOM established a 15-member committee with the appropriate expertise to determine the following:

1. if the integrated health care system represented by the FHCC in North Chicago has been beneficial in terms of access to, quality of, and cost of health care; mission readiness of Navy personnel; patient and provider satisfaction; clinical education and training; and research opportunities; and
2. whether the FHCC would be a good model for similar mergers around the country where VA and DoD medical facilities are in close proximity.

The committee membership includes experts in executive medicine (including former DoD and VA health care executives), clinical medicine and nursing, health care organization and management, health care quality, health information technology, graduate medical education, and health care program evaluation. Short biographies of the committee members and staff are found in Appendix A.

BOX 1-1
Statement of Work

The purpose is to conduct a study to evaluate whether the integrated Department of Defense/Department of Veterans Affairs (DoD/VA) James A. Lovell Federal Health Care Center (FHCC) located in North Chicago is more beneficial to DoD and VA than their independent facilities in serving the needs of their eligible populations. A panel that is comprised of independent, neutral, nongovernmental subject matter experts shall be convened to do the following, but is not limited to:

1. Establish criteria for near-term and longer-term assessment of the success of facility integration that can be used in follow-on assessments. Determine if success criteria would be different if the partner DoD health care facility was supporting operational units instead of basic/advanced training units, such as the Navy Health Clinic Great Lakes.
2. Evaluate whether performance benchmarks that DoD and VA have established in their executive agreement have been achieved.
3. Examine the lessons learned from similar mergers elsewhere in the federal and private health sectors that may be applicable to DoD/VA mergers.
4. Evaluate the most pressing concerns of the stakeholders,* and recommend ways to mitigate or eliminate these concerns.
5. Evaluate the specific impact of the merger on the level and quality of training received by active duty medical personnel and VA providers.
6. Prepare a written report with findings, conclusions, and recommendations for DoD and VA that will be available to the general public.

---

* Stakeholders include all groups affected directly and indirectly by the merger, such as the leadership of the merging units and their line of command/authority, the employees, active duty and civilian, eligible beneficiaries, local citizens, and labor unions.

The committee held five face-to-face meetings between February 2011 and March 2012, supplemented by conference calls and email exchanges. Two of the meetings were held in North Chicago, where the committee received presentations from the staff of the FHCC and area stakeholders affected by the integration effort. Stakeholders include leaders of the Navy Recruit Training Command, the affiliated medical school (Rosalind Franklin University of Medicine and Science), unions, patients, and veterans organizations. The presenters and their affiliations are listed in the Acknowledgments. The committee also toured the FHCC facilities for half a day, including naval branch clinics located on the naval base.

In the process of its deliberations, the committee created a framework (see Table 1-1) to guide its evaluation of the Lovell FHCC merger that

TABLE 1-1 Framework for Evaluating Department of Veterans Affairs and Department of Defense Health Care Collaborations*

National and Local Contexts	Organizational Capabilities and Readiness	Implementation Initiatives	Intermediate Outcomes First 2 Years	Long-Term Impact 3–5 Years
• Department of Veterans Affairs and Department of Defense (DoD) policies, goals, objectives • Number and location of facilities • Size and number of people served • Local health care market—public and private sectors • Local labor market • Other	• Shared vision • History of working together • Culture • Leadership • Information technology capabilities • Care management • Care improvement • Performance measurement • Training and human resources development • Financial reserves • Other	• Combining departments and services • Transferring personnel • Orienting employees • Communication/education • Developing policies • Developing shared electronic health records • Other	• Increased operational readiness for recruits • Expanding patient volume to critical mass to maintain competency • More in-house surgery—added posttraumatic stress disorder unit • Increased professional opportunities for staff • Residency opportunities • Healthcare Effectiveness Data and Information Set, DoD, Joint Commission benchmark measures • Employee satisfaction • Patient experience measures • Other	• Operating efficiencies • Costs per patient • Patient functional health status measures • Increased market share in local area • Other

* It is important to evaluate shared services, joint ventures, and partial and full mergers, etc., against their *own* stated goals and objectives in addition to those expected by external parties, including accreditation bodies, payers, and others.

may prove useful to assess future collaborations between the DoD and the VA, whether these take the form of shared service arrangements, joint ventures, or partial or full mergers. The five major categories for consideration include (1) national and local context, (2) organizational capabilities and readiness, (3) implementation initiatives, (4) intermediate outcomes, and (5) long-term impact. A detailed description of the conceptualization of this framework is found in Appendix B. The lessons learned from the VA/DoD joint ventures reported at the annual joint venture conferences are summarized in Chapter 5, and short profiles of the joint ventures and their reported lessons learned are in Appendix C. The committee was also informed by a commissioned paper authored by Thomas D'Aunno on the experiences of joint ventures and private-sector health care mergers (Appendix D).

2

History and Context

Although unique in certain aspects, the Captain James A. Lovell Federal Health Care Center (FHCC) is the latest development in a long history of cooperation between the health care systems of the Department of Defense (DoD) and the Department of Veterans Affairs (VA). A review of this history provides a better understanding of the drivers and goals of cooperative health care activities between the DoD and the VA and of the obstacles and constraints that joint activities have encountered that the Lovell FHCC model is expected to address.

FEDERAL HEALTH CARE

The U.S. government provides health care to several populations, primarily through the VA, the DoD, and the Departments of Health and Human Services (Indian Health Service), Homeland Security (Coast Guard), and Justice (Bureau of Prisons). This report addresses only the health care systems of the DoD and the VA, although lessons learned and recommendations in this report may well apply to joint service delivery efforts between and within the other agencies.

Military Health System

The Military Health System (MHS), which includes TRICARE, provides health care services to 9.6 million people, including 1.5 million active duty servicemembers, 2.1 million active duty family members, 5.1 million military retirees and their dependents, and 1.0 million reservists and their

BOX 2-1
TRICARE Prime and Other TRICARE Programs

TRICARE has a number of program options, depending on beneficiary category (e.g., active duty servicemember, active duty family member, military retiree, eligible retiree family member, survivor, qualifying former spouse, reserve members and family members, and retired reserve members and their families) and geographic location relative to military treatment facilities (MTFs) (TRICARE, 2012).* For purposes of this report, the important distinction is whether a TRICARE beneficiary (1) must enroll in TRICARE Prime at an MTF; (2) may enroll in TRICARE Prime at an MTF; and (3) may use an MTF on a space-available basis although not enrolled in TRICARE Prime.

Must Enroll in TRICARE Prime. Active duty servicemembers within the catchment of an MTF (which is within a 40-mile radius of the MTF) must enroll in TRICARE Prime at the MTF and receive all health care at the MTF unless referred out by their primary care manager. Therefore, all enlisted recruits and students at Naval Station Great Lakes are enrolled in TRICARE Prime at the Captain James A. Lovell Federal Health Care Center, as are active duty staff members who live within a 40-mile radius.

May Enroll in TRICARE Prime. Active duty family members, retirees ineligible for Medicare and their family members, survivors, and qualifying former spouses may enroll in TRICARE Prime rather than TRICARE Standard, TRICARE's fee-for-service option. The incentive for enrolling in TRICARE Prime, similar to a managed care plan or health maintenance organization, rather than TRICARE Standard or other options, is lower out-of-pocket costs. Active duty

family members.[1] More than 83 percent of DoD health care beneficiaries used TRICARE services in fiscal year (FY) 2010.

The MHS comprises 59 inpatient hospitals, 363 ambulatory care clinics, 281 dental clinics, and 255 veterinary facilities. It employs more than 139,000 people, including 32,000 officers, 54,000 enlisted personnel, and 53,000 civilians.

The care is provided either by military hospitals, called military treatment facilities (MTFs), or by non-DoD providers under contract, called TRICARE network providers. Those who enroll with an MTF, through TRICARE Prime, pay an annual enrollment fee but do not have to pay deductibles or copayments. Those who go to other providers, through TRICARE Standard, must pay deductibles and copayments but may choose

[1] The information and quotes in this section come from the Department of Defense (DoD, 2011a,b), unless otherwise indicated.

servicemembers, active duty family members, surviving children, and surviving spouses (the last for the first 3 years) pay no costs. Military retirees and their family members, qualifying former spouses, and surviving spouses (the last after 3 years) pay a modest annual enrollment fee ($260 for individuals, $520 for families in fiscal year 2012).

May Use an MTF on a Space-Available Basis. DoD beneficiaries not enrolled in TRICARE Prime may receive care at an MTF on a space-available basis. TRICARE Standard beneficiaries usually choose TRICARE Standard so they may use providers of their choice, but they must pay annual deductibles and copayments. However, they are not required to cost share if they receive services at an MTF. Retirees who become eligible for Medicare fall under the TRICARE for Life (TFL) option. TFL beneficiaries are not subject to deductibles or copayments but must take Medicare Part B, whereupon TRICARE becomes the secondary payer. If a Department of Veterans Affairs (VA) medical center treats a TFL beneficiary, it cannot be reimbursed because the VA is not authorized to bill Medicare.

Priority for Care at an MTF

1. Active duty servicemembers
2. Active duty family members enrolled in TRICARE Prime
3. Retirees, their family members, and survivors enrolled in TRICARE Prime
4. Active duty family members not enrolled in TRICARE Prime
5. All other eligible persons (CRS, 2009)

* SOURCE: See http://www.tricare.mil/tricaresmartfiles/Prod_856/TRICARE_Choices_At_a_Glance_ Brochure.pdf (accessed September 14, 2012).

their providers (if they are able to use an MTF on a space-available basis, they are not charged for a copayment) (see Box 2-1 for an explanation of TRICARE program options).

Although the number of MHS enrollees has been increasing in recent years, enrollment at MTFs, although required for active duty servicemembers, has been trending down, from about 4.2 million in 2004 to about 4.0 million in 2010. Meanwhile, enrollment in TRICARE Standard has increased from about 1.0 million in 2004 to 1.7 million in 2010.

Rising health care costs are a major concern. The budget has increased from $32 billion in FY 2004 to more than $49 billion in FY 2011, mostly due to the increase in average per capita costs ($3,500 a year in 2010, compared with $2,000 a year in 2002). While the use of inpatient and outpatient services at MTFs has changed little, the use of care purchased from network providers has been increasing substantially. The per capita costs of direct care are less on average than the costs of purchased care, which provides an incentive for the MHS to attempt to increase the proportion of DoD beneficiaries who are enrolled in TRICARE Prime. According to Dr. Jonathan Woodson, the assistant secretary of defense for health affairs, eliminating purchased care would save the MHS more than $16 billion per year (Kime, 2012).

The MHS faces an important obstacle in attracting beneficiaries to the direct care system of MTFs, however.

- Patients at military treatment facilities report more difficulty getting timely care than those who use TRICARE network providers (DoD, 2010, p. 24).
- Patients enrolled to TRICARE network providers report a higher satisfaction with (inpatient and outpatient) health care (DoD, 2010, p. 23).
- On average, enrollees to military treatment facilities see their assigned primary care manager less than half of the time (DoD, 2010, p. 23).
- Patients report higher satisfaction with inpatient medical care at MTFs than at TRICARE network hospitals, but lower satisfaction with inpatient surgical and obstetric care at MTFs than at TRICARE network hospitals.

The DoD has also been reducing the number of MTFs by closing small, less-efficient facilities. The number has decreased from 70 to 59 since 2004. These closures, the possibility of making the remaining MTFs more efficient by serving VA as well as DoD patients, and other cost trends provide an incentive for MHS facilities to seek cooperative arrangements with VA health care facilities.

Another trend is the shrinking share of the MHS workforce accounted for by active duty members, down from 58 percent (70,000 of the total workforce of 120,000) in 2004 to 49 percent (68,000 of the total workforce of 140,000) in 2010. This decline, coupled with the fact that about 12,000 are deployed at any given time, also provides an incentive for MTFs to cooperate with the VA to achieve more stable staffing arrangements (VA personnel do not move as part of their job). Collaboration also serves to sharpen the clinical skills of military providers because the VA serves a patient population with a broader range of acute and chronic medical, surgical, and psychiatric conditions and a higher acuity level.

Veterans Health Care System[2]

In 2012, the VA's Veterans Health Administration (VHA) expects to have more than 8.7 million enrollees. Nearly 6.3 million patients will actively use VA services for all or for a portion of their annual health care needs (VA, 2012). The VHA has more than 1,000 direct care sites, including 153 VA medical centers (VAMCs) that provide inpatient and outpatient services, 841 outpatient-only clinics, 133 long-term care facilities (called community living centers), 110 residential rehabilitation programs, and 300 counseling centers (VA, 2012). In FY 2010, the VHA experienced 680,000 inpatient admissions, 75.6 million outpatient visits, and 298,000 outpatient surgeries, at a cost of $47.5 billion. The workload projected for VA facilities in the FY 2011 budget was 87.0 million outpatient visits and 965,000 inpatient stays (U.S. House of Representatives, 2010, p. 38).

As a large integrated health care system, the VA is challenged to provide a comprehensive, full continuum of health services to veterans geographically dispersed across the United States, including in Alaska, Guam, Hawaii, and Puerto Rico. In addition, a large share of veterans (43 percent) lives in rural areas that have a shortage of public and private health care services.

More than 1.8 million women have served in the U.S. military and are veterans. Today, women constitute more than 15 percent of active duty forces and 18 percent of the National Guard and reserve components, and they account for 20 percent of new military recruits. In the decade between FYs 2000 and 2010, the number of women veterans enrolled in the VA health care system as patients doubled from approximately 150,000 to more than 325,000. In FY 2010, 292,000 women received health care services from the VA. The VA projects that by the year 2020, women will constitute 10 percent of the overall veteran population and make up 9.5 percent of VHA patients. While women veterans are still a small minority of VHA patients, their rapidly increasing numbers and gender-specific health needs are creating challenges for the VA's health system. VAMCs and MTFs have an incentive to combine health care services for active duty and veteran women to support a broader range of coordinated services and avoid referring patients to community health care providers for more specialized services such as mammography.

The VHA employs more than 86,000 health care providers, about 10,000 fewer than in 1995.

The VHA has academic teaching affiliations with 107 medical schools, involving 25,000 physicians, 35,000 residents and fellows, and 90,000 trainees. More than 65 percent of U.S. physicians and a near majority of other health professionals have received some training in a VA facility. The

[2] The information in this section comes from Ruschmeier (2011), unless otherwise indicated.

VHA also spends about $1.7 billion annually on clinical, basic, rehabilitation, and health services research.

NORTH CHICAGO BACKGROUND

This section reviews the history of the Navy and the VA health care facilities that combined to form the Lovell FHCC and the context in which the FHCC arose. A detailed history of issues encountered during implementation, and how they were resolved, is presented in Chapter 3. A cross-sectional description of the current FHCC is presented in Chapter 4.

Naval Hospital Great Lakes

The Navy opened a base in North Chicago in 1911 to train enlisted recruits from the Midwest. What is currently called the Naval Station Great Lakes (NSGL) went through boom cycles during and bust cycles after the two world wars, but the Korean conflict and the Cold War resulted in a substantial rebuilding of the recruit training facilities from the mid-1950s to the mid-1960s (Naval Station Great Lakes, 2012). The Naval Hospital Great Lakes (NHGL) was built in 1960. The 12-story, 825-bed building, known as 200H, was a tertiary facility with 850 beds, 11 operating rooms, and space for 16 clinics. It provided care for military personnel on the base and was the primary receiving hospital for sailors and Marines injured in the Vietnam War.

The 1993 Base Realignment and Closure (BRAC) Commission recommended closing the enlisted recruit training centers at San Diego, California, and Orlando, Florida, and consolidating all enlisted recruit training at North Chicago (BRAC, 1993). The consolidation of training meant that the NSGL would be processing in 30,000 to 40,000 recruits per year, each of whom must undergo medical intake and receive any needed medical and dental care to be found to be medically fit for deployment during the 8.5 weeks of basic training. The NSGL is also the location of many advanced training schools for about 22,000 enlisted personnel annually, as well as for the 29,000 military staff members and their families stationed at the base, for whom the Navy must provide health care.

To accommodate the expanded mission of the NSGL, the Navy launched an $860 million rebuilding program, known as the Recruit Training Command (RTC) Recapitalization Program, or RTC Recap, in 1997. (The RTC Recap was completed in July 2010.) The 200H would have been 40 years old in 2000 and in need of renovation or replacement. By this time, the Navy was staffing about 50 medical-surgical beds, which were about 50 percent occupied, and most of the building had been converted to outpatient clinic space.

The Navy had performed several studies to determine the optimal utilization and future state of the NHGL. A facility master planning study by the SRA Corporation in 2001 determined that the facility constraints of the NHGL were significantly impeding the delivery of quality health care. For example, the 40-year-old facility could no longer meet Joint Commission life safety standards without a substantial upgrading. DoD's military construction program planned to replace the 200H in FY 2007 at a cost estimated in 2001 to be $170 million (Cox and McCready, 2005).

In 1999, an internal VA study proposed closing all inpatient care at the North Chicago VAMC (NCVAMC) and converting it into an outpatient clinic. Local veterans' groups and the Illinois congressional delegation began to promote the possibility of combining inpatient care for both DoD and VA beneficiaries at the NCVAMC to justify keeping it open and to avoid the costs of building a new naval hospital. The Navy had the Center for Naval Analyses (CNA) analyze options that ranged from building a new hospital on the Navy base to partnering with the NCVAMC to take advantage of excess capacity in that facility. The most realistic options were either to build an ambulatory care center on the base and refer patients needing hospitalization to area hospitals, or to build a joint ambulatory care center next to the NCVAMC and use the facility for inpatient care. The advantages for the Navy of consolidation with the NCVAMC, in addition to avoiding the cost of building and maintaining a new hospital facility, included the lower cost of direct care compared with care provided by community facilities, the ability to keep injured and ill recruits in a military-like setting, and the opportunity for Navy clinicians to maintain their skills.

North Chicago Veterans Affairs Medical Center

The NCVAMC opened in 1926 on land obtained from the Navy. The initial mission of the 325-bed hospital was the care of long-term, chronic psychiatric patients who had served in World War I. From the beginning of the NCVAMC, it provided medical, surgical, and nursing services for the acute care needs of the inpatient population. In 1949, in the aftermath of World War II, the total number of hospital beds reached 2,500.

A new hospital building was constructed in 1978 and renovated in 1992 and 1996. Acute psychiatry facilities were modernized in 1996.

1970s: Expansion of Acute Care Capacity

Beginning in 1974, the NCVAMC began to return psychiatric patients to the community and to expand its acute care capacity. The overall number of beds fell from 2,500 in 1969 to 1,728 in 1978, reflecting a 35 percent decrease in psychiatric beds (from 1,313 to 849). By contrast, the number of general medical-surgical beds increased by 78 percent (from 388 to 689). In recognition of the shift away from psychiatric services, the NCVAMC was designated a general medical and surgical hospital by the VA in 1975. A 1978 General Accounting Office (GAO) report was very critical of this shift in mission, based on its modeling of demand, which found that the medical center would need only 105 beds in 1985 (GAO, 1978a).

In 1973, the NCVAMC proposed an affiliation with the Chicago Medical School, on the basis that the school would relocate from downtown to VA land adjacent to the hospital, and the medical center would maintain 450 to 500 acute care beds to enable training and education of medical school students and residents. The VA approved the affiliation, and the medical school, now part of the Rosalind Franklin University of Medicine and Science, moved to its present site in 1980.

1970s and 1980s: Abortive Attempts to Consolidate

In 1978, the GAO issued an in-depth report on obstacles to sharing of health resources between federal agencies (GAO, 1978b). In response, Senator Charles Percy of Illinois, chairman of the Senate Government Affairs Committee, introduced a bill to promote interagency sharing of health care resources that eventually became the VA/DoD Health Resources Sharing and Emergency Operations Act (Public Law 97-174) in 1982. After the Navy surgeon general testified at hearings on the bill that the NHGL had an average occupancy rate of less than 20 percent (120 of 656 beds), Percy asked the GAO to conduct a "review of the opportunities, the potential for savings and improved patient care, and the obstacles associated with sharing medical resources between the Veterans Administration Medical Center (VAMC), North Chicago and the Naval Regional Medical Center (NRMC), Great Lakes, Illinois" (GAO, 1980, p. 1).

The GAO found that, earlier in the 1970s, local VA officials had been interested in using the NHGL if a cross-servicing agreement could be reached, but that an effort to negotiate an agreement was never initiated. Instead, the VA spent $9.3 million on construction and equipment to upgrade the acute medical/surgical capability at the NCVAMC.

In late 1979, the Navy surgeon general and the VA's chief medical officer formed a working group of local, regional, and central office officials from both departments to explore the possibility of consolidating inpatient care at the naval hospital. The surgeon general suggested three alternatives:

1. Navy assumes the VA's workload on a reimbursable basis.
2. VA leases the Navy facility and provides services to Navy beneficiaries on a reimbursable basis.
3. Navy/VA operate jointly (GAO, 1980, Enclosure 1, p. 3).

The working group concluded that consolidating acute medical and surgical services at the naval hospital was possible and desirable. From the Navy's perspective, the benefits included

1. expansion of its services for its beneficiary population,
2. increased accessibility to care,
3. an opportunity for a portion of the local staff to remain in place during mobilization,
4. more efficient use of the existing facility, and
5. cost savings to the government and the Navy beneficiary population (GAO, 1980, Enclosure 1, p. 6).

From the VA's perspective, the naval hospital was more modern and better addressed the population's health care needs. The VA could close two 50-year-old psychiatric inpatient buildings that were expensive to maintain and operate and move the patients into the main hospital facility, Building 133, which was 20 years old, after renovation that would be less costly than upgrading the building to acute-care standards.

VA and Navy officials also noted that such a major sharing agreement could set a precedent and provide a model for additional VA/DoD sharing arrangements. The officials also pointed out, however, that the VA/DoD sharing act (Public Law 97-174) did not address a number of administrative and personnel issues that would have to be resolved.

- How would the consolidated hospital be managed? Who would control the joint medical/surgical service and ancillary service? Would the Chief of Medicine, for example, be from the VA or the Navy?
- With different employee pay and benefit systems, which agency would control the consolidated service arrangement?
- With dissimilar forms and records, which ones would be used?
- How would the upward mobility of VA employees working in the Naval facility be affected?
- How would union actions be addressed for VA employees working in the Naval facility?
- How would the Navy maintain command and control over military people working side-by-side with essentially civilian VA employees subject to different rules and regulations? (GAO, 1980, Enclosure 1, p. 17).

The same issues confronted the planners of the Lovell FHCC and, in some instances, had to be resolved by special legislation (see Chapter 3).

By the time the GAO reported on the situation, both the Navy surgeon general and the VA's chief medical officer had retired. Although the VHA regional director continued to favor a joint enterprise, the plan to use the NHGL to treat veterans was not implemented.

1990s: Department of Veterans Affairs Efforts to Rationalize Services in the Chicago Area

By the early 1990s, the VA health care system was encountering serious problems with quality of care and inpatient overcapacity. In 1991, the NCVAMC itself was in the national news when the VA inspector general reported that six deaths at the center were caused by poor care (*New York Times*, 1991). In 1992, inpatient surgery was discontinued at North Chicago and moved about 40 miles south to the Hines VA hospital.

Despite problems with inpatient surgery, Building 133 was renovated in 1996 at a cost of $139 million to consolidate all outpatient services except mental health in one building (DAC Bond, 2010). The renovation also included 150 medical and 25 acute psychiatric beds (Lovell FHCC, 2006). The GAO reported that the number of beds was not based on any analysis of need but on an assumption that if the beds were there, people would come. In fact, the NCVAMC suffered chronic overcapacity after the 1996 renovation (Lovell FHCC, 2006), which was an incentive to accept patients from the nearby naval base rather than face closure for lack of demand.

In 1995, the VHA adopted a new organizational structure. All veterans health care services in North Chicago were organized and regionally managed under the Veterans Integrated Service Network (VISN) 12, one of 21 VISNs nationwide. The VA had already begun the process of consolidating the VAMCs in some local areas, but the reorganization of services in the Chicago area was left to the new VISN director. There were four VAMCs in the area. Lakeside and West Side were 7 miles apart in the city. Hines was just west of Chicago. North Chicago was north in an outer suburb.

The GAO, at the request of the Illinois congressional delegation, began to report on developments in Chicago. In 1997, for example, the GAO reported that the VA could save $20 million a year in operating costs if there were three rather than four VAMCs in the Chicago area (GAO, 1997). In 1998, the GAO reported that, because of overcapacity, the VA could close one of the two downtown medical centers without reducing access. The same report noted that the average daily census at the NCVAMC had decreased from 470 in 1994 to 240 (27 medicine and 213 psychiatric) in 1997 and that the facility had closed 244 beds during that time period (GAO, 1998).

A committee representing the local stakeholders, including the medical schools, was unable to reach agreement on a restructuring plan. In response, the VHA chartered an internal committee composed of leaders and managers from outside of Chicago, headed by the director of the Central Arkansas Veterans Healthcare System. The committee considered six alternatives and, in September 1999, chose one that would save $188 million per year by consolidating most inpatient services at the Lakeside VAMC (U.S. House of Representatives, 1999). In its report, the *VISN 12 Delivery System Options Study*, the committee recommended that inpatient care at the NCVAMC be ended and shifted to Lakeside and that the center provide only outpatient care along with long-term and residential treatment (domiciliary) care. The VA undersecretary for health found that the committee's findings and recommendations provided a good foundation for further study, but were significantly limited because they did not account for (1) the geographic location of veterans living in VISN 12, (2) the modeling of future demand for health care services, (3) objective evaluation criteria to assess the value of each option, and (4) the lack of stakeholder input into the process.

Veterans groups in North Chicago strongly opposed the proposed changes, objecting to having to travel 60 minutes or more to Lakeside or Hines for hospitalization. Local unions representing NCVAMC employees also protested (Kuczka, 1999a). Senator Richard Durbin and Representative John Porter, the local congressman, told veterans that they would fight to keep the NCVAMC open (Kuczka, 1999b). The save-the-NCVAMC campaign was followed closely by the Chicago-area press (e.g., Flink, 1999).

1999–2000: Saving the North Chicago Veterans Affairs Medical Center

Within weeks of the leak of the VISN 12 options report in September 1999, Durbin and others in the Illinois congressional delegation developed a plan to save the NCVAMC. Rather than have the Navy spend millions of dollars to renovate or replace the 40-year-old NHGL, they proposed that the Navy use the nearby VA facility instead (O'Matz, 1999). In February 2000, Durbin was able to announce that agreement had been reached that the NCVAMC would provide psychiatric inpatient care and certain outpatient services to Navy personnel stationed at Great Lakes, and that the NHGL would provide certain surgical procedures and some diagnostic testing to veterans being seen by doctors at the NCVAMC. He characterized the agreement as "a first step toward what we hope will be a very positive partnership that is good for veterans, active-duty personnel and taxpayers" (Presecky, 2000).

Porter retired in 2000 and was succeeded by his longtime legislative assistant, Mark Kirk, who made saving the NCVAMC a major part of his election campaign. Soon after his election, Representative Kirk told local veterans in a meeting at the NCVAMC that the best way to keep the center open was to combine it with the NHGL, saying "that would obviate the need for a new naval hospital, it would decrease the cost for taxpayers, and it would ensure the survival of this institution" (*Chicago Tribune*, 2001). Kirk, a Naval Reserve officer, was assigned to the House Armed Services Committee, which helped him in working with the Navy to close a deal (Dunn, 2010). In June 2001, Kirk led a bipartisan group of congressional staffers on a tour of the NHGL and the NCVAMC to build further support for combining the facilities (Flink, 2001).

Local veterans groups favored a merger to save "their" hospital. At a rally at a Veterans of Foreign Wars post, for example, the head of the McHenry County Veterans Assistance Commission stated: "Surgery is their strong suit at Great Lakes; medical treatment is theirs at North Chicago. It would be a good thing for all of us" (Barnes, 1999).

The 2001 Veterans Integrated Service Network 12 Capital Asset Realignment for Enhanced Services Report

In response to the intense negative reaction of the various Chicago stakeholders to the 1999 VISN 12 options study, the House Committee on Veterans' Affairs Subcommittee on Health asked the VA to develop and adopt objective, measurable criteria for formulating and evaluating options for restructuring the delivery of health care (U.S. House of Representatives, 2000). In response to that request, the VHA developed an improved evaluation framework and study methodology for assessing facility needs, called the Capital Asset Realignment for Enhanced Services (CARES) process. CARES addressed the deficiencies in the original VHA internal committee methodology and incorporated the "all or none" decision-making model of DoD's BRAC process. The VA engaged Booz-Allen & Hamilton (BAH) to pilot the CARES process in VISN 12.

Meanwhile, as described above, the Navy was sponsoring studies of the follow-on to 200H, the obsolete NHGL building. Those studies explicitly considered alternatives that included shifting inpatient care to the NCVAMC.

BAH, using a private sector model to forecast demand through FY 2010, concluded that if no VAMCs had ever existed, that is, there was a clean slate, only two hospitals would be needed in the Chicago area, one near the existing West Side VAMC in downtown Chicago and the other 5–10 miles west of Hines. "We would not plan to construct an inpatient facility at North Chicago. . . . North Chicago is, however, a reasonable location for a multi-specialty ambulatory care clinic" (Booz-Allen & Hamilton, 2001, pp. 5–6). However, the four VAMCs did exist. BAH developed four options for the Chicago area, each featuring a different treatment of the West Side and Lakeside VAMCs. Each option treated the NCVAMC the same, however, allowing it 27 acute medicine and 30 acute psychiatric beds and suggesting a sharing agreement with the Navy.

> The nearby Naval hospital is in need of extensive renovation, and some consideration has been given to building a new one. With four empty acute wards and a state-of-the-art intensive care unit at the North Chicago VAMC, an opportunity exists for the VA and the DoD to share this underutilized acute care resource. Therefore, in Option A, as in all the options in the Southern Market, a sharing agreement between the VA and the DoD is proposed. If that agreement were reached, the acute medical and surgical workload provided by the Navy, currently estimated to be about two wards or 60 patients, when added to the VA acute care workload, would provide a critical mass of acute care beds sufficient to justify ongoing acute inpatient care.
>
> Even if a VA/DoD sharing agreement is not reached, all four options propose keeping a small acute medical service. With approximately 248 nursing home beds and approximately 100 psychiatric beds, acute medical beds will be needed on an ongoing basis to accommodate those long-term care patients who "decompensate." Given the size of this campus and the spectrum of services, the incremental cost of these added acute beds is relatively small and clinically appropriate. This option also preserves the affiliation with Chicago Medical School. (Booz-Allen & Hamilton, 2001, pp. 5–12)

Each of the four options recommended 57 acute care beds (27 medical and 30 psychiatry) at the NCVAMC, in part to serve the needs of patients in the 541 non-acute beds it recommended that the NCVAMC have (248 nursing home, 67 long-term psychiatry, 186 domiciliary, and 40 residential rehabilitation treatment program) (Booz-Allen & Hamilton, 2001, pp. 5–12). According to the BAH report, the NHGL's average daily census in its medical-surgical beds was 24 and in its acute psychiatric beds was 22, which BAH judged could be easily absorbed by the VA (Booz-Allen & Hamilton, 2001, pp. 8–20).

The VA secretary issued his decision on the restructuring of health care in VISN 12 in February 2002. The announcement focused on the decision to close inpatient care at the Lakeside VAMC and move all acute inpatient services to the West Side VAMC; the only reference to the disposition of inpatient and other services in North Chicago was the statement that "sharing opportunities between the North Chicago VA Medical Center and the adjacent Naval Hospital Great Lakes will be enhanced" (VA, 2002b). Before and shortly after the VA secretary's announcement, serious discussions were opened between the VA and the DoD on the futures of the NCVAMC and the NHGL.

2001–2002: Deciding on a Consolidated Federal Health Care Facility

By 2001, the director of the NCVAMC and the commanding officer of the NHGL were discussing how to proceed (Kuczka, 2001). The two facilities had done some sharing over the years. For example, in the late 1980s, the NHGL purchased a computed tomography scanner. The NCVAMC provided two technicians in return for use of the scanner. In the early 1990s, when the NHGL found it difficult for contracting and pay reasons to recruit psychologists, psychiatrists, pharmacists, radiologists, nurses, and other professionals, the NCVAMC agreed to hire 75 staff using its Title 38 authority to work at the hospital, although that arrangement was subsequently determined to be illegal by the Navy's judge advocate general (Harnly, 2005). In the mid-1990s, the NCVAMC was using the NHGL for total joint replacements, which tripled the volume of cases for the Navy orthopedic surgeons.

According to the VISN 12 CARES study, the VA and the DoD signed an agreement in March 2000 permitting active duty servicemembers and their dependents to receive specialty care at the VA and veterans to receive care at the NHGL (Booz-Allen & Hamilton, 2001, pp. 8–19). In 2003, 2–3 veterans per week were undergoing orthopedic and surgical procedures at the NHGL (Hagen, 2003).

In July 2001, the VA/DoD Health Executive Council became involved. It appointed a North Chicago VA–Great Lakes Naval Training Center Task Force to "explore short and long term options for improved coordination of health care delivery, including review of the possibility of establishing a joint medical facility serving both veterans and Navy personnel" (Mackay, 2002, p. 61). The task force was to report in the late spring of 2002 with the "facts and figures that are necessary to make a good business decision" (Chu, 2002, p. 33).

In February 2002, VA Deputy Secretary Leo Mackay and Secretary of the Navy Gordon England traveled to North Chicago to sign a "landmark" capital asset sharing agreement. The agreement was for the VA to transfer 48 acres to the Navy to build recruit barracks and a drill hall in exchange for which the Navy would purchase electricity and steam from a VA-sponsored cogeneration energy center (VA, 2002b).

In October 2002, the DoD and the VA agreed on the basic plan for structuring the VA/DoD health service system in North Chicago. According to the plan,

- the Navy would use the NCVAMC for inpatient mental health care.
- the VA would renovate the NCVAMC surgical suite, post-anesthesia care unit, and emergency department.

- the Navy would transfer its inpatient medical/surgical workload to the NCVAMC after the renovation.
- the Navy would construct a new Ambulatory Care Center on the NCVAMC campus for joint use (Cox and McCready, 2005).

According to the VA press release announcing the agreement, the Navy would

> construct a new ambulatory medical facility for outpatient services. The North Chicago VA Medical Center will provide comprehensive surgical care. The Navy, through partnership with North Chicago VAMC, will use the VA hospital for its inpatient medical and surgical needs. Additionally, Navy surgical teams will work at the North Chicago VAMC, enabling them to maintain their surgical competencies. (VA, 2002a)

William Winkenwerder, the assistant secretary of defense for health affairs, explained the purpose of the agreement as follows:

> With this agreement, the Navy gains a modern ambulatory care center at a cost less than building a new hospital. VA beneficiaries gain increased access to surgical care closer to their homes and families, and the overall operating expenses of both departments should be reduced. (VA, 2002a)

Summary Through 2002

A number of factors led to the effort to consolidate health care services provided by the Navy and the VA in North Chicago. A major factor in the proposed changes was driven by the national private and public health care delivery trend away from hospital care toward delivery of more services in the ambulatory medical, surgical, and psychiatric health care settings. Some other long-term health care, military, and political factors added pressure for change and others were events that helped to shape the changes that occurred. They included the following:

- The 1993 BRAC recommendation to close the naval training centers at San Diego and Orlando and consolidate all recruit training at the NSGL. This substantially increased the demand for health care services from DoD beneficiaries in North Chicago.
- The 1999 VA working group report on ways to address excess capacity in Chicago-area VAMCs, which recommended that the NCVAMC be converted into an ambulatory care center. That threat of closure provided an incentive to accept the NHGL's inpatient workload.

- Political pressure beginning in 1999 from local veterans organizations through the Illinois congressional delegation to keep the NCVAMC open.
- The 2001 VISN 12 CARES report, which recommended increased collaboration with the Navy to justify keeping the NCVAMC open.
- The 2001 report by the SRA Corporation on the need to replace the Navy hospital building, built in 1960, to meet Joint Commission life safety standards, which could be avoided by using the NCVAMC for inpatient and emergency services.
- Sustained oversight by and funding from the VA/DoD Joint Executive and Joint Health Councils beginning in 2001 for the establishment of a combined federal facility in North Chicago.
- The 2002 report by CNA on Navy health care options in North Chicago, several of which involved using the NCVAMC for inpatient care.
- Persistent congressional interest in piloting an integrated VA/DoD health care center at some location.

Some of the trends facilitating collaboration included the following:

- Shifts in beneficiary utilization. Demand for inpatient services was falling off sharply, reflecting changes in health care delivery, but that was offset by increases in the number of active duty enrollees due to the global war on terror, the number of veterans eligible for VA health care due to the Veterans Millennium Health Care and Benefits Act of 1999, and the demand from retirees and their dependents with the implementation of TFL in 2001.
- The reduced and constantly changing number of active duty providers resulting from deployments made after 2001, which would be mitigated by using VA providers who do not deploy.
- The need to maintain the clinical skills of active duty providers, which would be enhanced by treating a larger number of patients with a great range of high acuity medical conditions.
- The high and increasing cost of health care for DoD beneficiaries, which provided an incentive to expand direct care to avoid sending patients to more expensive community providers.

The main motivation for collaboration, however, was the confluence of the need to replace the NHGL and the constituent pressure to keep the NCVAMC open (Cox and McCready, 2005). In that context, a consolidation of services seemed to be a win-win solution. Developing a combined delivery structure would almost certainly reduce construction and operating costs, probably reduce the disruption of deployments of Navy clinicians, and possibly increase access and quality of care, patient satisfaction, medical education and research opportunities, and the ability of Navy clinicians to treat more complex cases.

REFERENCES

Barnes, D. 1999. McHenry County vets fear losing VA hospital. *Chicago Tribune*, November 19. http://articles.chicagotribune.com/1999-11-19/news/9911190240_1_veterans-hospital-world-war-ii-veteran-outpatient (accessed July 26, 2012).

Booz-Allen & Hamilton. 2001. *Capital Asset Realignment for Enhanced Services (CARES): VISN 12 service delivery options*. June 19. McLean, VA: Booz-Allen & Hamilton.

BRAC (Defense Base Closure and Realignment Commission). 1993 (July 1). *Report to the President*. Arlington, VA: BRAC.

Chicago Tribune. 2001. Kirk floats option to save VA center. March 24. http://articles.chicagotribune.com/2001-03-24/news/0103240201_1_veteran-population-ages-military-veterans-enrollees (accessed July 26, 2012).

Chu, D. 2002. *VA-DoD health care sharing by the Department of Defense and the Department of Veterans Affairs*. Hearing before the Health Subcommittee of the Committee on Veterans' Affairs and the Military Personnel Committee of the Committee on Armed Services, House of Representatives, March 7. Washington, DC: U.S. Government Printing Office. http://frwebgate.access.gpo.gov/cgi-bin/getdoc.cgi?dbname=107_house_hearings&docid=f:80528.pdf (accessed July 26, 2012).

Cox, K., and S. McCready. 2005. Current DoD/VA issues. PowerPoint presentation at the 2005 TRICARE Conference. http://www.tricare.mil/DVPCO/conf2005.cfm (accessed July 26, 2012).

CRS (Congressional Research Service). 2009. Military medical care: Questions and answers. RL33537, May 14. http://www.fas.org/sgp/crs/misc/RL33537.pdf (accessed September 14, 2012).

DAC Bond. 2010. Bond disclosure. http://pdfuri.com/north-chicago-veterans-affairs-medical-center (homepage: http://www.dacbond.com) (accessed August 3, 2012).

DoD (Department of Defense). 2010. *2010 Military Health System stakeholders report. Sharing knowledge: Achieving breakthrough performance*. http://health.mil/Libraries/Documents_Word_PDF_PPT_etc/2010_MHS_Stakeholders_Report.pdf (accessed July 27, 2012).

DoD. 2011a. *2011 Military Health System stakeholders report. The quadruple aim: Working together, achieving success*. http://health.mil/Libraries/Documents_Word_PDF_PPT_etc/2011_MHS_Stakeholders_Report.pdf (accessed July 27, 2012).

DoD. 2011b. *Evaluation of the TRICARE program FY 2011*. http://www.tricare.mil/hpae/_docs/TRICARE_2011.pdf (accessed August 3, 2012).

Dunn, J. 2010. The many sides of Mark Kirk. *Illinois Issues*, November. http://illinoisissues.uis.edu/archives/2011/01/kirk.html (accessed July 27, 2012).

Flink, J. 1999. Veterans speak out on altering VA hospital: Durbin hears pleas, vows to delay plans until rebuttal heard. *Chicago Tribune*, October 26. http://articles.chicagotribune.com/1999-10-26/news/9910260165_1_va-facilities-veterans-integrated-service-network-worl-war-ii-veteran (accessed July 27, 2012).

Flink, J. 2001. Kirk urges military hospital tie-in. *Chicago Tribune*, June 9. http://articles.chicagotribune.com/2001-06-09/news/0106090238_1_va-hospital-veterans-integrated-service-network-active-duty-personnel (accessed July 27, 2012).

GAO (U.S. General Accounting Office). 1978a. *Inappropriate number of hospital beds planned by Veterans Administration for Chicago area.* HRD-78-127. Washington, DC: GAO. http://archive.gao.gov/f0902b/106270.pdf (accessed July 27, 2012).

GAO. 1978b. *Legislation needed to encourage better use of federal medical resources and remove obstacles to interagency sharing.* GAO/HRD-78-54. Washington, DC: GAO. http://archive.gao.gov/f0902a/106271.pdf (accessed July 27, 2012).

GAO. 1980. *Sharing of federal medical resources in North Chicago/Great Lakes, Illinois area.* GAO/HRD-81-13. Washington, DC: GAO. http://archive.gao.gov/otherpdf2/113527.pdf (accessed July 27, 2012).

GAO. 1997. *VA health care: Lessons learned from medical facility integrations.* GAO/T-HEHS-97-184. Washington, DC: GAO. http://www.gao.gov/archive/1997/he97184t.pdf (accessed July 27, 2012).

GAO. 1998. *VA health care: Closing a Chicago hospital would save millions and enhance access to services.* GAO/HEHS-98-64. Washington, DC: GAO. http://www.gao.gov/archive/1998/he98064.pdf (accessed July 27, 2012).

Hagen, M. 2003. VA, Pentagon align health services: Improved care for vets, troops is goal. *Chicago Tribune*, July 2. http://articles.chicagotribune.com/2003-07-02/news/0307020177_1_gulf-war-vets-va-hospitals-health-care (accessed July 27, 2012).

Harnly, M. J. 2005. A qualitative analysis of resource sharing agreements between Naval Hospital Great Lakes and North Chicago Veterans Affairs Medical Center: The iron triangle theory of healthcare integration. Master's Thesis, Army-Baylor Program in Healthcare Administration, Fort Sam Houston, TX. http://www.dtic.mil/dtic/tr/fulltext/u2/a443921.pdf (accessed July 27, 2012).

Kime, P. 2012. DoD: Tricare beneficiaries should go to MTFs. *Army Times*, February 6. http://www.armytimes.com/news/2012/02/military-treatment-facilities-tricare-020612w/ (accessed July 27, 2012).

Kuczka, S. 1999a. Veterans rallying around hospital. *Chicago Tribune*, October 8. http://articles.chicagotribune.com/1999-10-08/news/9910080297_1_tollway-extension-rally-chicago-area (accessed July 27, 2012).

Kuczka, S. 1999b. Vets have an ally in hospital fight: Porter vows to battle for N. Chicago Center. *Chicago Tribune*, September 14. http://articles.chicagotribune.com/1999-09-14/news/9909140117_1_va-doctor-veterans-affairs-officials-world-war-ii-veteran (accessed July 27, 2012).

Kuczka, S. 2001. Pact likely for hospital, VA center. *Chicago Tribune*, October 30. http://articles.chicagotribune.com/2001-10-30/news/0110300206_1_va-facility-va-patients-veterans (accessed July 27, 2012).

Lovell FHCC (Captain James A. Lovell Federal Health Care Center). 2006. The joint initiative between the North Chicago VAMC and Naval Hospital Great Lakes. Presentation at the 2006 Military Health System Conference, January 31. www.tricare.mil/dvpco/bummed/NHGL%20NCVAMC%20BRIEF.ppt (accessed August 24, 2012).

Mackay, L. 2002. *VA-DoD health care sharing by the Department of Defense and the Department of Veterans Affairs.* Statement before the Health Subcommittee of the Committee on Veterans' Affairs and the Military Personnel Committee of the Committee on Armed Services, House of Representatives, March 7. Washington, DC: U.S. Government Printing Office. http://frwebgate.access.gpo.gov/cgi-bin/getdoc.cgi?dbname=107_house_hearings&docid=f:80528.pdf (accessed July 27, 2012).

Naval Station Great Lakes. 2012. CNIC/Naval Station Great Lakes: History. http://www.cnic.navy.mil/GreatLakes/AboutUs/History/index.htm (accessed July 26, 2012).

New York Times. 1991. U.S. tells how 6 died from poor care in hospital. http://www.nytimes.com/1991/04/10/us/us-tells-how-6-died-from-poor-care-in-hospital.html?src=pm (accessed July 27, 2012).

O'Matz, M. 1999. Navy urged to rescue VA hospital. *Chicago Tribune*, November 11. http://articles.chicagotribune.com/1999-11-11/news/9911110257_1_va-community-veterans-day-va-patients (accessed July 27, 2012).

Presecky, W. 2000. Navy, VA reach accord on vets' medical services; Great Lakes, N. Chicago Hospitals to provide care. *Chicago Tribune*, February 27. http://articles.chicagotribune.com/2000-02-27/news/0002270159_1_veterans-hospitals-va-study-delegation (accessed July 27, 2012).

Ruschmeier, E. 2011. VA health care overview: VA/DoD Liaison Sharing Office. Presentation at the 2011 VA/DoD Joint Venture Conference, October 18. http://www.tricare.mil/DVPCO/downloads/CJVC2011/VA%20Update.pptx (accessed July 27, 2012).

TRICARE. 2012. *TRICARE choices at a glance*. May. http://tricare.mil/mybenefit/Download/Forms/AtaGlance_Brochure.pdf (accessed September 17, 2012).

U.S. House of Representatives. 1999. *VA's capital assets realignment plan for enhancing services to veterans*. Hearing before the Subcommittee on Oversight and Investigation of the Committee on Veterans' Affairs, July 22. Washington, DC: U.S. Government Printing Office. http://frwebgate.access.gpo.gov/cgi-bin/getdoc.cgi?dbname=106_house_hearings&docid=f:62150.pdf (accessed July 27, 2012).

U.S. House of Representatives. 2000. *VA capital asset planning*. Hearing before the Subcommittee on Health of the Committee on Veterans' Affairs, April 5. Washington, DC: U.S. Government Printing Office. http://frwebgate.access.gpo.gov/cgi-bin/getdoc.cgi?dbname=106_house_hearings&docid=f:65441.pdf (accessed July 27, 2012).

U.S. House of Representatives. 2010. *Report to accompany H.R. 5822, Military Construction, Veterans Affairs, and related agencies appropriations bill, 2011*. Committee on Appropriations, July 22. Washington, DC: U.S. Government Printing Office.

VA (Department of Veterans Affairs). 2002a. VA and DoD agree on health care in North Chicago. Press release, October 18. http://www1.va.gov/opa/pressrel/pressrelease.cfm?id=523 (accessed July 27, 2012).

VA. 2002b. VA announces decision on realigning Chicago-area hospitals. Press release, February 8. http://www.va.gov/opa/pressrel/pressrelease.cfm?id=396 (accessed July 27, 2012).

VA. 2012. *VA congressional submission for FY 2013 funding and FY 2014 advance appropriations: Volume II, medical programs & information technology programs*. http://www.va.gov/budget/docs/summary/Fy2013_Volume_II-Medical_Programs_Information_Technology.pdf (accessed July 27, 2012).

3

Implementation

The Department of Veterans Affairs/Department of Defense (VA/DoD) Health Executive Council (HEC) executive decision memorandum (EDM) of October 2002 was only the beginning of a long and complicated process of consolidating federal health care delivery activities in North Chicago into a single federal health care facility (FHCC).[1] Some of the key decisions were made in the 2002 EDM, namely, that the Navy would close its hospital (Building 200H) and move inpatient services to the nearby North Chicago VA Medical Center (NCVAMC) building and outpatient services to a new, Navy-constructed ambulatory care center (ACC) connected to the NCVAMC hospital building. Other key decisions were made later, such as adopting a single chain of command, transferring civilians employed by the Navy to the VA, creating a unified financial system and jointly funded Department of the Treasury (Treasury) account for the combined facility, and creating a single interface with both the VA and the DoD electronic health record (EHR) systems. There were statements that VA and Navy providers would be working side by side, there would be a single standard of care regardless of beneficiary status, and the needs of both VA and Navy beneficiaries would be met seamlessly, but the steps it would take to achieve these goals were not clear at first.

---

[1] Initially, the proposed joint health care delivery initiative was called the federal health care facility, or FHCF. It began to be called a federal health care center in late 2007, in conjunction with plans to name the joint medical center after Captain James A. Lovell. "Federal health care center," or "FHCC," will be used in the rest of this report regardless of the time period. It should also be noted that while the Lovell FHCC name is singular, it comprises a number of buildings on the east and west campuses and three outlying outpatient centers.

THE IMPLEMENTATION PHASES

By 2006, the concept of a three-phase implementation process was adopted. Phase 1 was the shifting of inpatient mental health services from the Naval Hospital Great Lakes (NHGL) to the NCVAMC that had taken place in 2003. Phase 2 was the shifting of emergency services and inpatient medical, surgical, and pediatric services from the Navy hospital to the NCVAMC in 2006, after the NCVAMC's emergency department (ED) and surgical facilities were upgraded by the VA. Phase 3 was the shift of all Navy outpatient services to the new ACC building and other renovated spaces on the west campus of the Lovell FHCC, as well as the implementation of the FHCC as a single organization under a single chain of command in 2010.

Phase 1

In accordance with the October 2002 EDM, the Navy and the VA entered into a resource sharing agreement in which the Navy would discontinue acute inpatient psychiatric services at 200H and the NCVAMC would assume responsibility for the treatment of Navy patients in its acute mental health inpatient unit and lodge discharged mental patients in its psychiatric medical holding unit. According to the agreement, the Navy would compensate the NCVAMC for the services as a TRICARE network provider (i.e., at 90 percent of the CHAMPUS[2] maximum allowable charge for the specific diagnosis related group) and provide several psychiatric support staff (Harnly, 2005). The agreement was implemented in October 2003, when six patients were transferred to the NCVAMC (Kuczka, 2003).

In August 2004, the Navy and the VA signed another resource sharing agreement in which the Navy operates a blood donor processing center in the NCVAMC in return for providing the NCVAMC with blood products. The NCVAMC agreed to provide 3,242 square feet of unused laboratory space and utilities, in addition to staff to monitor the cooling equipment after hours. The Navy agreed to pay $40,000 for renovations and $46,600 in rent. In exchange, the NCVAMC agreed to buy 415 units of blood products annually at a cost that was approximately equal to the rent (Harnly, 2005). The arrangement has benefited the Navy because the space in which it was located at Building 81H on the Navy base was no longer adequate and would have cost more than $3 million to renovate; in return, the NCVAMC has benefited by paying less for blood products (Hassan et al., 2008).

Neither of the sharing agreements was free of problems at first. The Navy and the NCVAMC disagreed on the amount of air-conditioning that would be needed for the blood processing laboratory, and experience

[2] CHAMPUS stands for the Civilian Health and Medical Program of the Uniformed Services.

soon showed that more air-conditioning capacity was needed (Harnly, 2005). Although the Navy offered to operate the acute psychiatric unit, the NCVAMC preferred to provide the service and be reimbursed. The volume and acuity of patients and therefore the amounts of reimbursement were less than forecast, and, finding itself overstaffed and losing money, the NCVAMC sought more reimbursement, which the Navy was unwilling to pay (Harnly, 2005).

The NCVAMC held a press conference in November 2003 to announce that the transfer of mental health patients from the NHGL to the NCVAMC had begun. Representative Mark Kirk announced that construction on a $170 million joint VA/Navy health care facility next to the NCVAMC would begin in about 5 years. He told veterans at a Veterans Day ceremony the same day that "if the Navy moves into this facility, it can never close." NCVAMC director Patrick Sullivan said that the expanded volume of Navy patients would lead to the addition of inpatient surgical services in 2005 (Susnjara, 2003).

Phase 2

The second phase of the VA/DoD partnership was the moving of inpatient surgical and medical services and emergency services from the NHGL to the NCVAMC. The Navy could have sent its inpatient and emergency cases to community hospitals, but using the NCVAMC promised to be less expensive and would allow Navy clinicians to maintain their surgical skills. The move would enable the NCVAMC to have a large enough workload to offer inpatient surgery for the first time since 1992 and to upgrade and enlarge its ED, which would benefit its veteran enrollees (VA, 2002). Before 2006, veterans needing surgery had to be sent 45 miles or more to another VAMC (located either west of Chicago at Hines, in Chicago at the Jesse Brown VAMC, or in Milwaukee, Wisconsin) or referred to a community hospital.

The Navy providers were understandably concerned about moving surgical services to a VAMC where inpatient surgeries had not been performed for 20 years. When they toured the VAMC, they were concerned about the poor condition of the operating suites (Interviews[3]). The Navy was unwilling to expand the partnership unless appropriate renovations were done at the NCVAMC.

The VA worked with Congress to allocate $13 million in fiscal year (FY) 2004 construction funds to renovate the ED and construct a new surgical center because VA renovation projects were limited to $4 million (Chu, 2003). The number of ED examination rooms was increased from 6

[3] This indicates information provided by anonymous interviews with Lovell FHCC staff.

to 14; 4 new operating rooms and related facilities (e.g., recovery rooms) were built; and 4 existing operating rooms were renovated. The construction award was made in September 2004 and the project was completed in 2006 (U.S. Senate, 2005).

Meanwhile, the physician leaders of the NHGL and the NCVAMC began to work closely together to plan and implement the move of surgical services in 2006. Both leaders were able to remain throughout the implementation process, providing stable leadership to plan and launch the Lovell FHCC in 2010. In 2010, the NCVAMC chief of staff became the associate director for patient care/chief medical executive and the NHGL director became the assistant director for patient care/assistant chief medical executive. This continuity of clinical leadership is considered by the FHCC leadership to have been an important factor in achieving the degree of clinical integration that has been attained (the degree of clinical integration is discussed in Chapter 4).

In June 2006, after the ED, operating rooms, and intensive/critical care unit were upgraded, inpatient medical and surgical services for DoD beneficiaries were moved to the NCVAMC. Navy physicians provided inpatient surgery and pediatric services (the first time pediatrics had been offered at any VA health care facility). With the removal of all inpatient services in 2006, the NHGL was redesignated as the Naval Health Clinic Great Lakes (NHCGL).

Even before the inpatient services at the NHGL were transferred in 2006, there was a fair amount of clinical sharing. In July 2004, the Government Accountability Office (GAO) reported that

> VA provides inpatient psychiatry and intensive care, and outpatient clinic visits, for example, pulmonary care, neurology, gastrointestinal care, diabetic care, occupational and physical therapy, speech therapy, rehabilitation, and diagnostic tests to Navy beneficiaries. VA also provides medical training to Naval corpsmen, nursing staff, and dental residents. The Navy provides selected surgical services for VA beneficiaries such as joint replacement surgeries and cataract surgeries. In addition, as available, the Navy provides selected outpatient services, mammograms, magnetic resonance imaging (MRI) examinations, and laboratory tests. (GAO, 2004, pp. 16–17)

After the inpatient medical-surgical transfer, the reimbursement methodology for inpatient services was facility charges at the TRICARE network negotiated rate (Lovell FHCC, 2006). The VA paid the Navy about $295,000 and the Navy paid the VA $502,000 during FYs 2002 and 2003, which was estimated to be approximately $88,000 less than the VA and the Navy would have paid for the same services in the private sector, and having the VA provide acute mental health services in the 10-bed ward and the 10-bed medical hold unit saved the Navy about $323,000 per year (GAO, 2004, p. 17).

Governance of these collaborative activities was through an executive steering committee co-chaired by the NCVAMC director and the NHGL commanding officer. The executive steering committee worked through administrative, clinical, and mental health subcommittees (Lovell FHCC, 2006).

The VA/Navy merger process also benefited from a series of early Joint Incentive Fund (JIF) awards. In FY 2004, for example, the NHGL and the NCVAMC received JIF funds for two joint projects—mammography and a women's health clinic—to enhance access and quality of care for women veterans. The new women's health clinic, which offers mammography, ultrasound, gynecology, and case managers in one location, would not have been possible to sustain without the volume added by Navy beneficiaries. In FY 2005, the FHCC received JIF awards to purchase a magnetic resonance imaging (MRI) machine, start an oncology/hematology clinic, and build a high-capacity fiber optic cable to connect the facilities on the VA campus with the Navy clinics that would remain on the base. In FY 2006, there were awards to add a hospitalist and the capacity to perform digital radiography (picture archiving and communication system, or PACS), capitalizing on the new fiber optic connection between the campuses. (Additional JIF awards during Phase 3 are reviewed in Box 3-1.)

Phase 3

On May 26, 2005, William Winkenwerder, the assistant secretary of defense for health affairs, and Jonathan Perlin, the under secretary of veterans affairs for health, the co-chairs of the HEC, signed an EDM that approved construction of a Navy-funded ACC adjoining the North Chicago VA medical center hospital building (Building 133) and creation of a single-chain-of-command governance structure for a joint federal health care facility.

The approved costs included construction of the ACC, renovation of space in the VA hospital building for some of the outpatient clinics, and construction of a 562-car, 4-story parking garage and a 540-car surface parking lot. The total amount of $139.1 million was less than the $160.6 million originally proposed. It was achieved by reducing the size of the ACC through renovating additional space in Building 133 and by cutting additional administrative positions. The original cost also presumed that the ACC would be built on the south side of Building 133, which would have required demolition of a nursing home care unit (NHCU) and construction of a new $25 million NHCU elsewhere on the VA campus. The south site was preferred by the Navy because it was the largest, but scaling back the

BOX 3-1
Joint Incentive Fund Awards to North Chicago, Fiscal Years 2004–2007

Women's Health Clinic (FY 2004)
$852,000

Mammography Services (FY 2004)
$470,000

These JIF [Joint Incentive Fund] awards established a comprehensive women's health center to serve both female veterans and DoD [Department of Defense] beneficiaries. VA [Department of Veterans Affairs] hired gynecology staff (replacing a lost Navy physician billet), purchased digital mammography equipment and a stereotactic unit, and hired two wellness/case management nurses. A partial cost savings of $70,000 resulted during the fiscal year, for example, by paying less for stereotactic mammograms in the private sector (VA/DoD, 2008a, p. 29). The center was a significant expansion of services for veteran and DoD women.

Hematology-Oncology Program (FY 2005)
$685,000

A hematology-oncology program was added to include consultations, inpatient support, outpatient care, and a chemotherapy infusion center for VA and DoD beneficiaries. Neither the VA nor [the] DoD previously provided these services, and all patients had been referred to the local community for care. By combining services, access was improved and patients no longer needed to travel long distances to receive their care (VA/DoD, 2006a, p. 18).

Joint Magnetic Resonance Imaging (FY 2005)
$3,426,000

The award was to purchase a 3-Tesla state-of-the-art open-field MRI [magnetic resonance imaging unit] that was permanently housed in a modern MRI suite. The full-time fixed-site MRI, which became functional in March 2007, has reduced patient wait time and expensive referrals for contract care. It reduced delays in treatment and thus reduced the length of stay for acutely ill inpatients. This project included funding for a radiologist to perform interpretation of MRIs and [to] consult with providers (VA/DoD, 2006a, p. 18).

Clinical Fiber Optics (FY 2005)
$248,000

The project provided high-speed clinical connectivity between both facilities to transmit clinical images for the VA's PACS [picture archiving and communication system], VistA [Veterans Health Information Systems and Technology Architecture] imaging, and computerized patient record system (CPRS) (VA/DoD, 2006a, p. 18).

Hospitalist (FY 2006)
$403,000

The presence of the two hospitalists has enabled VA and Navy internal medicine, primary care, and specialty providers to increase capacity in the outpatient setting and to recapture and empanel more patients to the clinics. The program has shown a decrease in the average length of stay of patients while maintaining good clinical outcomes. It provides for the continuity of inpatient care, post-discharge planning and follow-up, and eliminates the uncertainty of who will be caring for patients on a day-to-day basis (VA/DoD, 2008a, pp. 28–29).

Digital Radiography (FY 2006)
$638,000

This project involves installing a PACS at NHGL [Naval Hospital Great Lakes] that will provide unlimited web-based access from NCVAMC [North Chicago Veterans Affairs Medical Center] as well as from within NHGL and its branch health clinics, and allow providers at both facilities greater access to patients' imaging studies. Additionally, this project will improve the NCVAMC PACS to include an upgraded memory for image archive, an updated software platform for PACS, and upgraded viewing stations. This will provide comparable imaging services at each facility with the availability for easy exchange of radiology information and images (VA/DoD, 2006b, p. 6).

Project Management Support (FY 2007)
$1,770,000

This award provided a dedicated contract staff for project management support of the steering group, the six national work groups, and a number of local joint committees engaged in planning the FHCC [federal health care center] (VA/DoD, 2006b, p. 6).

Enterprise Information Management/Information Technology Requirements at the Lovell Federal Health Care Center (FY 2008)
$11,000,000

This enterprise-level JIF project supported the development of the technical requirements for the basic interoperability capabilities that the Lovell FHCC staff would need to enter, edit, and retrieve patient information in both the VA and [the] DoD EHRs [electronic health record systems] simultaneously (VA/DoD, 2008b, pp. 17–18).

Enterprise Information Management/Information Technology Development at the Lovell Federal Health Care Center (FYs 2009/2010)
$100,020,000

This enterprise-level JIF project supported the work of VA and DoD IT staff and private contractors to develop new interoperability software to enable the Lovell FHCC staff to enter, edit, and retrieve patient information in both the VA and DoD EHRs simultaneously (VA, 2010a, pp. 1G–4G).

Interim Pharmacy Solution at the Lovell Federal Health Care Center (FY 2010)
$1,000,000

This enterprise-level JIF award supported the interim solution to the lack of interoperability between VA and DoD EHRs that would have created unacceptable patient safety risks. The interim solution was to hire five licensed pharmacists to manually check for potential drug-drug and drug-allergy interactions in both EHRs for every prescription (VA/DoD, 2011, p. 57).

footprint of the ACC meant it could be built on the east site, obviating the need to replace the NHCU.

The decision to downsize the ACC by half, to 201,000 square feet, had another impact. It affected decisions on which and how many clinics to combine instead of to maintain as separate Navy and VA clinics (discussed below). It drove a decision to adopt the VA's Consolidated Mail Order Pharmacy (CMOP) program so that the pharmacy dispensing space in the ACC could be downsized, which became a problem when the DoD decided against letting the FHCC use the CMOP. The reduced size of the pharmacy space also made it more difficult to implement a manual workaround when the IT solution to enable orders portability between the DoD and the VA EHR systems was not ready in time (discussed below).

In addition to a lower-cost construction project, the proposal contained a substantially revised governance structure. At the March 2005 meeting of the HEC, the VA and Navy planning group had proposed a dual command and reporting structure in which the NCVAMC director and the NHGL commanding officer would be coequals, each reporting to his or her respective department. Under them would be consolidated directorates for clinical services, patient services, and administration, each headed by coequal associate directors. There would be a single medical staff working within a matrix system under a single set of bylaws. This partnership was considered to be a step toward the ultimate goal of full integration. The HEC, at the urging of Vice Admiral Donald Arthur, the Navy surgeon general, directed the planning group to plan a fully integrated organization under a single-line-of-authority governance structure.

The revised governance EDM listed the pros and cons for what it called the federal health care model, in which all services currently provided by the Navy and the VA in North Chicago would be located within a single organizational structure under a single chain of command. The single chain of command would be a VA senior executive service director and chief executive officer and a Navy captain deputy director and chief of operations, who would report to a board of directors under the HEC. The EDM identified the pros of establishing a single organization, as it would

- increase the range of specialty care services available to VA and DoD beneficiaries,
- meld the medical staff into one body for clinical oversight,
- create a single standard of care for all beneficiaries and thus provide a seamless patient care environment, and
- reduce redundancies and thus reduce operating costs.

The cons were a prescient listing of the challenges that were subsequently encountered during the implementation. The creation of a combined health care center would require

- significant communication efforts among all senior members of the DoD, the Navy, and the VA to support the development and implementation of the combined federal health care organization;
- each parent organization to accept a significant reorganization resulting in a loss of autonomy over its respective personnel and assets;
- the crossing of cultural borders when personnel from one organization were supervised by the other organization's personnel for daily functions;
- the establishment of an interdepartmental process for resolution of disputes; and
- the development of support systems (e.g., acquisition, information, budgeting, human resources) that would meet the standards and reporting requirements of the VA, the Navy, and the DoD.

The working group identified areas in which issues would have to be addressed, some of which might require legislative relief or changes in one or both departments' policies, regulations, or business rules. These included personnel management, information management/information technology (IM/IT), budgeting, eligibility, and pharmacy. To identify these and explore the options for resolving any differences, the HEC chartered six national task groups:

1. Leadership
2. Finance and budgeting
3. Human resources
4. IM/IT
5. Clinical
6. Administration

In 2007, another task group, for communications, was established to inform stakeholders about and involve them in the integration process.

The task group members were national and local subject matter experts and were co-chaired by a VA official and a Navy or a DoD official. In all, more than 100 individuals served as members of task groups.

Each task group was charged with

- identifying all policies, directives, regulations, and laws (e.g., Titles 5, 10, and 38 of the U.S. Code) specific to each department's operations in the task group's subject area that would have to be changed or dropped to allow integration of NCVAMC and NHGL health care operations in the FHCC;
- developing a timeline for the full implementation of the operational plan, including milestones and activities; and

- developing recommendations of ways to overcome any barriers to full implementation of the FHCC.

On October 17, 2005, Winkenwerder and Gordon Mansfield, the VA deputy secretary, announced the joint agreement during a press conference in North Chicago. A local newspaper headline was "Navy, VA do hospital deal; Sailors, vets to get care under 1 roof" (Gibbard, 2005). In a press release, Winkenwerder said that the process of combining the two health centers would be "difficult," but the benefit would be "the continued provision of accessible, high quality health care for active duty and veteran patients that benefits taxpayers through the reduction of costs by reducing duplication between these two health care delivery systems." He also said that the collaboration would "improve the seamless delivery of care to patients, from entry into the armed forces through veteran status" (Ellis, 2005).

THE TASK GROUP PROCESS

The national task groups began to meet periodically, usually quarterly, either in North Chicago or in the Washington, DC, area. They were mirrored by local task groups that met more often, usually biweekly but sometimes weekly. The national leadership task group (LTG) met biweekly by telephone to address governance and other organizational and management issues and to oversee the progress of the other task groups. The LTG and some of the other task groups held periodic 2-day retreats and, once or twice per year, all the national task groups met in retreat for several days. There was also a series of cross–task group meetings to address issues that affected two or more task groups.

The procedure was for each task group to develop an EDM for HEC approval for each of the issues in its jurisdiction that could not be decided under local authority. The EDMs were to present options, usually three but sometimes two or four, with pros and cons for each option, and to recommend one option for HEC consideration and decision. The plan was to use the approved EDMs to develop a concept of operations as the basis for a business plan and then for detailed standard operating procedures.

Developing the EDMs was generally a lengthy process involving numerous revisions as they were circulated locally, then at the regional level (Veterans Integrated Service Network [VISN] 12 and Navy Medicine East [NME]), then at the national level (typically involving multiple offices within the VA, the Navy, and the DoD, and on matters involving legislation, the Office of Management and Budget [OMB]), and the Executive Office of the President. Most of the EDMs were not signed until July 2008, more than 3 years after the start of the process.

The EDM process was intended to identify operational differences in the departments' policies and procedures and resolve them at the lowest level possible. As it turned out, many aspects of the FHCC required higher-level approval, usually changes in the standard procedures or program policies of one department or the other, or of both. The task groups spent a great deal of time trying to identify who needed to be consulted at the regional or national level, or both, and getting them to the table to make decisions. In some cases, the LTG had to appeal to the HEC to intervene to obtain needed decisions when there was agreement to disagree between the departments. When funding was involved, the department comptrollers and the OMB had to approve. Ultimately, legislative authority was required to resolve some matters, which had to be worked out with the Armed Services committees or the Veterans' Affairs committees of the House and Senate, or all four of them, and sometimes also with the House and Senate Appropriations Subcommittees for Defense and Veterans Affairs. Despite strong support for VA/DoD health care collaborations by Congress, full legislative authority required to create, staff, and fund the FHCC was not received until the National Defense Authorization Act for FY 2010 (NDAA 2010[4]) was signed on October 28, 2009, less than a year before the FHCC was officially established on October 1, 2010. This created a great deal of uncertainty during most of the planning process, which began in earnest in 2005, about whether the FHCC would be considered to be a military treatment facility (MTF) so that cost sharing would not have to be required from DoD beneficiaries; whether the ownership of the ACC and equipment in the Navy hospital could be transferred to the VA to operate and maintain; what the status of Navy civilian employees would be; and what the funding mechanism would be.

ISSUES AFFECTING THE INTEGRATION PROCESS[5]

The task groups were oriented by a video teleconference in September 2005 and began work. All the task groups met in Washington, DC, for several days in December 2005 to report on issues, recommend solutions and plans of action, and set milestones for Phase 3 leading to the launching of the FHCC in 2010. Early on, the task groups classified issues they identified as "big rock" EDMs, "critical" EDMs, or issues that could be settled without an EDM. Big rocks were issues that were deemed to be key

[4] National Defense Authorization Act (NDAA), Public Law 111-84. http://www.intelligence.senate.gov/pdfs/military_act_2009.pdf (accessed August 6, 2012).

[5] This section of Chapter 3 provides a detailed account of implementation issues encountered at the Lovell FHCC. Table 3-2 summarizes the implementation issues likely to be encountered in creating other integrated VA/DoD health care centers, based on the Lovell FHCC experience.

to success but difficult to resolve and potentially requiring higher-level sign-off, if not legislation.[6]

Governance was a big rock, because the proposed line of authority from the FHCC director to a board of directors appointed by an interdepartmental group (the HEC) was something that would clearly have to be approved at the national level. Another big rock was the ability to treat DoD beneficiaries the same as they would be treated at the NHGL or at any other MTF; that is, they would not have to pay deductibles and copayments.

Other big rocks included the transfer of Navy civilians to the VA, ACC ownership, funding and reconciliation arrangements between the VA and the DoD, joint pharmacy, treatment of other health insurance, joint asset management, joint acquisition and contracting, joint credentialing, interagency IT network trust, and the safe exchange of patient care data between the VA and the DoD IT systems able to support an integrated VA/DoD health care facility with multiple care locations (Hassan et al., 2008).

Many of the issues were resolved by EDMs approved by the HEC co-chairs, or by other means, such as memoranda for the record, after being thoroughly vetted by many individuals at multiple levels in the VA, the Navy, the DoD, and the OMB—local, regional, and national. Four big rocks, however, required legislative relief, which was not achieved until the passage of NDAA 2010 in October 2009, nearly 2 years after the package of legislative proposals was sent to Capitol Hill. These were the transfer of civilian personnel from the DoD to the VA, ownership of the ACC facility, the scope of benefits for DoD beneficiaries, and a mechanism for joint funding of the FHCC.

The Vision of a Federal Health Care Center

The local leaders of the leadership task group—the director of the NCVAMC[7] and the current commander of the NHGL/NHCGL[8] as well as key members of their staffs—had a consistent vision of the way the Lovell FHCC should function to achieve its mission of providing seamless health care to all patients, regardless of their status as VA or DoD beneficiaries or providers. The vision was to have, to the fullest extent possible, one

[6] The "big rocks" are enumerated in Hassan et al. (2008).

[7] Patrick Sullivan has been the director of the North Chicago Veterans Affairs Medical Center since 2003 and was the associate director for the previous 6 years.

[8] There have been three commanders since 2003: Captains Michael H. Anderson (2003–2006), Thomas McGue (2006–2010), and David Beardsley (2010–present). A new commander will be appointed in 2012. Both McGue and Beardsley were posted to North Chicago to work with their predecessors several months before taking command in an effort to preserve continuity of leadership.

set of standards and a single set of processes for meeting those standards. For example, the local leadership wanted a single set of medical bylaws and quality of care standards. They pushed for single systems for finance (e.g., purchasing, logistics and inventory, payroll, assets), personnel and human resources management, facilities management, appointment scheduling, medical records and other IM systems, credentialing, workload measurement, performance measures, and inspector general inspections. They wanted a single operating fund and budget so that the FHCC staff did not have to determine which department's funds were being used and for what purpose in daily operational decision making. They envisioned a combined medical staff organized in single departments and clinics under one chief medical officer, operating under a single set of bylaws and with one standard of care for all patients.

Governance

The governance goal was to create a unified management and accountability structure for an organization that was to be neither VA nor Navy but a blending of the best of both. The intent was to achieve efficiencies by reducing redundancies and to deliver seamless care to servicemembers and their family members whether they are active duty or veterans or transitioning from active duty to veteran status.

As noted above, in 2005, the VA/DoD North Chicago–Great Lakes Task Force had proposed coequal directors, each reporting to his or her respective department, with coequal associate directors but a unified medical staff. The HEC directed the group to establish a single line of authority, a task made easier when the Navy surgeon general offered to have the Navy take the deputy director position. The EDM also created a board of directors appointed by the HEC to which the VA director and the Navy deputy director would report. The Navy surgeon general called it a "hybrid organization with new paradigms and practices" that would have a changed relationship with the parent organizations, VISN 12 and the Bureau of Medicine and Surgery (BUMED) (Arthur, 2006, p. 5).

This approach was not feasible because it violated the principle of unified executive authority. The department secretaries could not delegate their authority to an entity outside their departments. Congress would have had to create a new executive branch agency, which was not a solution desired either by it or by the administration. Accordingly, the governance EDM was revised in 2007 to comply with existing authority under 38 U.S.C. § 8111 and 10 U.S.C. § 1104.

The revised governance EDM established what it called an integrated governance model. It might have been called the lead agency model, because it made the Lovell FHCC director directly responsible to the VA rather than to a joint board of directors. The Navy deputy director was dually designated as the commanding officer of military personnel for military matters, including the exercise of the Uniform Code of Military Justice authority. An extensive executive sharing agreement between the department secretaries would be used to spell out how the FHCC would operate in an integrated fashion to provide seamless care to both VA and DoD beneficiaries. The intent was to have an organization that would seamlessly serve both DoD and VA beneficiaries yet be fiscally and operationally accountable for each agency's assets and costs.

Instead of a board of directors, there would be an advisory board with a similar membership, for example, senior representatives from the Veterans Affairs Central Office, the Department of the Navy BUMED, the Naval Education Training Command, VISN 12, and the NME. There would also be a stakeholders' advisory council and a local management council of senior VA and DoD staff. Dispute resolution would be handled first by the departments' respective chains of command, then—if necessary—by the Joint Health Care Facility Operations Steering Group, then by the HEC, and then by the Joint Executive Council (JEC).

Initially, the plan was to organize all operations of the Lovell FHCC through three directorates—Clinical Care, Patient Services, and Facility Support (administration)—which was the standard VA model. Over time, three more directorates were established: first a Dental Directorate (medical and dental are separate commands in the Navy and the dental program for the 50,000 recruits and students each year was a very large program to manage in its own right); then a Resources Directorate (carved out of Facility Support); and finally a Branch Clinics Directorate (the medical program for 50,000 recruits and students each year was also a very large program to manage). Three directorates were headed by a VA associate director and a DoD assistant director, and three were headed by a DoD associate director and a VA assistant director. The expanded number of directorates recognized certain realities—the size and organization of the Navy dental program for recruits and students and the special, time-critical mission of the Navy branch health clinics in ensuring medically fit recruits—and it provided more high-level slots for two organizations that were retaining all those they had employed before the merger. The resulting organization chart is complicated and somewhat unorthodox (see Figure 3-1). It has a bold line for "management authority from executive agreement (EA)" from the command suite to the VA (the command suite box includes the VA director and Navy deputy director). Another line—denoting an "operational line of authority"—connects the VA director to the VA via the VISN and the Veterans Health Administration. A similar line—denoting "military reporting relationship & accountability"—connects the Navy deputy director to the DoD via NME and BUMED. The command suite is connected to the Navy

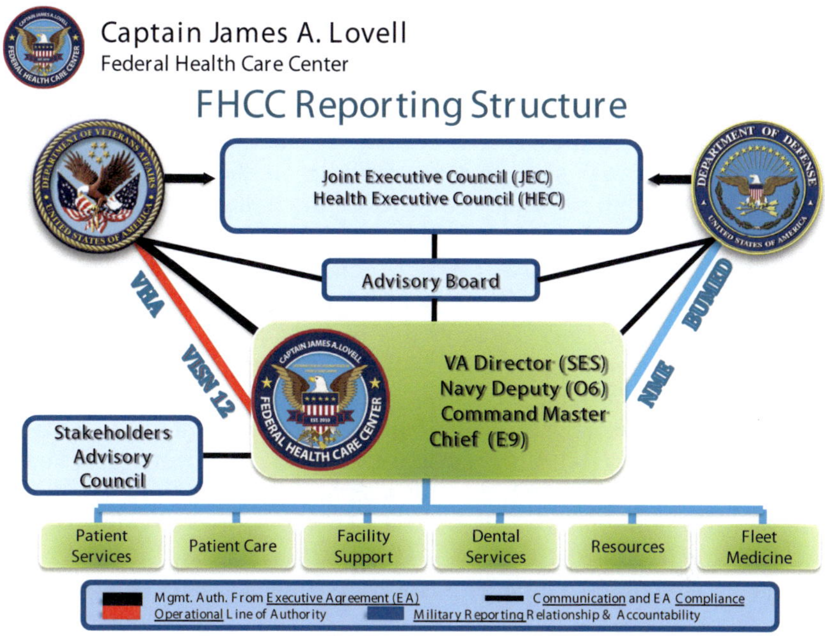

FIGURE 3-1 Lovell Federal Health Care Center leadership organization chart. SOURCE: Lovell FHCC staff, October 2012.

by a dotted line—denoting "communication and EA compliance." The Advisory Board and Stakeholders Advisory Council also have bold line relationships with the command suite and, in the case of the Advisory Board, to the DoD and the VA for communication and compliance with the EA.

Scope of Beneficiary Services

Another critical issue was the status of DoD beneficiaries. A primary goal of creating the Lovell FHCC was to have a single organization delivering health care to the beneficiaries of both the DoD and the VA to achieve efficiencies and seamless service delivery. The benefits of the 25,000 VA beneficiaries using the NCVAMC were not to be affected by the creation of the FHCC. The problem was that TRICARE Prime enrollees and other TRICARE beneficiaries (when they use an MTF on a space-available basis) are not charged deductibles or copayments, but they are subject to copayments and, in some cases, deductibles if they use a non-MTF facility, such as a VAMC. In fact, from 2006, when all inpatient and emergency services for Navy beneficiaries moved to the NCVAMC, until 2010, when the FHCC opened, Navy patients used the NCVAMC through the TRICARE network, which required copayments for all patients except active duty servicemembers and their family members.[9] This joint venture arrangement involved a third party in a vendor relationship between the VA and the DoD in what was supposed to become a single, merged organization.

The NHCGL was serving approximately 50,000 Navy recruits and students annually. In addition, the NHCGL catchment area contained approximately 59,000 DoD beneficiaries, of whom approximately 19,000 were enrolled at the NHCG. Most of the 19,000 enrolled beneficiaries were TRICARE Prime beneficiaries but some (approximately 500) were TFL and other direct care patients. Most of the 40,000 non-enrolled beneficiaries were non-Prime beneficiaries who could receive care on a space-available basis.

The vision of the Lovell FHCC planners was to serve all these TRICARE patient categories as if they were still using an MTF, that is, without imposing any cost-sharing requirements. It was feared that copayments would interrupt the continuity of care when DoD beneficiaries seen in the ACC (which could be designated as an MTF as long as the Navy retained ownership) were referred to inpatient care or to those specialty clinics located in the VA building. Copayments would also have to be administered by the TRICARE managed care support contractor, which does not become involved when a DoD beneficiary uses an MTF. There was another practical consideration. A DoD analysis of the impact of copayments predicted a 50 percent or greater reduction in DoD beneficiaries seeking treatment at the FHCC because it would no longer benefit them to travel there when they could get private care closer to home for the same or lesser copayments (DoD, 2010). The joint venture was already experiencing a fall-off in demand from TFL beneficiaries for this reason in the period leading up the launching of the FHCC in 2010 (Interviews). The initial strategy was to obtain dual designation as an MTF and a VAMC. However, department lawyers ruled that, because the law (Title 10 U.S.C.) refers to MTFs as "facilities of the uniformed services," they must be under the direct control of the secretary of defense, which would not be the case with the FHCC.[10]

In response, the scope of beneficiary benefits in the EDM (originally the dual designation EDM) laid out three options. Option 1 was to change

---

[9] Military retirees may also qualify for free care as veterans, for example, for a service-connected disability or for all care if they are rated 50 percent disabled or higher.

[10] There are uniformed services in three departments: the Department of Defense (DoD) (the Air Force, the Army, the Navy, and the Marines); the Department of Homeland Security (the Coast Guard and the commissioned corps of the National Oceanic and Atmospheric Administration); and the Department of Health and Human Services (the commissioned corps of the Public Health Service), although only the DoD currently has health facilities, that is, military treatment facilities (MTFs) (the Public Health Service stopped running hospitals in 1981).

TRICARE regulations to allow TRICARE Prime enrollees and their family members to receive care at the FHCC without deductibles or copayments as before. Non-enrolled beneficiaries could also receive free inpatient medical, surgical, and pediatric services provided in the VA building if they were referred there by their DoD primary care providers. Option 2 was to seek legislative relief to allow the FHCC to be "MTF-like"—able to serve all DoD beneficiary groups without cost sharing. Option 3 was to have the VA part of the FHCC continue to be a TRICARE network provider, the arrangement in force since 2006 when all inpatient and emergency services for DoD beneficiaries were shifted to the NCVAMC.

The problems with Option 1 were that (1) the number of non-enrolled beneficiaries would be limited by the number of DoD primary care providers required to refer them to non-MTF care, and (2) TFL beneficiaries would have to be charged because the VA is not permitted to bill Medicare, the first payer for these beneficiaries enrollees. The problem with Option 2 was the uncertainty that the departments, the OMB, and Congress would agree to authorize the FHCC to operate as though it were an MTF. Also, the departments would have to pay for the expenses of TFL beneficiaries that otherwise would have been paid by Medicare. The problem with Option 3 was not only that it required cost sharing from non-enrolled beneficiaries but also that it would have involved the TRICARE managed-care support contractor, which created a vendor rather than a direct relationship between the DoD and the VA.

The LTG recommended and the HEC co-chairs agreed to pursue Option 2, with Option 1 as a fallback if authorizing legislation was not passed. The draft bill introduced by Senator Dick Durbin in September 2008 would have "deemed" the Lovell FHCC to be an MTF "for the purposes of eligibility for health care." When Durbin resubmitted the bill in June 2009, the language was changed to say the FHCC "may be treated" as an MTF "for the purposes of eligibility for health care," and this language was retained in the version of the bill that became law (NDAA 2010). Although sponsors of the bill thought the language would eliminate the requirement for cost sharing by DoD beneficiaries (Bean, 2009; Durbin, 2009), the language of the law did not explicitly exclude it. The solution was to have the secretary of defense publish a notice in the *Federal Register* waiving TRICARE deductibles, cost shares, and copayments for eligible beneficiaries seeking care at the FHCC as part of the 5-year DoD/VA Medical Demonstration Project. The notice specifically noted that the waiver was "consistent with current policies and procedures followed at all MTFs" (DoD, 2010, p. 59238). The notice was put on a fast track for publication and appeared three days before the October 1, 2010, advent of the FHCC.

The main downside of the inclusive benefit policy was the loss of Medicare reimbursement for TFL patients because the VA is prohibited from billing Medicare. The loss was estimated to be between $85,000 and $100,000 per year (the higher amount if use by TFL patients increased because of the lack of copayments). The DoD and the VA agreed to split the lost revenue from dual-eligible TFL beneficiaries through the financial reconciliation process (TFL beneficiaries must elect to be a VA or DoD beneficiary during each episode of care, which could be tracked for cost allocation purposes).

Transfer of Ownership of the Ambulatory Care Center Facility

Another big rock issue was the planned transfer of the Navy-built ACC to the VA. The intent was to have a single organization maintain and repair the buildings on the VA campus, rather than to have two organizations maintain and repair buildings that are interconnected physically and operationally. It made the most sense to have the VA own the ACC because it was already maintaining all other facilities and equipment on the VA campus. The VA would also be providing the utility infrastructure for the new facility. The main argument against the transfer of the ACC was its status if the FHCC did not meet expectations and was dissolved. Another argument emerged when it became questionable whether the FHCC would be designated as an MTF.

The facility ownership EDM, developed by a working group of VA, Navy, and DoD personnel, presented two options. Option 1 was to have the Navy transfer custody and accountability for the new ACC and parking facilities to the VA to achieve unified oversight over and responsibility for the FHCC facilities on the VA campus, which would require legislation. Option 2 was for the Navy to retain ownership of and responsibility for the new facilities, which would not require legislation. It would also make it much less complicated if the FHCC did not work out as planned.

Under Option 1, the responsibility for funding maintenance and repairs and purchasing equipment would be more equitably distributed between the two departments through the financial reconciliation process that was being developed by the financial task group. Each department would pay for the facilities in proportion to its usage of the Lovell FHCC (the financial reconciliation model developed for the FHCC is discussed below).

There was consensus that the new facilities should be transferred to the VA, but current law did not make it easy. The Navy did not have authority to transfer property to any agency other than the other military services. The General Services Administration had authority to transfer a facility that was declared to be surplus, but even assuming a new facility could be declared surplus, the VA would have had to reimburse the Navy for the full value of the facility unless the OMB granted an exemption. The EDM working group drafted proposed legislation granting the Navy the authority to transfer the ACC and related facilities to the VA.

The EDM recommended and the HEC co-chairs approved Option 1 and the seeking of legislation authorizing the transfer of ownership from the Navy to the VA. Draft legislation was vetted up both the DoD and the VA chains of command and worked out with Durbin, who introduced it as an amendment to the NDAA 2009 in September 2008, but it was introduced too late in the congressional process to be adopted. The legislation was reintroduced several more times as the Captain James A. Lovell Federal Health Care Center Act before it was passed as part of the NDAA 2009. Although the legislation was revised in conference, the substance of the section on transfer of property stayed the same. The DoD secretary was authorized, but not required, to transfer the Navy-built facilities and related medical personal property and equipment to the VA without reimbursement, and the VA secretary was authorized to transfer the facilities back to the DoD without reimbursement "in [the] event of lack of facilities integration."

By this time, the Navy had decided to retain ownership for the time being (the Navy still owned the facilities at the time this report was drafted). One impetus for this was the uncertainty about whether some DoD beneficiaries would be charged copayments and deductibles if the Lovell FHCC was not deemed to be an MTF. If the ACC was an MTF, it could serve DoD beneficiaries without copayments, and no beneficiaries, except TFL, would have to pay copayments to use the VA facilities if they were referred by their primary care providers (this was Option 1 in the scopes of beneficiary benefits EDM, which was the fallback option if legislative authority for the transfer of property was not granted).

Personnel

Another big rock was achieving a single personnel system for all civilian employees. Having a single personnel system would help unify the new organization. It would also avoid a situation that had been encountered in the VA/DoD joint ventures, that is, employees of the DoD and the VA working side by side performing the same jobs but receiving different pay, benefits, incentive bonuses, and other perquisites, which was bad for morale and productivity.

The NHCGL employed 533 civilians under the authority of Title 5. The original plan was to use a mechanism called "transfer of function" to move the Navy civilians into the VA's Title 38 personnel system without loss of pay and benefits; however, transfer of function can only be used within, not between, executive departments. Ultimately, the transfer of civilians from the Department of the Navy to the VA had to be authorized by legislation. The alternative to legislative relief was to let go the former NHCGL civilians through reduction-in-force actions and rehire them through regular competitive procedures, which would have caused a number of difficulties.

The legislation (NDAA 2010) authorized the DoD and the Navy secretaries to transfer functions required for successful operation of the Lovell FHCC and the VA secretary to accept them. Transferred employees would maintain their rate of total compensation (including physician comparability allowances); not have to undergo the 1-year probationary period normally required of VA employees if they had served the probationary period under Title 5; and, for 2 years, keep collective bargaining rights under Title 5.[11] The FHCC had also previously stipulated that no civilian would lose his or her job in the integration.

There were complications:

- Only 40 percent of Title 5 DoD civilians had occupational titles that also existed in Title 38, which meant that 60 percent of them had to be placed in new occupations that were comparable in duties and pay.
- Some NHCGL employees in hard-to-recruit professions were receiving special additional pay, which the VA had to match.
- Some NHCGL workers were employed through personal services contracts (PSCs), which the VA does not have authority to use. The contracts totaled more than $16 million a year, nearly $11 million of which was dedicated to pay more than 100 staff in the dental clinics on the Great Lakes Navy base. The use of the PSCs gave the Navy more flexibility in meeting the ups and downs in the number of recruits and students over time. The solution was to allow the Navy to maintain the PSCs using the Navy Medical Logistics Command (NMLC) rather than to try to convert the contractors to civil service positions.
- Several IM/IT staff members remained Title 5 employees because access to certain computer systems is restricted to DoD employees. Ultimately, the Navy retained 14 NHCGL civilian positions for this reason.

The personnel transfer issue affected two other issues: security clearances and IM/IT access cards.

[11] For example, DoD civilians have the right to appeal adverse personnel actions to the Merit Systems Protection Board, but Department of Veterans Affairs (VA) employees do not.

Security Clearance Policy

To achieve the Lovell FHCC vision, the hope was to have one security clearance policy for all FHCC staff to allow seamless access to IM/IT systems. The Navy's policy for access to patient records was stricter than the VA's and used different security clearance procedures and ways of paying for it. As a practical matter, the time and expense needed to achieve secret-level security clearances for all FHCC personnel, as required by the Navy for access to patient records, would have crippled the effort to launch the FHCC on schedule.

The VA's security clearance system is based on the public trust model and does not require secret clearances. Most VA employees receive either a special agreement check or the National Agency Check with Inquiries (NACI) using the SF85P form—VA executives and managers and IT personnel are subject to two higher levels of security clearance (minimum background investigation or background investigation), using the more extensive SF86 form. The VAMC pays for the costs of the checks.

The Navy's security clearances are based on the national security model, ranging from confidential, to secret, to top secret, and Navy policy on access to information protected by the Privacy Act requires a secret clearance and the SF86 form. The Navy, not the individual facility, pays the costs of the Access National Agency Check with Inquiries (ANACI),[12] about $350 for military servicemembers and $427 for DoD civilians in FY 2011 (GAO, 2012a).

Also, non–U.S. citizens were barred from access to patient information by the Navy except on an individual waiver basis. Approximately a dozen active duty sailors and 10 Navy contractors at the NHCGL were noncitizens requiring an individual waiver. The NCVAMC, in contrast, employed many more noncitizens—about 100—as medical students, interns, residents, and physicians, which would have overwhelmed the individual waiver process. However, the FHCC's joint teaching mission depends on students, interns, and residents—many of them noncitizens—having access to patient records.

The matter was slow to be resolved because the Navy was reluctant to lower its standards.[13] On the other hand, it did not seem to make sense

[12] An "Access National Agency Check with Inquiries" is used for the initial investigation for federal employees at the confidential and secret access levels. It consists of employment, education, residence, reference, and law enforcement agency checks, as well as a national agency check, which includes data from military records and from the Federal Bureau of Investigation's investigative index (GAO, 2012b).

[13] This is one of a number of instances in which the department involved—the VA, the Navy, or the DoD—was reluctant to set a precedent by granting the FHCC an exception. This in turn limited the extent to which the FHCC could achieve internal consistency in its policies and procedures.

to require everyone at the FHCC to obtain a secret clearance just to access the DoD's EHR system, which does not contain classified information. The situation became more amenable to solution when the Navy's medical records were moved from the Navy computer system enclave to the Military Health System (MHS) computer system enclave under DoD jurisdiction, because the MHS uses the public trust model used by the VA. At that point, the departments agreed to resolve the minimum level of clearance needed to access the medical IT systems of the DoD through a memorandum of agreement (MOA) rather than an EDM.

The impasse was eased further when legal counsel advised that a secret clearance is not legally required to access information protected by the Privacy Act. However, the Navy insisted on requiring all FHCC employees to undergo an ANACI investigation. The MOA, not signed until October 20, 2010, required an SF86 form and an ANACI investigation of all VA personnel but allowed interim access for a year while the investigations were conducted. U.S. citizens and permanent residents who had completed a NACI investigation by October 1, 2010, were allowed access to the DoD system until they successfully completed the ANACI process. U.S. citizens and permanent residents who arrived after October 1 had to undergo the SF86/ANACI process but would be given interim access after a favorable fingerprint check and confirmation that the Office of Personnel Management (OPM) had scheduled an investigation. The solution to the need for foreign students, interns, and residents to have access to patient records was to continue the VA's policy of requiring NACI investigations and to allow local authorities to grant access to the clinical applications in DoD's Armed Forces Health Longitudinal Technology Application (AHLTA) EHR system to the extent required by each individual's duties.

Implementing the ANACI clearance process was a substantial undertaking. The VA was not set up to process more than 900 ANACI clearances, even on a phased basis. Lovell FHCC staff assisted the VA in reducing the submission time of ANACI requests to OPM from several months to a few weeks.

Access Cards

To provide seamless, coordinated, and safe care, VA employees need a way to access AHLTA and other DoD electronic information systems. Similarly, active duty personnel need a way to access the VA's Veterans Health Information Systems and Technology Architecture (VistA) EHR and other information systems, for example, the financial management, decision support, and acquisition and contracting systems. Each agency uses access cards to control access to their computer systems. Again, the DoD has stricter policies. The DoD does not allow anyone outside the DoD to have a common access card (CAC). The solution was to enable employees with CACs to access VA systems and to allow VA employees to use their personal identity verification (PIV) cards to access AHLTA (but not other DoD systems), which took some time to negotiate and required expensive software and hardware changes and updates.

The changeover was briefly interrupted when the VA decided to upgrade the security code of its PIV cards nationally, without realizing the impact this would have on the logistics of having everyone at the Lovell FHCC obtain AHLTA-enabled PIV cards by October 2010. The upgrading was delayed.

Interagency Information Technology Network Trust

The plan was to connect the two department computer systems with a wide bandwidth fiber optic cable so that everyone could access both systems through his or her computer. As noted above, a JIF-funded fiber optic cable was installed between the campuses to allow this to happen. Each department had protocols, however, for allowing access to their computer systems, called "interagency IT network trust." The alternative was to have two computer rooms and networks and two computers on each desktop. The problems were the stricter standards for "dot.mil" than for "dot.va" systems, programs, and applications, and the high level of review and approval that would be needed in each department to upgrade the VA systems to dot.mil standards and establish a gateway between the systems. On the DoD side, for example, the Defense Information Systems Agency had to agree that adequate interagency trust was achieved, and final sign-off authority at the DoD was at the deputy secretary level.

Interagency Funding Mechanism

Another goal of the Lovell FHCC integration was to have a unified financial system. Part of this goal was to fund the FHCC in a way that was not categorical, for example, "these are VA dollars that must be used for this but not for that," and "these are DoD dollars that can be used only for these purposes." Other aspects of what the FHCC planners called the "unified financial vision" are presented below.

The Lovell FHCC could not receive funds directly from the DoD or the VA for the same reason it could not be run by a board of directors. This would make it an independent federal agency, which was not the intent. The first alternative was to explore whether the JIF could serve as the funding vehicle. Congress had established the JIF as a Treasury fund to which the departments could contribute funding for joint venture projects. Although the NHGL/NHCGL and the NCVAMC had received a number of JIF projects to fund joint services and infrastructure, they were expected by the DoD and the VA to be self-sustaining within 2 years. There was resistance from both the executive and the legislative side to expanding the purpose of the JIF so substantially from its original purpose and scope.[14]

Ultimately, Congress established a separate Treasury fund for the Lovell FHCC, called the Joint Medical Facility Demonstration Fund (JMFDF). The demonstration fund was established on the financial accounting ledgers of the VA, and the VA and the DoD were authorized to transfer funds that are authorized and appropriated specifically for the FHCC in amounts determined by a formula agreed to by the two department secretaries. This is tighter control than Congress exercises over the JIF, to which the departments are directed to contribute "at least" $15 million per year each and to use the funds until expended (i.e., "no-year" money). The Armed Services committees are requiring annual authorization of 1-year funding of DoD contributions; the VA committees are authorizing funding that can be used over a period of 2 years. This difference in congressional policies had an upside; it allowed the FHCC to be funded by the VA during the first few months when the DoD appropriation was held up by a continuing resolution (CR) in Congress.

Ambulatory Care Center Building and Equipment Ownership

The original plan was to transfer the Navy-built ACC to the VA immediately, which, it was determined, would require legislation to permit. Subsequently, the Navy decided to hold off on transferring the building because of concern about losing MTF status for the ACC when it became apparent that the entire Lovell FHCC would not be designated as an MTF. The legislation (NDAA 2010) states that the Navy *may* transfer the building to the VA at any time during the 5-year demonstration period. The legislation also included procedures for transferring the building back to the Navy if it was decided not to continue the FHCC during or after the demonstration period. Keeping the ACC under Navy ownership also avoided a VA requirement that the pharmacy be equipped with ballistic glass.[15] At

---

[14] "The purpose [of the DoD-VA Health Care Sharing Incentive Fund] is to provide seed money for creative sharing initiatives at facility, regional and national levels to facilitate the mutually beneficial coordination, use, or exchange of health care resources, with the goal of improving the access to, and quality and cost effectiveness of, the health care provided to beneficiaries of both departments" (DoD/VA, 2009).

[15] According to the VA's security handbook, at the time the ambulatory care center was constructed, "Windows and walls of pharmacy dispensing must meet the U.L. Standard 752 for Class III Ballistic Level" (VA, 2004). This requirement was continued in the 2010 update of the handbook (VA, 2010b).

the time this report was drafted, there were no active plans to transfer the ACC to the VA.

Financial System and Reconciliation

The accounting system may seem to be a trivial part of such a substantial organizational effort, but the vision of the Lovell FHCC was for each partner to pay for its share of the health care provided by the FHCC. This required the development of an accounting system meeting both departments' needs. Such an accounting system did not exist. After much discussion at different levels and a summit meeting of the VA chief financial officer, the BUMED deputy chief of resource management, and the director of health budgets and financial policy in the Office of the Assistant Secretary of Defense for Health Affairs, the decision was made to adopt the VA's Financial Management System (FMS) as the basis for a unified financial system.

Once the FMS was chosen, it became logical to adopt other VA administrative systems compatible with it, such as the VA decision support, payroll, and logistics systems. The key question was whether the VA's Decision Support System (DSS), a managerial cost accounting system, could accurately allocate costs to the services provided to VA beneficiaries and DoD beneficiaries so that each department could be charged appropriately.

The DSS was developed by adapting commercial software to interface with and be populated by VistA and other VA databases to provide data on costs of goods and services for patients down to the encounter and laboratory test level. According to the VA,

> DSS provides a mechanism for integrating expenses, workload, and patient utilization. DSS information supports process and performance improvement by measuring quality of care, clinical outcomes, and financial impact.[16]

The problem was that the DSS did not accept financial and workload data from DoD systems in a manner that could be used for both the workload and costing portions of the financial reconciliation process. First, the departments had to agree on how to measure workload. Accordingly, workload data documented in VistA (for example, VA primary care, inpatient care, and the combined VA/DoD specialty care) are obtained from the VA's Allocation Resource Center (ARC) on a quarterly basis and provided to the DoD's Office of Health Affairs (OHA). This workload is then imported into Centers for Medicare & Medicaid Services (CMS) tables to determine

---

[16] See http://www.virec.research.va.gov/DataSourcesName/DSS/DSSintro.htm (accessed October 14, 2012).

the relative value unit (RVU), relative weighted product (RWP), and dental weighted value (DWV) workload values. The workload statistics documented in DoD systems (such as the branch health clinics and the DoD primary care clinic) are obtained by the OHA from DoD's M2 system, which determines enhanced CMS values for all MTFs (Lovell FHCC, 2010b).

For the cost allocation portion of the financial reconciliation process, the Defense Medical Human Resources Systems-internet (DMHRSi) is used to document and capture labor costs for active duty personnel, DoD contractors, and the few remaining DoD civilian positions. DMHRSi labor costs are then mapped into the DSS, which allows all FHCC costs to be contained within it. The FHCC's health care business office processes DSS costs for the quarterly financial reconciliation and provides that output to the OHA for final processing. The FHCC, the OHA, and other stakeholders are presently developing an automated reconciliation process, as outlined in the financial reconciliation EDM.

In order to meet the requirements of the Economy Act, there was a need for budget reconciliation such that each department would pay only for the amount of care provided to its beneficiaries while functions unique to one department should be funded only by that department (Opsut, 2011). The latter are called mission specific pass-throughs (MSPTs), for example, recruit medical and dental care for the Navy and veterans nursing home and long-term care for the VA. The approach adopted was to divide all care into 10 "buckets" (categories); determine the total cost of each of the categories using the DSS; use the industry standard workload measures to determine the proportion of workload accounted for by each department's beneficiaries in each category; multiply the proportion times the total cost in each category to get each department's costs; and sum the costs across the 10 categories to determine each department's total costs (see Table 3-1 for the 10 categories and workload measures). The MSPT costs are then added to determine the final bill.

Applying this model to FY 2009 data from the DSS and DoD's cost accounting system found that services to VA beneficiaries cost $119.6 million (including $36,000 from DoD providers) and services to DoD beneficiaries cost $60.3 million (including $8.3 million from VA providers). Once the Navy's higher MSPT costs for the branch medical clinics were added in, the total costs were nearly split, $196.9 million for the VA versus $187.1 million for the DoD.

Historical trends are being used to fund the Lovell FHCC for the first 3 years (FY 2011–FY 2013), after which the reconciliation methodology will be used to determine each department's costs. It is too early to tell if utilization patterns will shift enough to substantially change total costs or their allocation between the departments, or both. If utilization declines

TABLE 3-1 Workload Categories and Measures

Categories	Workload Measures
Non–mental health inpatient	MS-RWPs adjusted for length of stay
Mental health inpatient	Bed days
Outpatient	Work + practice RVUs
Same-day surgery	Work + practice RVUs + APCs
Emergency department	Work + practice RVUs + APCs
Outpatient laboratory	Work + practice RVUs
Outpatient radiology	Work + practice RVUs
Outpatient pharmacy	Actual costs
Prosthetics	Actual costs
Dental	Actual costs

NOTE: APC = ambulatory payment classification; MS-RWP = Medicare severity relative weighted product; RVU = relative value unit.

while fixed costs stay the same, it will be difficult for the Lovell FHCC to be more economical than its predecessor organizations.

Purchasing of Supplies

The choices were to use the Navy supply system, the VA supply system, or both. The preference was to use one system for the Lovell FHCC to best support the unified administration of the FHCC rather than two systems side by side. The decision was to use the VA system because it was compatible with the FMS that was going to be used (the VA's).

The VA's Great Lakes Acquisition Center (GLAC) also had an advantage because of its higher contracting limit than that of the National Naval Medical Center Portsmouth ($100 million versus $10 million), although supplies might be more expensive through the VA because the DoD purchases in larger quantities. There was also a concern whether the GLAC had the capacity to keep the Navy recruit clinics supplied on a timely basis. Another issue was how to supply non-NHCGL medical activities (e.g., Naval Hospital Corpsman School, Naval Drug Screening Laboratory, Naval Institute for Dental and Biomedical Research).

After a year's experience using the GLAC, the FHCC is drafting a revised acquisition and contracting EDM recommending that the NMLC and the Naval Facilities Engineering Command (NFEC) be added to the GLAC as sources of supplies and services. The NMLC was already being used for the PSCs for personnel working in the branch clinics on the east campus, because the VA does not have authority for PSCs and converting the contractors to federal civil service employees would have been much more costly. The recommendation to allow the use of the NFEC results from the need to have a mechanism for repairing the branch health clinics, which are Navy facilities on Navy land (the EA specifies that each department is responsible for maintaining its own buildings).

Asset Management

Like other administrative functions, the Lovell FHCC planners hoped to use one asset management system rather than two programs to enhance accountability and efficiency. The DoD and the VA each had an automated program for asset management. DoD's asset management program was and still is the Defense Medical Logistics Standard Support (DMLSS) automated information system, a Web-based program that was deployed in 2001. The VA's system is the disk operating system (DOS)-based Generic Inventory Package (GIP).[17] The administrative task group recommended using the VA asset management system for the same reason they had recommended using the VA's systems for personnel, acquisition and contracting, payroll, and decision support, namely, because it interfaced with the VA's FMS, the financial system chosen for the FHCC.

At the time the asset management EDM was being developed, the VA was developing a new automated asset management program as a component of its Financial and Logistics Integrated Technology Enterprise (FLITE) program (VA OIG, 2010).[18] The new asset management program will be a customized version of MAXIMO, a commercial, Web-based asset management software program, and will replace the GIP. However, the MAXIMO program was not ready for use in October 2010, and the FHCC has had to continue to use the GIP. The former Navy personnel were unhappy because the DOS commands used in the GIP are much clumsier to use than DMLSS's point-and-click system and some of the prices are higher (Interviews). The FHCC has submitted a revised asset management EDM recommending that the use of the DMLSS be explored, and a VA/DoD work group was chartered in September 2012 to explore the feasibility of using the DMLSS at the FHCC and, potentially, at other joint venture sites.

Pharmacy

The Lovell FHCC vision was to have a single pharmacy, with a single drug formulary, rather than to have VA and DoD pharmacies with different formularies operating side by side in the ACC, to simplify administration, reduce personnel costs, and avoid a perception of unequal benefits between

[17] The VA also has a separate specialized prosthetics inventory program.

[18] The Financial and Logistics Integrated Technology Enterprise program, except for the MAXIMO module, was canceled in 2010 for lack of progress.

VA and DoD beneficiaries. The decision to have one pharmacy was also driven in part by space considerations. The pharmacy area and number of outpatient windows had been reduced when the size of the ACC was halved, on the assumption that refills would be provided by mail using the VA's CMOP.

Other issues that had to be addressed were the following:

- **Pharmacy security.** VA regulations require that pharmacy windows and walls be bullet proof. The DoD requires that every patient be counseled when filling a prescription, and opposed having a window at the dispensing counter. Redesigning the pharmacy area to include a room for counseling that met the VA's ballistic standards—typical of VA pharmacies—would have reduced the pharmacy's already minimal storage area by a third, cut the number of automation units from three to two, and increased construction costs. An impasse was avoided when the Navy decided to retain ownership of the ACC.
- **Choice of formulary.** Because of differences in populations served, the VA and the Navy had different formularies. Lovell FHCC planners would have preferred to create a new FHCC formulary—including pediatric and women's medications—which combined and reduced overlaps between the VA and the DoD core formularies, but after much discussion, the outcome was to continue to use the VA formulary for VA patients and a combination of the VA formulary and the current Navy formulary for DoD beneficiaries.
- **Choice of prime vendor.** The Lovell FHCC hoped to use the DoD or the VA pharmaceutical prime vendor that offered the best terms to maximize purchasing power and economies of scale. This would have required the FHCC to stop using the current VA or DoD prime vendor, which might have violated the contract. The decision was made to have a single prime pharmacy vendor in 2012, after existing VA and DoD contracts expired and a new combined contract could be competed.
- **CMOP access for all DoD beneficiaries for prescription refills.** The Lovell FHCC wanted to use the VA's CMOP service for DoD beneficiaries to save money and also to reduce waiting time at the space-limited pharmacy. The DoD does not participate in the CMOP and did not wish to set a precedent by making an exception for the FHCC.[19] There was hope that the tri-service integration

[19] The DoD experimented with the use of the Consolidated Mail Order Pharmacy (CMOP) at three MTFs in FY 2003. The Government Accountability Office reported that drug costs using the CMOP were 3.9 percent less than the DoD's, but this saving was offset by the ad-

of health care services in the National Capital Area would set a precedent, but that did not work out when it was determined that the CMOP would not be cost effective there. It was also possible that permitting DoD beneficiaries to use the CMOP would require legislative action. The CMOP option for DoD beneficiaries was dropped, although the FHCC continues to seek permission to use it (Interviews).

- **Pharmacy inspection.** The Lovell FHCC hoped to have a single inspection process for the pharmacy rather than separate inspections by the VA and the Navy. The departments did not agree, and both are inspecting the pharmacy.
- **Use of Navy pharmacy technicians as technician checkers at the FHCC or just at Navy branch clinics.** The clinical task group (CTG) hoped to rotate Navy and civilian pharmacy technicians who completed military pharmacy training through the Lovell FHCC, satellite, and three Navy branch clinic pharmacies. This would reduce the number of licensed registered pharmacists needed to staff the three Navy branch clinics by up to five and also would maintain the operational readiness of Navy pharmacy technicians for deployment to combat operations.[20] However, VA pharmacy regulations do not allow the use of technician checkers, and the Joint Commission would have to expand its current waiver allowing MTFs to use technician checkers to the FHCC. The recommendation was to use pharmacy technicians only at the Navy branch clinics, which did not require any rule changes and still contributed to the operational readiness of the Navy pharmacy technicians.
- **Ensuring patient safety.** Using two EHR systems for the same patient population raised the specter of patient injury because of negative drug interactions or allergic reactions occurring when the provider and pharmacist using one EHR system is unaware of prescriptions or allergies entered into the other EHR system. For this reason, the CTG had prefaced its pharmacy options with a caveat that everything depended on orders portability for

---

ministrative costs of maintaining the pharmacies at the MTFs. The DoD did not want to close the MTF pharmacies, which are necessary for filling initial prescriptions and are convenient for the MTF's TRICARE Prime users. It was concerned that if it closed the MTF pharmacies, at least some beneficiaries would join the growing percentage of beneficiaries using retail pharmacies—the most expensive option for the DoD—instead of using the CMOP (already, from 2001–2004, the percentage of pharmacy benefit customers using retail pharmacies rather than the MTF pharmacies or TRICARE's mail order pharmacy program had increased from approximately 26 to 42 percent) (GAO, 2005).

[20] Navy pharmacy technicians (Navy Enlisted Classification HM-8482) are qualified to prepare and dispense prescribed pharmaceuticals (U.S. Navy, 2011, p. 168).

> pharmacy because of its critical role in ensuring patient safety. Orders portability for pharmacy—the ability to enter a prescription into either the DoD EHR system or the VA EHR system and have it appear in the other system simultaneously so that potential drug interactions and allergies could be recognized—was one of the basic IM/IT requirements that was supposed to be operational by October 1, 2010. As it became clear that this would not be achieved and would pose an unacceptable threat to patient safety, an interim workaround solution had to be developed.[21] Funded as a $1 million JIF project for 1 year, the plan involved hiring seven to nine additional pharmacists to perform manual checks and finding room for them to work. Ultimately, only five pharmacists were needed, but the pharmacy space is still very crowded. Since then, the project has been extended past 1 year.

When the DoD and the VA secretaries agreed in March 2011 to develop jointly a single EHR system to replace their legacy systems (AHLTA and VistA, respectively), they decided to complete the undelivered IM/IT solutions for the Lovell FHCC as part of the new joint EHR system development process. This included orders portability for pharmacy (also orders portability for consults and referrals). The new EHR system is being developed in stages, but the pharmacy is in the initial development group, with the FHCC designated as the primary development site. The current schedule is for it to be ready for use in 2014.

Patient Records

The vision of the Lovell FHCC was for VA or Navy beneficiaries to be treated by either VA or DoD providers (depending on availability) so that care was seamless from the patient's perspective. This meant that Navy providers would have to be able to access and update the patient records of VA beneficiaries they treated in VistA (the VA's EHR system) and VA clinicians would have to be able to access and update the patient records of DoD beneficiaries in AHLTA (the DoD's EHR system) as well as in VistA. There was also a need for information recorded in VistA for Navy patients (e.g., inpatients, those using the ED, and those seeing VA specialists) to be replicated in AHLTA, so that their medical operational readiness could be determined and their medical records would be complete when they left for new assignments beyond North Chicago. Orders for laboratory and radiol-

[21] The events leading to the delay of orders portability for pharmacy and other computer software interoperability solutions are described in more detail in the next section, on information management systems.

ogy tests, for prescriptions, and for consultations and referrals and their results needed to be viewable in both systems regardless of the system in which they were entered, a capability called orders portability. As discussed above, orders portability for pharmacy was especially important to prevent drug interactions and allergic reactions.

As of 2006, when the Lovell FHCC's IM/IT systems were being planned, VA and DoD providers had limited access to each other's patient information. The two departments had developed two interim solutions for sharing clinical information: (1) the Bi-directional Health Information Exchange (BHIE), a program that enables VA and DoD providers to view clinical data from each other's EHR system, and (2) the Clinical Data Repository/Health Data Repository (CHDR), a program that enables VA and DoD clinical data repositories to share computable pharmacy and drug allergy data. The BHIE was initially implemented in 2005, and the CHDR was at the field-testing stage in 2006.

NHCGL and NCVAMC providers had dual icons on their computer screens for accessing the two EHR systems; however, there were significant limitations to the functionality of the two programs (DoD, 2011). Providers had to log on to each EHR system separately. VA provider access was on a read-only basis, which meant that information on inpatient, emergency, and specialty provider encounters on the west campus had to be entered into AHLTA separately. The information only pertained to "active dual consumers," that is, military retirees also eligible for VA health care, not active duty servicemembers who had not yet retired, such as the recruits, students, and staff at Great Lakes (although arrangements could be made—and were—to flag recruits and other active duty servicemembers at Great Lakes as active dual consumers). The ability to look back, that is, see information from earlier encounters, was limited. In addition, CHDR/BHIE functionality was not expected to be reliable enough in 2010 to meet the tempo of health care delivery at the Lovell FHCC, especially for the recruits for whom medical status had to be current on a daily basis (Maldonado and Poulin, 2012). As the pharmacy discussion (above) indicates, the CHDR was not considered reliable enough for patient safety and an interim manual workaround was instituted and is still in place. The BHIE is still considered to be too awkward and too slow to use in patient encounters (Interviews).

From the beginning, the CTG recommended having one patient record system or a single-user interface to both systems (VistA and AHLTA) for entering and retrieving patient clinical information. The CTG concluded that it would not be realistic to expect a single EHR system to be ready by the time the FHCC opened in 2010. Given the continuing existence of VistA and AHLTA, the focus was on achieving interoperability, that is, finding a user-friendly front-end or back-end software bridge between the two systems so that clinicians could log onto either system and see, enter, and update patient information in both systems simultaneously (Brewin, 2007). Single entry into and simultaneous access to both systems would not only be more efficient, it would promote continuity and coordination of care and help reduce errors that might affect patient safety.

The departments agreed with the need for interoperable EHR systems when the Lovell FHCC was launched in 2010. Development of interoperability solutions—beginning with the identification of system requirements to meet the needs of the clinicians and the identification of sources of funding for development—began in earnest in late 2007. A proposal for JIF funds was developed for $11 million for support for 2–2.5 years of a joint local program management office and a joint enterprise-level (i.e., national-level) office for systems development (Hassan et al., 2008). The proposal, which was funded, was justified in part on the basis that the interoperability solutions—although expensive to develop—could be used by all VA/DoD joint health care ventures (VA/DoD, 2009, p. 46) and could potentially be exported to all other VA and DoD facilities to provide a seamless medical record from active duty to veteran status. The $11 million was for developing the requirements, not the solutions. Funding for the latter was estimated to be $100 million over 3 years.

A tiger team was dispatched several times to North Chicago to identify the technical requirements for critical interoperability solutions—including a single sign-on solution that would allow providers to log in once to see clinical data from both AHLTA and VistA (including the medical readiness status of active duty servicemembers).

When the JIF funds became available, contracts were awarded to complete the specifications for solutions that would meet the Lovell FHCC's baseline functional requirements when it started up in 2010. The CTG had come up with various lists of critical functional requirements. Certain items were common to those lists:

- Single patient registration in AHLTA and VistA
- Single medical sign-on to access AHLTA and VistA
- Single entry into either AHLTA or VistA that allows the user to
    - enter and view the results of laboratory, radiology, and pharmacy orders, and order and view consults and referrals, and have them appear in the other system while preventing duplication (i.e., orders portability)
    - read test results and progress notes originating from either system and enter or revise them once and have them appear in both systems
    - be assured that the records are for the same patient, regardless of the application, a function called "context management"

- Medical operational readiness status, for example, the ability to enter readiness data into VistA that is viewable in AHLTA throughout the world

In addition to single patient registration, single sign-on, and orders portability processes and support for the DoD operational readiness system, the contractors also worked on requirements for outpatient appointment scheduling and for producing data on clinical costs and workload needed for financial reconciliation. The requirements for these six capabilities were completed in July 2009 in the form of business requirements documents for each.

The next step was to obtain the $100 million needed to develop the interoperability capabilities, which were supposed to be ready by June 2010, leaving 90 days to ensure that they were stable before the FHCC opening. A proposal to use the JIF mechanism to provide the $100 million was submitted in mid-2009 and it had to be reviewed by the OMB and the congressional appropriations committees before it was approved in August 2009. By this time, the likelihood of completing the set of initial EHR system capabilities by October 2010 was fading, and the departments began to prioritize among them. In July 2009, the DoD notified Congress that the departments were seeking to have three of the key capabilities ready by October 2010: (1) single patient registration, (2) single sign-on with context management for clinical users, and (3) the "first phase" of orders portability for laboratory, radiology, pharmacy, and consultations and referrals. In October 2010, they expected to be just beginning the development of applications to support the Navy's operational readiness requirements, in the process of developing the requirements for producing financial reconciliation data, and exploring a joint appointment scheduling system (U.S. House of Representatives, 2009). In its annual report, the JEC also reported that single patient registration, single sign-on, and orders portability were the three necessary initial capabilities for implementing the Lovell FHCC, noting that the $100 million in JIF funding was not approved until August 2009, "leaving little time for IT design, development, testing, information assurance, and deployment" (VA/DoD, 2011, p. 41). However, the EA between the departments signed in April 2010 specified that single patient registration, single sign-on, and orders portability would be ready on opening day, as well as documentation of medical and dental operational readiness of recruits and other active duty servicemembers (DoD/VA, 2010, Attachment A).

The funding plan was for the departments to deposit $25 million each in the JIF funds in FY 2009 and another $25 million each in FY 2010, for a total of $100 million. The VA and the DoD began the contracting process using the FY 2009 funding in August 2009. The VA was able to deposit and use the FY 2010 funding, but the DoD could not because its appropriations bill had not been passed and the DoD was operating under a CR. This delayed DoD funding of work on orders portability until January 2010. DoD funding was further held up by a congressional committee pending submission of a report on joint medical IT.

By early 2010, it was evident that orders portability for laboratory, radiology, pharmacy, and consultations and referrals were probably not going to be ready by October, and that a "Plan B"—a workaround solution—was going to be necessary for the pharmacy to assure patient safety. In February, the VA's chief information officer told Congress that single patient registration, single sign-on, and orders portability for laboratory, pharmacy, and radiology would not be ready until the end of November 2010 (and orders portability for consults not until later in 2011), which would delay the move of the Navy's outpatient clinics to the ACC (U.S. House of Representatives, 2010, p. 39). At that time, "significant concerns regarding the ability to deliver IT capabilities in such a compressed time frame were elevated to the Deputy Secretaries of Defense and Veterans Affairs" (VA/DoD, 2011, p. 41). They assigned the Interagency Program Office (IPO) to oversee and coordinate the Lovell FHCC IM/IT development effort. The IPO developed a joint interagency master schedule and established an executive committee of top national and local VA and DoD IT officials that met biweekly. The VA and the DoD controlled the funding, however, and proceeded to develop the interoperability capabilities on parallel tracks, which made it difficult for the IPO to coordinate the development process (Filippi, 2011). The IPO reported later that it encountered long lead times because of the separate review processes within each department and the need to adjudicate differences (IPO, 2012, p. 6).[22]

The main stumbling block in developing orders portability for pharmacy was the need to have sequential prescription numbers that are the same in both EHR systems, which could not be achieved without making changes in AHLTA and VistA. The departments, however, had agreed that no changes would be made in those legacy systems. This left a gap in IT capability, because the orders in VistA would not be consistent in AHLTA, and vice versa. "This gap created several unacceptable patient safety risks that could only be overcome by having licensed pharmacists manually input the necessary functions that will be performed automatically when the IT solution is deployed" (VA/DoD, 2011, p. 57). The departments agreed to provide $1 million through the JIF to fund up to seven pharmacists for a year as a workaround until orders portability for pharmacy could be de-

[22] The DoD and the VA revised the Interagency Program Office charter in October 2011 to make it "the single point of accountability for [i.e., have the authority to manage] the development and implementation of the integrated electronic health record" (DoD/VA, 2011).

veloped, which was estimated to be ready by the last quarter of FY 2011. This arrangement has been extended beyond 1 year until the pharmacy capability of the joint VA/DoD integrated EHR (iEHR) system is developed, currently scheduled to occur in 2014 (the iEHR, the next generation EHR system being developed jointly by the VA and the DoD to replace VistA and AHLTA, is described at the end of this section).

Meanwhile, the schedules for the other capabilities proved to be too ambitious and were not met. Each department was developing solutions for its own system and testing them in laboratory conditions rather than in a live environment (GAO, 2011, p. 21). In some cases, the two department solutions did not work well together when field-tested in North Chicago. For example, each department selected a different commercial program for single sign-on with context management, and it proved to be difficult for the two programs to work together through DoD's firewall and server. Mostly, it just took longer than expected to develop the various capabilities and then longer than expected to implement them because of unexpected glitches. As Lovell FHCC IT leaders put it, "integration was dependent on the computer systems functioning as planned" (Poulin et al., 2012). Unfortunately, things did not always go as planned.

The single patient registration and single sign-on with context management capabilities were delivered to the Lovell FHCC on December 13, 2010, and were operational by the end of the month, except for delays in access to single sign-on for some users and limitations on context management because of inconsistent family member codes between the DoD and the VA and other problems. Because of continuing problems with using two single sign-on with context management programs at Lovell, the IPO recently decided to use just one of the two programs for use in the iEHR system (Brewin, 2012).

Orders portability for laboratory and radiology were also delivered in December 2010, but user testing found that additional testing and development were required (IPO, 2011). Limited use of orders portability for radiology and laboratory was deployed in March 2011, but the Lovell FHCC decided to delay implementation of orders portability for laboratory until radiology was running smoothly—that is, achieving a rate of 90 percent matching of patients with images—which was achieved by the end of 2011 (GAO, 2011). Orders portability for laboratory was deployed initially in a few clinics in January 2012, after remaining software defects, complete user account and laboratory test mapping, and patient registration issues were resolved.

Current Status of Information Management/Information Technology for Patient Care

As of June 2012, when this report was written, the status of IM/IT for patient care was as follows:

- **Single patient registration.** Deployed on December 13, 2010. Operational after fixes to accommodate batch processing of recruit classes.
- **Single sign-on with context management.** Deployed on December 13, 2010. Operational after fixes to deal with inconsistent family member codes used by the DoD and the VA. Continuing problems aligning DoD and VA versions of the program. Due to be replaced by a single program as part of the iEHR system.
- **Orders portability for pharmacy.** This capability turned out to be too complex to develop by the end of 2010. In March 2011, when the DoD and VA secretaries decided to jointly develop a single EHR system (the iEHR), they elected to use the iEHR's orders portability solutions for pharmacy and for consultations and referrals at the Lovell FHCC rather than continue to attempt to develop an interoperable solution using the legacy systems, VistA and AHLTA. In the interim, five registered pharmacists are conducting manual checks of prescriptions for potential drug interactions and allergies at a cost of approximately $700,000 per year.
- **Orders portability for radiology.** User testing in December 2010 found that further development was needed. It was initially deployed in June 2011 and fully operational by the end of 2011.
- **Orders portability for laboratory.** User testing in December 2010 found that further development was needed. Deployment was delayed until January 2012, after orders portability for radiology was implemented and made fully operational.
- **Orders portability for consultations and referrals.** This capability is complex to develop and, early in 2010, it was postponed until later in 2011, in favor of making single patient registration, single sign-on, and orders portability for laboratory, radiology, and pharmacy ready for the opening of the Lovell FHCC. Along with orders portability for pharmacy (see above), the DoD and VA secretaries decided in March 2011 to cancel the effort to make consultations and referrals interoperable between the two legacy EHR systems and instead to develop a single joint solution as part of the iEHR system. This would have delayed the capability for several years. Subsequently, given the urgent need for this capability at the Lovell FHCC, an effort to develop an interoperable solution for the

FHCC has been reestablished. As of September 2012, consult and referral interoperability was being phased in.

Plans for a Joint Department of Veterans Affairs/Department of Defense Electronic Health Record System

In 2010, the VA and DoD secretaries began to meet every two months to discuss progress on developing a joint disability evaluation system to replace their separate systems and interoperability between their EHR systems, and the situation at the Lovell FHCC was an explicit agenda item. In early 2011, aware of major problems in the effort to develop interoperability software for use at the FHCC, they decided to halt the upgrade programs for their respective EHR systems, AHLTA and VistA, and instead develop a new EHR system for joint use, dubbed the iEHR.

Aware of the ongoing needs at the Lovell FHCC, they decided to follow through on the software programs that were in advanced development for the FHCC, namely, the programs for radiology and laboratory orders portability. The two programs in early development, which were orders portability for pharmacy and consults and referrals, were stopped in favor of developing a single joint solution for them as part of the iEHR. Recognizing the need at the Lovell FHCC, the pharmacy solution was chosen to be one of the first several products of the iEHR development process, with the FHCC as the alpha test site. The goal is to have an operational pharmacy program for the FHCC in 2014. Meanwhile, the FHCC will continue its workaround arrangement for ensuring patient safety from harmful drug interactions and allergies. At the time this report was drafted, there were discussions about restarting the development of an interoperable capability for consults and referrals because of the lack of a workable temporary workaround such as that for pharmacy.

Among the early decisions on the structure of the iEHR was one to adapt Janus, a user interface developed for the joint venture in Hawaii, which allows clinicians at the Honolulu VAMC and the Tripler Army Hospital, which provides inpatient care for veterans, to read a patient's records in both systems. In December 2011, the Lovell FHCC began testing Janus in its clinics. In its current form, it is read-only, but it does pull the information into a single view rather than requiring a provider to look at information in the VA and the DoD EHR systems separately. The plan is to further develop Janus so that patient information can be entered and updated, as well as viewed, in real time.

Credentialing and Privileging Clinical Providers

The VA and the DoD database software packages that are currently used to credential independent licensed and licensed non-independent health care providers—VetPro and the Centralized Credentials and Quality Assurance System (CCQAS), respectively—are not interoperable, although each is designed to meet the same Joint Commission standards. FHCC planners preferred to have a single system wherever possible for efficient operation of the FHCC. In this case, however, there was early agreement that both credentialing systems had to be maintained because information about active duty providers had to be in CCQAS when they transferred to their next duty station, and information about VA providers had to be in VetPro for the same reason. In addition, CCQAS includes information about adverse actions, training, and other types of information not tracked in VetPro. In 2003, the VA and the DoD piloted a common interface to the two systems at several VA/DoD joint ventures. An evaluation determined that the interface, while technically feasible, was not cost effective unless nearly 1,000 providers per year were processed (the Lovell FHCC was expected to have approximately 565 providers) (DoD/VA, 2008, p. 56).

Because it was determined that use of a single credentialing system did not meet VA and DoD organizational requirements, and that using an interface to create interoperability was not cost effective, Lovell FHCC planners proposed and the HEC co-chairs approved using CCQAS for active duty providers and VetPro for civilian providers and establishing a combined credentialing office in which staff would be cross-trained to use both systems. This solution was functional but less efficient than staffing a single system.

The Navy proposed having the active duty providers be privileged by the senior Navy captain acting as the commanding officer (CO) of the NHCGL as well as the deputy director of the Lovell FHCC. The VA director of the FHCC would in turn accept or deny the privileges granted by the deputy director, based on the Inter-facility Credentialing Transfer Brief (ICTB) provided by the Navy. This would have required a change in VA policies, which at the time did not accept ICTBs from other agencies and instead verified all information directly with the primary sources. This approach was seen as inconsistent with the single-chain-of-command concept and the staff integration concept of the medical bylaws. The credentialing EDM recommended and the HEC co-chairs approved the option where the FHCC director is the credentialing and privileging approval authority for DoD and VA providers at the FHCC with input from the deputy director. The deputy director privileges the active duty providers for Navy, not for FHCC, purposes. Granting of Navy privileges by the deputy director acting as the CO of the NHCGL is required to maintain readiness for deployment and to meet the Navy mission requirements.

Scope of Practice for Advanced Practice Nurses and Navy Hospital Corpsmen

One of the Navy's main concerns about participating in the creation of the Lovell FHCC was ensuring that the consolidated health care system would not degrade military operational readiness. One area of concern was maintenance of the clinical proficiency of active duty nurse practitioners and other advanced practice nurses (APNs), hospital corpsmen, and other allied health professionals. The problem was the difference between VA and DoD policies on privileging health professionals other than physicians, psychologists, podiatrists, optometrists, dentists, and chiropractors.

The VA will privilege APNs, audiologists, pharmacists, and social workers only if their state licenses allow for independent practice. Other VA health professionals—for example, physician's assistants (PAs), dietitians, marriage and family therapists, occupational therapists, and physical therapists—function under a scope of practice and protocols approved by the medical staff, but they are not a part of the medical staff. In contrast, the Navy privileges APNs, audiologists, pharmacists, and social workers, as well as dietitians, marriage and family therapists, occupational therapists, physical therapists, and speech-language pathologists—and PAs supervised by a physician—and recognizes them as part of the medical staff. The Navy will also grant privileges on a waiver basis even if the provider's state license does not allow independent practice.

When asked by Congress about obstacles to integration at the Lovell FHCC, the Navy surgeon general identified one of them as VA policies on credentialing of ancillary health workers:

> The VA and how they credential is different than what we do in DoD because very few VA providers, perhaps none, but very few VA providers are operationally oriented or deploy. But I have to make sure my providers maintain their operational medical skills so that when I tap them to deploy to an operational area they are full up. So I have to make sure that we have the credentialing issues that are taken care of and that we are going to solve problems that I may have in the Navy. (Robinson, 2009, p. 31)

On this issue, the CTG could not reach consensus and the VA and the Navy agreed to disagree. The VA wanted to use VA privileging policies for all providers at the Lovell FHCC, arguing that a scope of practice arrangement would maintain the clinical skills required for military operational readiness; the Navy wanted to privilege APNs, hospital corpsmen, and other health professionals as permitted by Navy policies. The Navy's position was that independent practice was needed to develop the critical thinking skills that such health professionals would need when deployed where there are no physicians to consult. The VA's position was consistent with the vision of an integrated organization under a single chain of command. Ultimately, agreement was reached on an alternative, approved by the HEC co-chairs, in which active duty health professionals who could not be privileged according to VA policies would be able to practice at the Lovell FHCC with the clinical proficiencies required to maintain Navy privileges included in their scope of practice.[23]

Another obstacle to maintaining operational readiness was posed by the lack of active duty nurses in the inpatient wards and the ED. These positions had been lost in 2006 when inpatient and emergency care was moved to the NCVAMC. The Navy wants hospital corpsmen to gain experience in inpatient and emergency settings but that requires supervision by an active duty nurse. The workaround was an agreement that hospital corpsmen can be supervised on a daily basis by VA nurses and meet Navy requirements as long as they have an active duty nurse mentor who meets with them regularly.

Corpsmen, especially those with advanced training that qualifies them as independent duty corpsmen (IDCs), carry out certain functions that are reserved to registered nurses and to PAs in the civilian sector. To forestall resistance from VA physicians and nurses to allowing IDCs to perform medical and nursing procedures, the Lovell FHCC provided training to familiarize VA staff with the skill sets of corpsmen and to underscore the need to allow them to practice those skills to develop and maintain the clinical proficiencies they will need when deployed to posts where they are the only medical professionals.

Collection of Other Health Insurance

The VA and the DoD have different processes for billing other insurance companies. Although governed by different laws, in both cases any monies collected must be deposited in the department's appropriation system. The Lovell FHCC planners hoped to adopt one billing process and deposit the collected funds in the FHCC's account for budgeting and spending without regard to the source of the funds.

The NCVAMC was using VISN 12's central billing office, located in Madison, Wisconsin, for billing and collecting from insurance programs. The NHCGL performed its own collections. The options were to (1) have the VISN 12's central billing office in Madison perform billing and collections for the Lovell FHCC using the VA's reimbursement rates; (2) have the Lovell FHCC perform the billing and collections using the VA's reim-

[23] The proficiencies are included in clinical privilege sheets appended to Navy BUMED (Bureau of Medicine and Surgery) Instruction 6320.66E (Appendix H for APNs and Appendix G for other allied health specialists).

bursement rates; or (3) have the FHCC perform the billing and collections using the DoD's and the VA's reimbursement rates and processes. Option 1 was preferred because Option 2 would have required the FHCC to hire and train additional staff and Option 3 would have required running two systems, which would be less efficient and more prone to error. Option 1 also bypassed the question about whether legislation would be needed for the DoD to deposit collections in a non-DoD account.

The decision was to adopt Option 1, that is, to have the VA perform all the billing and collections through VISN 12's billing center in Madison, using VA reimbursement rates but providing a discount for services provided to certain DoD beneficiaries, such as foreign military servicemembers training in the United States. The EA, invoking NDAA 2010, specifies that all monies collected from other insurers by the Lovell FHCC will be deposited in the JMFDF.

Cultural Integration

The Lovell FHCC planners recognized the existence of—and the importance of overcoming—differences in the organizational cultures of the Navy and the VA to achieve success in creating an integrated health care delivery system. There was also recognition that the beneficiary groups and other stakeholders would have concerns about potential negative impacts affecting them with the creation of the FHCC. Some Navy personnel worried that the FHCC would encumber their mission of medically processing recruits and ensuring they were medically fit for deployment, while some veterans worried that they would receive lower priority than active duty servicemembers in obtaining services (Interviews).

The 2005 governance and sitting EDM talked about the need for a communications plan to address the concerns of those affected by the integration effort. The Lovell FHCC leadership's presentation at the February 2006 VA/DoD joint venture conference began by quoting the eight steps to achieve organizational change from *Leading Change*, the 1996 book by Harvard Business School professor John P. Kotter (Lovell FHCC, 2006):

1. Establishing a sense of urgency,
2. Creating the guiding coalition,
3. Developing a vision and strategy,
4. Communicating the change vision,
5. Empowering employees,
6. Generating short-term wins,
7. Consolidating gains and producing more change, and
8. Anchoring new approaches in the culture.

The presentation then reported on how each of the steps was being addressed. For example, a sense of urgency and the creation of a guiding coalition of the Navy and the VA were traced to the impact of the 2001 reports that identified the need for a new Navy facility and the underutilization of the NCVAMC inpatient facility. The vision was total integration, and the strategy for promoting the adaptation of the two organizational cultures to each other by 2010 was the three-phase approach. Communicating the vision included the establishment of a marketing task group. The membership of NHGL and NCVAMC personnel on the national task groups was the example of empowering employees. Short-term wins included cost avoidance from shifting inpatient mental health (Phase 1) and inpatient medicine, surgery, and pediatrics (Phase 2) to the NCVAMC rather than building and maintaining a new Navy hospital. Other short-term wins were the Navy's use of NCVAMC space for its new blood donor processing center (instead of renovating the building it had been using on the Navy base) and the winning of six JIF awards to expand services. The example of consolidating gains and producing more change was the effort to address cultural differences.

As mentioned earlier, a communications task group was added to the six original task groups in 2007 and renamed the communications and organization culture task group in 2008. The group's assignment was to conduct an assessment of the local, regional, and national stakeholders, including the staff and beneficiaries of the NHGL and the NCVAMC, and then to develop a communications plan and marketing strategy to inform each audience about the benefits of an integrated FHCC. The initial steps included a quarterly newsletter, an FHCC website, and all-employee meetings. The FHCC's logo and motto—"Proud to Partner: Excellence in Federal Health Care!"—were developed early in the process (Lovell FHCC, 2006).

The VA's National Center for Organizational Development (NCOD) and the Naval Postgraduate School were engaged to assess Phase 2, survey employee attitudes, conduct focus groups with patients and employees, identify barriers to collaboration, and hold offsite retreats of VA and DoD personnel (Lovell FHCC, 2009). The NCOD surveyed VA and Navy staff in May 2006, September 2007, and February 2008. The goal of these assessments was "to identify what is currently working well and what opportunities currently exist to enhance integration efforts for all staff" (Lovell FHCC, 2010a).

There was a considerable effort by the human resources task group to keep employees, especially the Navy civilians who were going to be transferred to the VA, informed about their status. Fourteen hundred civilian employees of the NHCGL and the NCVAMC received letters at the end of August 2009 stating their job titles and locations; the remaining 600 civilians received letters confirming that they had jobs at the Lovell FHCC, although its location had not been determined. VA and DoD human resources specialists were available at the NHCGL the week following the notification letters to answer questions, and several frequently asked questions documents were issued that provided answers to anticipated concerns. There were at least three sets of town hall meetings in 2009 and 2010.

The joint strategic planning conferences held periodically to plan the Lovell FHCC explicitly considered the cultural aspects of merging programs and departments. There were conscious efforts to invite key stakeholders in the VA, the Navy, and Congress to tour the nascent FHCC resulting from the first two phases of the integration process. The HEC received periodic briefings on cultural blending initiatives. The Navy surgeon general and the VA secretary testified before Congress on the challenges of merging the two organizations (Robinson, 2009; Shinseki, 2009).

The first Stakeholder Advisory Committee (SAC) meeting was held in July 2010. The SAC members included community representatives and representatives of veterans service organizations, the Navy line commands and the Navy ombudsman at the NSGL, the TRICARE regional office and managed care support contractors, VISN 12 representatives, the Rosalind Franklin University of Medicine and Science, and a congressional liaison. In August 2010, a final round of leadership meetings and mini-retreats of VA and DoD staff was held to keep employees informed and discuss cultural issues.

Despite the efforts to forge identification of the employees at the NHCGL and the NCVAMC with the Lovell FHCC rather than with the Navy or the VA, not everyone was happy with the change. Not all Navy personnel, including those transferred to the VA personnel system, thought that the FHCC was a good idea. From their point of view, the fast-paced mission of preparing recruits for deployment has not changed, but achieving it has become more complicated and time-consuming. The main problem for the branch clinics on the Navy base is the need to manually obtain and enter patient information into AHLTA (the DoD EHR system) from VistA (the VA EHR system) when recruits, students, and Navy staff receive emergency, inpatient, or specialty medical services on the west campus. In addition, IT support, laboratory services, and supply, which have been centralized, are seen as less responsive than when they were part of the NHCGL.

Legislative Process

The six task groups formed in 2005 were instructed to identify any laws, regulations, policies, and procedures that would have to be revised or dropped to enable the VA and the Navy to integrate their health care centers in North Chicago. The approach was to minimize legislative changes and rely as much as possible on existing law, specifically, 38 U.S.C. § 8111, "Sharing of Department of Veterans Affairs and Department of Defense Health Care Resources."

Certainly there was room for optimism that Congress would revise the statutes where needed. Congress had repeatedly encouraged greater cooperation in delivering health care between the DoD and the VA in laws, conference committee reports on VA and DoD bills, and by requesting annual and ad hoc reports on the state of VA/DoD sharing. The NDAA 2002[24] had mandated a series of demonstrations of mechanisms to facilitate VA/DoD sharing and created the JIF award program. The appropriations committees had approved $13 million in 2004 to renovate the NCVAMC surgical suite and ED, and $135 million in 2007 to construct the ACC and related facilities. In 2008, they had allowed the VA and the DoD to funnel an additional $100 million through the JIF program to develop software to enable the two EHR systems to work together at the Lovell FHCC.

The Lovell FHCC planners gradually identified the minimum set of legislative changes that would be required to implement the FHCC. The lack of authority to transfer Navy civilians to the VA was evident early on. It also became evident that the governance model in which the FHCC reported to a DoD/VA committee under the HEC would require legislation to implement. In that case, the departments changed the model in 2007 so that the FHCC director reported to the VA, because legislation to create what in effect would be a new federal agency did not seem likely to pass. There was no acceptable way for the Navy to transfer the ACC to the VA under existing legislation (discussed above). The planners hoped to avoid the need for legislation to create a joint fund for the FHCC by using the JIF mechanism, which was resisted by VA and DoD comptrollers and by the congressional appropriations committees, so legislation establishing a new Treasury account was required. Finally, legislation would be needed to designate the FHCC as an MTF to enable it to provide health care to DoD beneficiaries without charging deductibles and copayments required if they used non-MTF facilities.

In 2008, the congressional affairs offices of the VA and the DoD worked with members of the Illinois delegation to draft language permitting the transfer of personnel from the Navy to the VA, allowing the transfer of ownership of the ACC from the Navy to the VA, designating the Lovell FHCC as an MTF, and establishing a JIF-like mechanism to allow the department to fund the FHCC jointly. In September 2008, Senator Dick Durbin introduced an amendment to the NDAA for FY 2009 (NDAA

---

[24] NDAA for Fiscal Year 2002, Public Law 107-107 (December 28, 2001). http://www.dod.gov/dodgc/olc/docs/2002NDAA.pdf (accessed August 6, 2012).

2009[25]), but the process of passing the bill was too far along to include the FHCC provisions. Instead, when the NDAA 2009 was passed by Congress, it included a section on "Guidelines for Combined Medical Facilities of the Department of Defense and the Department of Veterans Affairs" that required the DoD and VA secretaries to execute a binding operational agreement on nine areas:

1. Governance
2. Patient priority categories
3. Budgeting
4. Staffing and training
5. Construction
6. Physical plant management
7. Contingency planning
8. Quality assurance
9. Information technology

Although the NDAA 2009 allowed the DoD and the VA to negotiate an operational agreement for a combined facility, it did not explicitly confer additional legal authority regarding beneficiary benefits, ACC ownership, employee transfers, or a joint funding mechanism. In June 2009, Senators Durbin and Daniel Akaka reintroduced legislation in the new Congress with the four specific authorities needed for the Lovell FHCC to function with hopes that it would pass as part of a DoD supplemental appropriations bill. The fast-track initiative failed and the bill became part of the regular NDAA process. One area that required considerable negotiation was the transfer of personnel. The draft language was designed to "protect" the Navy civilians moving into the VA personnel system by specifying that they would not lose pay or seniority or be subject to a probationary period if they had already completed this as a DoD employee. Although the departments agreed on the language, the union representing Navy civilians at Great Lakes—the American Federation of Government Employees—opposed the language because the Navy personnel would lose the right under the VA's Title 38 personnel system to appeal to the Merit Systems Appeal Board (Robinson, 2009, p. 98). The Durbin-Akaka bill extended collective bargaining rights under Title 5 to transferred employees for 2 years, at which time the VA secretary, in consultation with the DoD and Navy secretaries, would determine whether the appeal rights should be terminated, revised, or retained.

---

[25] NDAA, S. 3001, January 3, 2008. http://www.gpo.gov/fdsys/pkg/BILLS-110s3001enr/pdf/BILLS-110s3001enr.pdf (accessed August 6, 2012).

The DoD was also concerned about using the JIF program as the funding mechanism, because it wanted to control how much and when the funding would be spent (the JIF legislation says each department has to contribute "at least $15 million a year" which becomes "no year" money—that is, there is no limit on what a department can contribute and it does not have to be spent the same year) (Robinson, 2009). The departments had already stretched the intent of the JIF program in using it to provide the $100 million for interoperable IT solutions for the Lovell FHCC. The Durbin-Akaka bill provided for a Treasury fund under the VA to which the DoD and the VA could transfer funds for the FHCC, and it stipulated that the funds would be available for 1 FY, except for 2 percent, which could be carried over into a second year.

After a fair amount of behind-the-scenes negotiating in the executive branch, and then between the House and the Senate, which had passed different versions of the NDAA 2010, the Department of Defense-Department of Veterans Affairs Medical Facility Demonstration Project was passed as part of the NDAA 2010 and signed into law on October 28, 2009. The House had not included a Lovell FHCC section in its bill but acceded to the Senate language with certain modifications and additions. The final bill did not refer to the Captain James A. Lovell FHCC because the name had not been approved through customary procedures. The final version directed the DoD and VA secretaries to submit a copy of the EA required by the NDAA 2009 to Congress at least 7 days before finalizing it. It also directed the GAO to review and assess progress annually. The legislation renamed the Treasury fund the "Joint Department of Defense-Department of Veterans Affairs Medical Facility Demonstration Fund," and said that DoD and VA funds for the joint fund had to be specifically authorized and appropriated for that purpose. It specified that the first priority for care would be given to active duty servicemembers. The department secretaries were required to submit a final report to Congress after 5 years, describing and assessing the demonstration and recommending whether or not to continue it.

In the meantime, the Lovell FHCC planners began to draft an EA covering the nine areas specified in the NDAA 2009. The EA draft went through nearly 70 iterations while it was reviewed up the two department chains before being signed by the three secretaries (VA, DoD, and Navy) on April 23, 2010. At the same time, the Lovell FHCC began drafting an executive sharing agreement (ESA) to prepare for the possibility that the joint Treasury fund might not be ready, or the appropriations for it passed, by October 1, 2010. In fact, the FHCC was operated under the ESA for the first 9 months because the defense appropriations bill for FY 2011 was not passed and the DoD had to operate under a CR. This meant that the requirement in the NDAA 2010 that funds be specifically appropriated for the FHCC could not be fulfilled.

SUMMARY OF IMPLEMENTATION CHALLENGES

The experience of the planning and implementation of the Lovell FHCC provides many examples of the issues that arise—and how they can resolved—when the VA and the DoD decide to serve their respective beneficiary populations by combining their medical centers. Some of the significant issues that had to be addressed to implement the Lovell FHCC are listed in Table 3-2. This history is ripe for the evaluation of lessons learned that should be considered in designing any future FHCCs. Some of the solutions developed by the Lovell FHCC might be adopted by future FHCCs. Many of them are compromises or time-consuming workarounds necessitated by differing policies and procedures of the VA, the DoD, and

TABLE 3-2 Issues Likely to Be Encountered in Creating an Integrated Department of Veterans Affairs/Department of Defense Joint Health Care Center

Implementation Issue	Discussion
Joint governance	The desire to have a joint governance structure must be reconciled with the requirement that a federal health care center (FHCC) be assigned to, and the director/chief executive officer to come from, one department or the other. The requirement that the ranking active duty military officer, if he or she is not the director, exercise the Uniform Code of Military Justice and other command responsibilities is another irreducible complication in achieving a single chain of command.
Beneficiary benefits and copayments	Although the intent at the Lovell FHCC was to treat everyone equally, this was not totally achieved. Because the Navy's boot camp for enlisted recruits is at Naval Station Great Lakes, there was an agreement, which was specified in the 2010 National Defense Authorization Act (NDAA), that active duty servicemembers are to receive first priority in scheduling appointments and receiving services. This is most evident at the west campus pharmacy, where active duty beneficiaries go to the head of the line, making some veterans unhappy (see Chapter 4). The FHCC planners also wanted Department of Defense (DoD) beneficiaries to be exempt from cost sharing, as they are at military treatment facilities (MTFs). Congress allowed the FHCC to be an MTF for eligibility purposes, but only during the 5-year demonstration, and the DoD secretary had to issue a ruling that cost sharing would not be required as part of the 5-year demonstration. A more permanent arrangement will have to be worked out if FHCCs become standard programs rather than demonstration projects.

TABLE 3-2 Continued

Implementation Issue	Discussion
Joint funding mechanism and reconciliation model	The solution in North Chicago was to create a Department of the Treasury (Treasury) fund under the Department of Veterans Affairs (VA) where the departments could pool their funds and to develop a reconciliation process based on workload measures to apportion responsibility between the Navy and the VA for funding after the fact. The reconciliation methodology could be a model for future FHCCs, but the VA decision support system does not routinely track industry standard workload measures (e.g., relative value units and relative weighted products) that, therefore, have to be determined manually as a workaround. Also, the Treasury fund is only authorized for the 5-year demonstration in North Chicago and would have to be extended by Congress to additional FHCC sites. In addition, the reconciliation methodology has not yet been put to the test; the FHCC funding is based on historical levels during the first 3 years.
Employee status	It is desirable for several reasons to have all employees in the same personnel system. In a VA/DoD FHCC, active duty personnel will always be in a separate personnel system. However, civilians can be put under one department or the other, if Congress approves. Nonetheless, differences regarding job descriptions, compensation, and collective bargaining rights must be resolved. At this time, the authority to transfer Navy civilians to the VA is only granted for the 5-year demonstration in North Chicago and would have to be extended to any additional sites by Congress.
Joint workforce planning	The VA and the military department (the Navy in the case of the Lovell FHCC) must agree on staffing levels and a mechanism for revising them during the year in response to shifts in workload. The situation is complicated at the Lovell FHCC because the Navy personnel rotate out after 2 or 3 years and are often deployed once or twice during their rotation at Great Lakes.
Joint electronic health record (EHR) system	Although joint use of the DoD and the VA EHR systems was considered to be a prerequisite for seamless health care delivery at the Lovell FHCC, attempts to develop a minimum set of software capabilities (e.g., single patient registration, single sign-on, and single order entry and results retrieval) by the opening of the Lovell FHCC were not successful. In fact, the lack of integration of the DoD and the VA EHR systems has caused time-consuming workarounds to ensure that patient information is the same and current in both of them and integrated health care delivery has been inhibited. The Lovell FHCC experience was a major factor in the decision of the DoD and the VA secretaries to cancel updates of their legacy EHR systems and jointly develop a single EHR system for use by both departments. Having a single EHR system designed to meet the needs of both departments would greatly facilitate integrated health care delivery.

continued

TABLE 3-2 Continued

Implementation Issue	Discussion
Information technology (IT) network trust, security, and computer system access	Ideally, there would be network trust so that users of one computer system would be automatically allowed access to the other. The VA "dot.gov" system does not meet the DoD's "dot.mil" security standards and it would be very costly to bring it up to DoD standards. The Navy relented on requiring a secret-level security clearance to access the DoD EHR system when the VA agreed to have all VA personnel undergo a more intensive security investigation. The departments also could not reach agreement on using a single access card and more than 1,000 VA employees had to be issued special access cards, a process that could not be completed by October 1, 2010.
Credentialing and privileging	It was not cost effective to operate a common interface for the VA and DoD credentialing verification systems at the Lovell FHCC, even though both are based on the same Joint Commission standards. As at the Lovell FHCC, future FHCCs would have to staff and operate both systems unless the departments agreed to develop a single, joint system similar to what the Lovell FHCC decided to do in the case of the incompatible EHR systems. Although there was agreement that the FHCC director, a career VA employee, would be the final privileging authority, the deputy director, as the ranking active duty officer, must also privilege active duty clinicians for certain military purposes.
Privileging and supervision of active duty advanced practice nurses (APNs), hospital corpsmen, and independent duty hospital corpsmen (IDCs)	The DoD has more permissive privileging rules than the VA because it deploys registered nurses and hospital corpsmen with advanced training to assignments in locations where they must perform independently of physicians. The solution at the Lovell FHCC was for the VA to agree to a scope of practice that included the specific functions that APNs and IDCs are expected by the DoD to perform, which are broader than the VA's usual scope of practice for these positions. Supervision of corpsmen is also an issue. The Navy requires them to be supervised by an active duty nurse, which inhibits staff integration. The workaround at the FHCC was to allow corpsmen working on the west campus to be supervised by civilian nurses in their daily work as long as there is an active duty nurse mentor.
Procurement	There was agreement that the Lovell FHCC would use the VA procurement system, but experience has shown that it would be more cost effective if the Navy facilities command could be used for certain base operations. It is also more cost effective to use personal services contracts (PSCs) for staffing the east campus branch clinics, given that the workload there varies, but the VA does not have authority to use them. The FHCC would like the VA to obtain authority from Congress to use the PSCs. Meanwhile, despite the agreement to use the VA logistics system, the Navy logistics command is administering the PSCs on the east campus.

TABLE 3-2 Continued

Implementation Issue	Discussion
Pharmacy formulary	It might be more efficient to have one formulary, but the decision for the Lovell FHCC was to maintain two of them. If the two departments could agree on a common formulary, it also might lead to lower prices because of their combined demand.
Mail order pharmacy	The Lovell FHCC saved space in the ambulatory care center by deciding to rely on the VA's Consolidated Mail Order Pharmacy (CMOP) for prescription refills, but the DoD does not want to allow DoD beneficiaries to use this program. The resulting backup at the FHCC pharmacy has been a major consumer dissatisfaction issue. This question—whether or not to use the CMOP for DoD beneficiaries—should be settled before designing the pharmacy space in future FHCCs.
Military operational readiness	The issue is finding a way to document the current individual medical readiness of active duty servicemembers who obtain emergency, inpatient, or specialty services on the east campus. Because of the lack of interoperability between the VA and the DoD EHR systems, entries in the VA EHR system used at these west campus locations are not simultaneously recorded automatically in the DoD EHR system. This problem is being addressed by the development of the integrated EHR system, the iEHR.
Law enforcement and security	The Lovell FHCC expected to integrate the Navy and the VA police forces, but efforts have been stymied by the Posse Comitatus Act, which generally prohibits active duty servicemembers from arresting civilians. In August 2012, permission was granted for the Navy masters-at-arms to attend the 8-week VA Police Academy in Little Rock, Arkansas, after which they will be able to carry lethal and nonlethal weapons as they participate in patrolling the west campus of the FHCC.

the affected military service (in this case, the Navy) that could be addressed more effectively at the enterprise level. Others may be unique to North Chicago, for example, the priority given to active duty servicemembers because of the demands of the recruit training mission.

REFERENCES

Arthur, D. 2006. Written statement of Vice Admiral Donald C. Arthur, Surgeon General of the Navy, before the Subcommittee on Military Quality of Life and Veterans Affairs of the House Appropriations Committee (also before Senate Appropriations Subcommittee on Defense on May 3, 2006). http://www.med.navy.mil/bumed/comms/Pages/Congressional Testimony.aspx (accessed August 7, 2012).

Bean, M. L. 2009. Speech of Hon. Melissa L. Bean of Illinois in the House of Representatives, June 24. *Congressional Record*. Pp. E1620–E1621.

Brewin, B. 2007. Navy eyes front-end system for joint health facility. *GovernmentHealthIT*, February 26. http://www.govhealthit.com/news/navy-eyes-front-end-system-joint-health-facility-0 (accessed October 14, 2012).

Brewin, B. 2012. Defense and VA tap vendor to save clinicians from multiple log-ons. *Next Gov.com*, May 21. http://www.nextgov.com/health/2012/05/defense-and-va-tap-vendor-save-clinicians-multiple-log-ons/55832/?oref=ng-dropdown (accessed August 7, 2012).

Chu, D. 2003. Testimony of the under secretary of defense for personnel and readiness at the House Committee on Veterans' Affairs hearing to discuss the report of the President's Task Force to Improve Health Care Delivery for Our Nation's Veterans. June 17. Washington, DC: U.S. Government Printing Office. http://democrats.veterans.house.gov/hearings/schedule108/jun03/6-3-03/6-3_6-17-03.pdf (accessed September 17, 2012).

DoD (Department of Defense). 2010. TRICARE copayment waiver at Captain James A. Lovell Federal Health Care Center Demonstration Project. *Federal Register*, September 27, pp. 59237-59238. http://edocket.access.gpo.gov/2010/pdf/2010-24092.pdf (accessed August 7, 2012).

DoD. 2011. DoD-VA integrated electronic health record pharmacy solution: Request for information. Solicitation Number: TMA-0007-iEHR. https://www.fbo.gov/utils/view?id=3af028f1d3bd70860228f8256bca9ef0 (accessed August 7, 2012).

DoD/VA (Department of Veterans Affairs). 2008. *Fiscal Year 2003 National Defense Authorization Act Department of Defense and Department of Veterans Affairs Demonstration Projects: Final report. July.* http://www.tricare.mil/DVPCO/downloads/DSS%20Consolidated%20Final%20Report%20v%202.31%20formatted.doc (accessed August 7, 2012).

DoD/VA. 2009. *DOD/VA Joint Incentive Fund guide*. November. vadodrs.amedd.army.mil/jif/JIFGuideFinal.doc (accessed August 21, 2012).

DoD/VA. 2010. Executive agreement for the Department of Defense-Department of Veterans Affairs Medical Facility Demonstration Project Federal Health Care Center. April 23. http://tricare.mil/tma/congressionalinformation/downloads/2010310/111-288%20Section%201701(d)(1)%20FHCC%20EA.pdf (accessed September 6, 2012).

DoD/VA. 2011. Department of Defense and Department of Veterans Affairs Interagency Program Office (IPO) charter. http://www.tricare.mil/tma/ipo/documents/IPO.pdf (accessed August 15, 2012).

Durbin, R. 2009. Lovell Health Center one step closer to completion. Press Release, June 23. http://durbin.senate.gov/public/index.cfm/pressreleases?ID=f993baba-956b-4ba1-9d1b-e3e4382a70d7 (accessed August 7, 2012).

Ellis, K. 2005. *Navy partners with North Chicago Veterans Affairs Medical Center.* America's Navy, Story Number NNS 051024-09. http://www.navy.mil/submit/display.asp?story_id=20692 (accessed August 7, 2012).

Filippi, D. 2011. Testimony of Debra M. Filippi, former Director, DoD/VA Interagency Program Office, before the House Veterans Affairs Committee Hearing on H.R. 2383, H.R. 2243, H.R. 2388 and H.R. 2470. http://veterans.house.gov/prepared-statement/prepared-statement-debra-m-filippi-former-director-us-department-defenseus (accessed August 15, 2012).

GAO (U.S. Government Accountability Office). 2004. *VA and DoD health care: Resource sharing at selected sites*. GAO-04-792. Washington, DC: GAO. http://www.gao.gov/new.items/d04792.pdf (accessed August 7, 2012).

GAO. 2005. *Mail order pharmacies: DOD's use of VA's mail pharmacy could produce savings and other benefits*. GAO-05-555. Washington, DC: GAO. http://www.gao.gov/assets/250/246841.pdf (accessed August 7, 2012).

GAO. 2011. *VA and DoD health care: First federal health care center established, but implementation concerns need to be addressed.* GAO-11-570. Washington, DC: GAO. http://www.gao.gov/new.items/d11570.pdf (accessed August 7, 2012).

GAO. 2012a. *Background investigation: Office of Personnel Management needs to improve transparency of its pricing and seek cost savings.* GAO-12-197. Washington, DC: GAO. http://www.gao.gov/assets/590/588947.pdf (accessed August 7, 2012).

GAO. 2012b. *Security clearances: Agencies need clearly defined policy for determining civilian position requirements.* GAO-12-800. Washington, DC: GAO. http://gao.gov/assets/600/592371.pdf (accessed August 7, 2012).

Gibbard, M. D. 2005. Navy, VA do hospital deal: Sailors, vets to get care under 1 roof. *Chicago Tribune*, October 18. http://articles.chicagotribune.com/2005-10-18/news/0510180212_1_va-hospital-va-deputy-secretary-va-facility (accessed August 7, 2012).

Harnly, M. J. 2005. A qualitative analysis of resource sharing agreements between Naval Hospital Great Lakes and North Chicago Veterans Affairs Medical Center: The iron triangle theory of healthcare integration. Master's Thesis, Army-Baylor Program in Healthcare Administration, Fort Sam Houston, TX. http://www.dtic.mil/dtic/tr/fulltext/u2/a443921.pdf (accessed August 7, 2012).

Hassan, T., R. Kline, and M. A. Cardinali. 2008. Federal Health Care Center Great Lakes. Presentation at the 2008 VA/DoD Joint Venture Conference, Honolulu, Hawaii, March 5. http://www.tricare.mil/DVPCO/Hawaii/2008%20JV%20Conf%20-%20FHCC%20Great%20Lakes.ppt (accessed August 7, 2012).

IPO (Interagency Program Office). 2011. *DoD/VA Interagency Program Office annual report to Congress 2010.* http://www.govexec.com/pdfs/033111bb1.pdf (accessed August 7, 2012).

IPO. 2012. *DoD/VA Interagency Program Office annual report to Congress 2011.* http://tricare.mil/tma/congressionalinformation/downloads/FullyInteroperableElectronicPersonalHealthInformationDoDDVA.pdf (accessed July 31, 2012).

Kuczka, S. 2003. VA hospital gets Navy patients; Great Lakes sends 6 to North Chicago. *Chicago Tribune,* November 8, 2003. http://articles.chicagotribune.com/2003-11-08/news/0311080208_1_va-facility-va-campus-navy-patients (accessed October 5, 2012).

Lovell FHCC (Captain James A. Lovell Federal Health Care Center). 2006. The joint initiative between the North Chicago VAMC and Naval Hospital Great Lakes. Presentation at the 2006 Military Health System Conference, January 31. www.tricare.mil/dvpco/bummed/NHGL%20NCVAMC%20BRIEF.ppt (accessed August 24, 2012).

Lovell FHCC. 2009. Captain James A. Lovell Federal Health Care Center. Presentation by Patrick Sullivan and Captain Thomas E. McGue at the 2009 VA/DoD Joint Venture Conference, June 3. http://www.tricare.mil/DVPCO/downloads/20090625/Breakout4cJVUpdateGreatLakesNorthChicago.ppt (accessed October 5, 2012).

Lovell FHCC. 2010a. *Captain James A. Lovell Federal Health Care Center concept of operations.* October 1. Provided to the Committee on Evaluation of the Lovell Federal Health Care Center Merger by the Lovell FHCC.

Lovell FHCC. 2010b. *FY 2011 business plan, April 5.* Provided to the IOM Committee on Evaluation of the Lovell Federal Health Care Center Merger by the Lovell FHCC.

Maldonado, F. A., and D. M. Poulin. 2012. IT news from James A. Lovell Federal Health Care Center. Presentation at the 2012 annual meeting of the Healthcare Information and Management Systems Society, New Orleans, Louisiana, February 23. http://69.59.162.218/HIMSS2012/Venetian%20Sands%20Expo%20Center/2.23.12_Thu/Marco%20Polo%20803/Thu_1300/157-11_Donna_Poulin_Marco%20Polo%20803/157MaldonadoPoulin.pdf (accessed August 7, 2012).

Opsut, R. 2011. Reconciling financial liability for the North Chicago Federal Health Care Center. Presentation by Dr. Robert Opsut, TRICARE Management Agency, DoD, to the IOM Committee on Evaluation of the Lovell Federal Health Care Center Merger, Washington, DC, February 25.

Poulin, D., C. Foster, and J. Nelson. 2012. Lovell Federal Health Care Center lessons learned. Presentation by LCDR Donna Poulin, LCDR Chuck Foster, and Mr. Joseph Nelson at the Tri-Service Medical Information Management Symposium 2012. http://cdn.govexec.com/media/gbc/docs/pdfs_edit/052112bb1.pdf (accessed August 7, 2012).

Robinson, A. M, Jr. 2009. Statement of Vice Admiral Adam M. Robinson, Jr., Surgeon General of the Navy, United States Navy. Transcript of Hearing on the Defense Health Program appropriations for FY 2010 held by the Senate Appropriations Defense Subcommittee, March 18. Washington, DC: U.S. Government Printing Office. http://www.gpo.gov/fdsys/pkg/CHRG-111shrg48290/pdf/CHRG-111shrg48290.pdf (accessed August 7, 2012).

Shinseki, E. 2009. Statement of Secretary of Veterans Affairs Eric K. Shinseki at Update on the State of the U.S. Department of Veterans Affairs. Hearing before the Committee on Veterans' Affairs, U.S. House of Representatives, October 14. http://www.gpo.gov/fdsys/pkg/CHRG-111hhrg53434/html/CHRG-111hhrg53434.htm (accessed September 7, 2012).

Susnjara, B. 2003. VA hospital's future gets a boost. *Daily Herald*, November 11. http://www.jsosolutions.com/archive/kirkforcongress/inthenews_DailyHerald111103.htm (accessed September 7, 2012).

U.S. House of Representatives. 2009. *Examining the progress of electronic health record interoperability between the U.S. Department of Veterans Affairs and U.S. Department of Defense.* Hearing before the Subcommittee on Oversight and Investigations of the Committee on Veterans' Affairs, July 14. Washington, DC: U.S. Government Printing Office. http://www.gpo.gov/fdsys/pkg/CHRG-111hhrg51872/pdf/CHRG-111hhrg51872.pdf (accessed August 7, 2012).

U.S. House of Representatives. 2010. *U.S. Department of Veterans Affairs Office of Inspector General and Office of Information Technology budget requests for fiscal year 2011.* Hearing before the Subcommittee on Oversight and Investigations, Committee on Veterans' Affairs, February 23. Washington, DC: U.S. Government Printing Office. http://fr webgate.access.gpo.gov/cgi-bin/getdoc.cgi?dbname=111_house_hearings&docid=f:55228.pdf (accessed August 7, 2012).

U.S. Navy. 2011. *Manual of Navy enlisted manpower and personnel classifications and occupational standards, Volume II, Navy enlisted classifications (NECs).* January. http://www.public.navy.mil/bupers-npc/enlisted/detailing/personnelreadiness/Documents/NECVol2.pdf (accessed August 7, 2012).

U.S. Senate. 2005. *Military construction and Veterans Affairs, and related agencies appropriations for fiscal year 2006.* Hearing before the Subcommittee on Military Construction and Veterans Affairs, and Related Agencies, Committee on Appropriations, March 8. Washington, DC: U.S. Government Printing Office. http://frwebgate.access.gpo.gov/cgi-bin/getdoc.cgi?dbname=109_senate_hearings&docid=f:99875.wais (accessed August 7, 2012).

VA (Department of Veterans Affairs). 2002. VA and DoD agree on health care in North Chicago. VA press release, October 18. http://www.va.gov/opa/pressrel/pressrelease.cfm?id=523 (accessed September 4, 2012).

VA. 2004. *Security and law enforcement.* VA handbook 0730/1. http://www1.va.gov/vapubs/viewPublication.asp?Pub_ID=96 (accessed August 7, 2012).

VA. 2010a. *FY 2011 congressional budget submission, Vol. II, medical programs & information technology programs.* http://www.va.gov/budget/docs/summary/archive/FY-2011_VA-BudgetSubmission.zip (accessed August 7, 2012).

VA. 2010b. *Security and law enforcement.* VA handbook 0730/2. http://www.va.gov/vapubs/viewPublication.asp?Pub_ID=488&FType=2 (accessed August 7, 2012).

VA/DoD. 2006a. *VA/DoD Joint Executive Council FY 2005 annual report.* http://www.tricare.mil/DVPCO/downloads/VADoD2005.pdf (accessed August 7, 2012).

VA/DoD. 2006b. *VA/DoD Health Executive Council executive decision memorandum, Second call for Joint Incentive Fund (JIF) projects.* http://www.tricare.mil/DVPCO/downloads/JIF-Projects-2006-2.pdf (accessed August 7, 2012).

VA/DoD. 2008a. *VA/DoD Joint Executive Council FY 2007 annual report.* http://www.tricare.mil/DVPCO/downloads/VA%20DoD%202007%20Annual%20Report%20FINAL%203-14-08.pdf (accessed August 7, 2012).

VA/DoD. 2008b. *VA/DoD Joint Executive Council FY 2008 annual report.* http://www.tricare.mil/DVPCO/downloads/VA%20DoD%20Joint%20Executive%20Council%20Annual%20Report.pdf (accessed August 7, 2012).

VA/DoD. 2009. *VA/DoD Joint Executive Council FY 2009 annual report.* http://prhome.defense.gov/docs/2009%20VA%20DoD%20Joint%20Executive%20Council%20Annual%20Report%20and%20Joint%20Strategic%20Plan.pdf (accessed August 7, 2012).

VA/DoD. 2011. *VA/DoD Joint Executive Council FY 2010 annual report.* http://www.tricare.mil/DVPCO/downloads/2010%20JEC%20Annual%20Report%20to%20Congress%20(signed).pdf (accessed August 7, 2012).

VA OIG (VA Office of the Inspector General). 2010. *Audit of the FLITE Strategic Asset Management Pilot Project.* #09-03861-238, September 14. http://www.va.gov/oig/52/reports/2010/VAOIG-09-03861-238.pdf (accessed August 15, 2012).

4

Initial Results of the Integration Demonstration

This chapter analyzes the initial results of the effort to merge the health care centers of the Navy and the Department of Veterans Affairs (VA) in North Chicago into a single integrated health care center that improves access, quality of care, and cost effectiveness; maintains military operational readiness; maintains patient and staff satisfaction; and improves research and training opportunities. Before examining data on these outcomes, however, the chapter documents the organizational results of the merger, especially the degree of integration achieved.

These are initial results because the Captain James A. Lovell Federal Health Care Center (FHCC) had been in operation only for a year and a half when this report was drafted and is still a work in progress. For example, the electronic health records (EHRs) of the Lovell FHCC beneficiaries are not yet fully integrated, which means that inefficient workarounds are required to ensure patient safety, let alone deliver improved care through better coordination. In addition, the bulk of the effort to launch the Lovell FHCC was spent planning and implementing the basic administrative systems necessary to operate the new organization, such as payroll, accounting, computer access, and credentialing. The leadership of the Lovell FHCC plans to focus more attention in the next several years on opportunities to better integrate clinical services (Interviews).

DEGREE OF INTEGRATION

Although the term "integration" has been widely used to describe the consolidation of the North Chicago VA Medical Center (NCVAMC) and the Naval Hospital Great Lakes (NHGL), it was never formally defined. Dictionary definitions of integration range from the process of joining entities together[1] to the process of blending into a functioning whole.[2] These definitions could apply to very different situations, for example, the simple collocation of DoD and VA clinics in the same building that share a laboratory versus a more ambitious unification of like clinics that are jointly staffed and serve both Department of Defense (DoD) and VA beneficiaries. According to the Lovell FHCC's concept of operations, the planning assumptions supported the more expansive concept of integration. The assumptions included the following:

- There is total integration—a single chain of command exists with single departments.
- There are unified operating systems whenever possible.
- There is one standard of care.
- There is a single medical staff.
- There is seamless transition from active duty to veteran status.
- The two organizational cultures must blend into one.
- The integrated facility has flexibility to adjust staffing based upon mission requirements (Lovell FHCC, 2010a, p. 15).

Although the vision of the FHCC planners was total organizational integration, including single operating systems, blended staff, and seamless care delivery regardless of beneficiary status, the implementation history in North Chicago reveals the limits to and the costs of integration, as well as some of the beneficial outcomes that might be realized from the creation of the FHCC. The limits pertain to differences between the beneficiary populations in terms of health needs and eligibility; differences in the departments' missions in North Chicago (i.e., preparing recruits for deployment versus meeting the health needs of veterans); the limited ability of the two EHR systems to interface to allow an integrated patient record; and the need to continue to meet different standards and reporting requirements of the agencies (the VA, the Navy, and the DoD). The costs pertain to the extra time it takes to meet the requirements of two reporting chains; the duplication of functions that could not be unified; and the need to develop and maintain interoperability capabilities between separate systems (e.g., EHR systems, accounting systems, credentialing systems, drug formularies). The

[1] "1. To make a whole by bringing all parts together; unify; 2a. To join with something else; unite; 2b. To make part of a larger unit" (*American Heritage College Dictionary*, 3rd ed., Boston, MA, Houghton Mifflin, 1997).

[2] "To form, coordinate, or blend into a functioning or unified whole: unite" (*Webster's Ninth New Collegiate Dictionary*, Springfield, MA, Merriam-Webster Inc., 1987).

benefits were expected to be increased access to care (in terms of a greater range of services for both DoD and VA beneficiaries); better quality of care (in terms of coordination and continuity of care and access to a greater range of specialties for consultation and referral); lower operating costs (because of reduced duplication of both administrative and clinical functions and economies of scale); greater patient and staff satisfaction; and more research and training opportunities.

In this section of the chapter, the extent of integration—defined as the blending of previously separate entities into a cohesive whole—is explored. The degree of integration will be analyzed along three dimensions: (1) functional integration, (2) physician integration, and (3) clinical integration.

- *Functional integration* is "the extent to which key support functions and activities (such as financial management, human resources, strategic planning, information management, marketing, and quality improvement) are coordinated across operating units so as to add the greatest overall value to the system" (Shortell et al., 2000, p. 31).
- *Physician integration* is "the extent to which physicians and the organized delivery systems with which they are associated agree on the aims and purposes of the system and work together to achieve mutually shared objectives" (Shortell et al., 2000, p. 67).
- *Clinical integration* is "the extent to which patient care services are coordinated across people, functions, activities, and sites over time so as to maximize the value of services delivered to patients" (Shortell et al., 2000, p. 129).

Functional Integration

Administrative services are combined and integrated to some extent at the Lovell FHCC, although the need to adhere to the different business rules and procedures of the DoD and the VA requires a certain amount of duplication and limits the realization of optimal operating efficiencies. In addition, some services, or product lines, are provided at the regional or the national level by one department or the other. For example, human resources (HR) services for the NCVAMC were provided by the Veterans Integrated Service Network (VISN) 12. In that case, the FHCC was able to establish an integrated local HR office. In other cases, integration was not possible. For example, the DoD has a national contract to provide appointment call center services at the military treatment facilities (MTFs), which means that there are separate call centers at the FHCC for DoD and VA beneficiaries. In any case, under the terms of the National Defense Authorization Act of 2010 (NDAA 2010), the FHCC cannot cut staff, even though efficiencies from the integration might require fewer staff. In addition, the FHCC has not been under pressure initially to reduce costs because it is receiving the same funding—with inflation adjustments—that it did before the integration during the first several years of operation.

In early September 2009, more than a year in advance of the launching of the FHCC, the communication staffs of the Naval Health Clinic Great Lakes (NHCGL) and the NCVAMC were functionally integrated in a single Department of Communications and Public Affairs. The department was charged with meeting Navy, VA, and Lovell FHCC communication needs and designing and implementing a single, comprehensive communication plan to address the concerns of all the stakeholders (VA, 2010a). In October 2009, education and training programs were functionally integrated in a single Department of Education and Training (Fouse and Faber, 2011). In October 2010, the remaining administrative offices were combined under the Resource Directorate (Offices of HR, Financial Management, Information Resources Management, and Information Security) and the Facility Support Directorate (Offices of Communications and Public Affairs, Managed Care Operations, Protective Services, Patient Administration, Facilities Management, and Logistics). There is a single Office of Performance Improvement in the executive office. The intent was for the operations within these offices to be integrated, that is, to have one set of policies and procedures for the entire FHCC. However, as is documented in Chapter 3, the degree to which integration is possible has been circumscribed by differences in policies and procedures between the parent departments to which the FHCC must continue to adhere. For example, the departments could not agree to have one of the two inspectors general conduct inspections on behalf of both departments, so the Office of Performance Improvement must manage two inspection processes. Although there is a single HR office, there are separate units for VA and DoD personnel.

Physician Integration

The clinical task group recommended from the start that Navy active duty and VA physicians be unified through the development of a single set of medical staff bylaws and organization into single departments under a single chief medical executive. It became evident, however, that it made sense to create a separate organization for dental services because of the volume of dental work and the size of the dental staff, which also conforms to the Navy practice of having separate medical and dental commands. There is a single head of the dental directorate, a Navy captain, with a civilian VA deputy. Most of the dental services are provided at the United States ship (USS) Weeden Osborne Dental Clinic, a branch health clinic on the Navy base, because nearly 75 percent of the recruits require dental work to become operationally ready for deployment (VA, 2010b). Of the 644,700 dental visits during the first year of the FHCC, 5,700 (less than 1 percent) were by veterans at the dental clinic on the west campus; the rest were at the east campus branch health clinics.

Although the clinical staffs were not officially combined until October 1, 2010, the chief medical officers of the NCVAMC and the NHCGL were already fully engaged in merging the medical staffs, a goal that they strongly supported. The merger of inpatient services in 2006 had some active duty and VA clinicians working together in advance of moving all the active duty clinicians to the west campus (Interviews). The NCVAMC and the NHCGL executive committees of nursing services began meeting jointly in May 2010 (Fouse and Faber, 2011).

Clinical Integration

Acute Inpatient Mental Health Services

The first major step toward creating an FHCC in North Chicago was to have the NCVAMC provide acute mental health services to DoD as well as to VA beneficiaries. The first DoD beneficiaries were admitted in October 2003 under a resource sharing agreement in which VA providers treated Navy mental health patients in the NCVAMC acute mental health inpatient unit and, in return, the Navy paid for the services and provided several psychiatric support staff. The NHGL was able to close its inpatient psychiatric unit and reduce overall staffing.

The NCVAMC continued to provide acute inpatient mental health services to Navy recruits and to other DoD beneficiaries on a reimbursement basis until the Department of the Treasury (Treasury) fund for the FHCC became operational in 2011. The arrangement—for example, VA providers treating VA and DoD beneficiaries—continues, although it is now paid for seamlessly from the joint Treasury fund. Beginning in fiscal year (FY) 2013, a behind-the-scenes reconciliation process will allocate costs between the VA and the DoD in proportion to their respective workloads.

Inpatient Medical, Surgical, and Pediatric Services

The next step in the integration process was to centralize all inpatient medical and surgical services for adults and children at the NCVAMC. In this case, the range of services available to VA beneficiaries was expanded because the NCVAMC did not offer inpatient surgery, only some types of outpatient surgery. Previously, VA patients needing inpatient surgery had to be referred to other area VA facilities or to community hospitals. In addition, VA and Navy inpatient beneficiaries benefit from the availability of consultations with a broader range of specialists than would have been available if the Navy had built a separate hospital.

In June 2006, after four existing operating rooms were renovated and four new operating rooms with recovery beds were constructed in a vacant ward, the NHGL closed its 22 inpatient beds and became the NHCGL (VA/DoD, 2007). Under a resource sharing agreement, DoD beneficiaries needing inpatient medical, surgical, or pediatric care were admitted to the NCVAMC (obstetrical cases are still referred to the community). VA nurses and technicians staffed and operated the nursing units, but Navy physicians who admitted patients could follow them and Navy surgeons could operate on veterans as well as on DoD beneficiaries. The NCVAMC was reimbursed as a TRICARE network provider. Because the NCVAMC was not an MTF, however, DoD beneficiaries were subject to copayments that they did not have to pay to receive services at the NHGL.

Surgical services were essentially integrated before the FHCC came into being formally on October 1, 2010, but on that date a single line of authority, with a single head of the department of surgery under a single chief medical executive, was formally established. The funding arrangement also changed. All inpatient services—mental health, general medical, surgical, and pediatric—are funded by the joint Treasury fund, and beginning in FY 2013, a reconciliation process will allocate costs between the VA and the DoD in proportion to their respective workloads. In addition, as part of the 5-year demonstration project, DoD beneficiaries are not being charged for copayments, just as if they were going to an MTF.

The surgical services offered at the FHCC currently are general surgery, dermatology, otolaryngology, gynecology (women's health), ophthalmology, orthopedics, podiatry, and urology (Lovell FHCC, 2012b). Physicians are both active duty servicemembers and VA civilians, and in many cases they treat both VA and DoD beneficiaries.

Emergency and Urgent Care Services

The NCVAMC emergency department (ED) was renovated and expanded from a 6-bed open floor plan to a 15-private-room configuration at the same time as the new surgical suites were constructed. In October 2006, all emergency services for DoD beneficiaries were transferred to the NCVAMC, and the NHGL (now the NHCGL), closed its ED. DoD beneficiaries benefited from having access to an ED staffed by board-certified emergency physicians in place of the internists who staffed the NHGL ED. Like DoD inpatients, they also had access to consultations from a greater range of specialties. VA beneficiaries benefited from having access to an expanded and more up-to-date ED, including privacy and gender-specific considerations for female patients. Originally, emergency/urgent care services for DoD beneficiaries were reimbursed to the NCVAMC as a TRICARE network provider. Currently, services for both DoD and VA beneficiaries are paid for from the joint Treasury fund and the costs will be allocated between the departments through the reconciliation process.

Women's Health Clinic

A new Women's Health Center was built as part of the ambulatory care center (ACC). This clinic was designed to serve both women veterans and DoD beneficiaries. The center provides comprehensive primary care and gender-specific services in a separate, self-contained clinic space to provide an environment that is secure and supportive. Using Joint Incentive Fund (JIF) monies, the VA hired gynecology staff (replacing a lost Navy physician billet); purchased digital mammography equipment and gender-specific equipment, such as a stereotactic biopsy device and a culposcopy unit; and hired two wellness/case management nurses. Without the combined veteran and military beneficiary populations, the VA would not have had the critical volume to support onsite mammography services or been able to maintain accreditation.

Dental Services

Tentative plans to combine the dental clinic for Navy staff at the NHGL (Building 200H) with the VA dental clinic on the west campus were abandoned when the square footage of the ACC was cut in half. Instead, the Navy dental clinic was moved to the Zachary and Elizabeth Fisher Medical and Dental Clinic on the east campus, which also provides medical care to active duty staff. There is no sharing of services, although the VA clinic does not have specialists such as endodontists and periodontists who are part of the staff at the USS Osborne. This is because the dentists at the USS Osborne are already booked to capacity to ensure that the recruits are ready for deployment.

Ancillary Services

In 2003, rather than renovate and expand its blood donor center to accommodate increasing volume, the NHGL agreed to renovate unused space in the NCVAMC for a new blood donor center. Renovating space in the NCVAMC saved $3 million in new construction costs. In lieu of paying for rent and utilities, the NHGL agreed to provide the NCVAMC approximately 415 units of blood products annually, worth approximately $47,000, or the equivalent of $14 per square foot (Harnly, 2005).

Other ancillary services, such as laboratory and radiology, were centralized as part of the move into the ACC that began in December 2010.

Outpatient Services

After inpatient and emergency services were consolidated at the NCVAMC in 2006, the renamed NHCGL continued to provide outpatient services for DoD beneficiaries at the former hospital building until December 2010, when the clinics were moved to the new ACC.

Discussion

Initially, the Navy was going to build the ACC for its beneficiaries and the VA was going to continue to provide outpatient services to veterans from its existing facilities (VA/DoD, 2002). Soon, however, the concept of integrating at least some outpatient services or clinics was adopted, in which both VA and DoD beneficiaries would be treated by either VA or Navy providers, depending on who was available. It was recognized that some services were unique to each department and should not be integrated. For example, the NCVAMC had long-term residential programs for veterans, such as the nursing home, the domiciliary, and residential rehabilitation treatment programs, which were not available to DoD beneficiaries. It was also agreed that the NCVAMC would staff and operate the inpatient mental health unit; the inpatient medical, surgical, and pediatric nursing units; and the ED. The Navy, for its part, had clinics in place on its base to medically process in and provide efficient health care for a large volume of enlisted recruits and students, and it did not make sense to move or to integrate them, except for ancillary services. It also did not make sense to create a joint pediatric clinic because the VA does not have pediatric beneficiaries.

Prior to the integration of outpatient services in late 2010 and early 2011, the NHCGL offered 20 outpatient medical clinics in 200H and the NCVAMC offered 24 medical specialties and subspecialties (Table 4-1) that were candidates for clinical integration. Although the consistent vision of local leaders was to unify clinical as well as administrative staff—to "allow a patient who could be a veteran, active duty servicemember, or family member to be treated by a Navy surgeon, a VA nurse, and a Navy technician" (DoD/VA, 2008)—pragmatic considerations dictated different degrees of staff and clinic integration in outpatient services. One factor was the reduced size of the ACC, which necessitated greater use of space in the VA hospital building (Interviews). Plans to integrate primary care services and dental clinics were changed because it no longer made sense to move or expand the existing VA primary care and dental clinics to serve both populations (Interviews). Instead, the Navy has a separate primary care

TABLE 4-1 Projected Fiscal Year 2011 Lovell Federal Health Care Center Full-Time-Equivalent Clinical Providers by Specialty (North Chicago Veterans Affairs Medical Center)/Clinic (Naval Health Clinic Great Lakes)

Specialty/Clinic	NCVAMC	NHCGL
Audiology	6.09	1.00
Cardiology	1.40	0.95
Dermatology	0.13	1.90
Endocrinology	1.97	
Family Practice		6.00
Gastroenterology	3.63	
General Surgery	2.11	2.90
Gynecology	1.05	2.00
Immunizations		1.00
Infectious Disease	0.23	
Internal Medicine	19.15	5.95
Mental Health Clinic	49.01	11.00
Nephrology	0.70	
Neurology	2.64	0.50
Occupational Therapy	0.98	
Oncology	0.89	
Ophthalmology	1.40	1.00
Optometry	1.88	1.00
Orthopedic	3.15	3.90
Otolaryngology	0.55	1.90
Outpatient Nutrition		2.00
Pediatric		3.89
Physical Therapy	5.95	8.00
Podiatry	1.43	2.00
Primary Care Employee Health	1.00	
Pulmonary Disease	2.50	
Rheumatology	1.00	
Substance Abuse		3.00
Urology	1.10	0.90
Total	109.94	60.79

NOTE: This table pertains to the clinical personnel (e.g., physicians, psychologists, podiatrists, audiologists, nutritionists, and physical and occupational therapists) at the NHCGL's 200H facility who moved to the ambulatory care center on the west campus, not the clinical personnel in the branch health clinics who remained on the east campus (i.e., at Naval Station Great Lakes) or Veterans Administration personnel providing veteran-only services (e.g., long-term care, domiciliary care, and residential rehabilitation). It also does not include inpatient and emergency room providers. NCVAMC = North Chicago Veterans Affairs Medical Center; NHGL = Naval Hospital Great Lakes.
SOURCE: Lovell FHCC, 2010b.

clinic in the new ACC building, and all dental services for DoD beneficiaries remained on the east campus. Another factor was the provision in the executive agreement (EA) that VA providers can be seen by DoD providers, and vice versa, only if there is excess capacity. At the time of the integration of outpatient services, only dermatology and otolaryngology had excess capacity and were fully integrated in terms of staff and patients for regular scheduling purposes; other clinical services were shared on an ad hoc basis when there were openings.

The plan that evolved and was eventually implemented resulted in a variety of organizational arrangements for outpatient services. As mentioned already, some of the health delivery sites on the Navy base continued to do what they did before, the main difference being that the Navy civilians working there became VA employees and administrative and some clinical support services (e.g., laboratory) were centralized. These branch health clinics include the USS Red Rover, which screens recruits for medical and dental problems as they arrive and provides immunizations, eyeglasses, and women's health services; the USS Weeden Osborne, which provides dental services to recruits, a large percentage of whom have dental deficiencies; the USS Tranquility, which provides medical services to recruits and active duty members of the Recruit Training Command (RTC) staff; and the Fisher Clinic, which provides primary medical and dental care to the active duty staff at the Naval Station Great Lakes (NSGL).

As already noted, the primary care clinics remain separate and are staffed separately by DoD and VA providers. In the DoD primary care clinic (and the pediatric clinic), DoD providers treat DoD beneficiaries and use the Armed Forces Health Longitudinal Technology Application (AHLTA) to document visits while VA providers treat veterans and use the Veterans Health Information Systems and Technology Architecture (VistA). Having the DoD primary care clinic use AHLTA ensured that information affecting deployability, such as immunizations, would be available immediately, especially if the interoperability solutions under development were not operational when the FHCC became operational. The existing VA primary care clinic was little affected because providers did not need to access or document information in AHLTA except for dual eligible retirees. DoD providers treating dual eligible beneficiaries could view their VA health records through the Bi-directional Health Information Exchange, although this is a time-consuming process and is not always done (Interviews).

The women's clinic has both DoD and VA providers, but DoD providers treat DoD beneficiaries and use AHLTA while VA providers treat veterans and use VistA. The women's clinic is integrated in another way, however, because it also provides primary care and onsite radiology.

In addition to space considerations, the different policies concerning outpatient scheduling and standards of the VA and the Bureau of Medicine and Surgery (BUMED) also support having separate primary care clinics. For example, the VA requires an appointment within 7 days, and BUMED requires one within 14 days.

Many VA clinicians were part-time (see Table 4-1) at the NCVAMC, available only several times a week. The Navy had a full-time gynecologist, orthopedist, otolaryngologist, dermatologist, and urologist. Although only dermatology and otolaryngology are formally integrated, DoD beneficiaries are seen by VA specialty providers and vice versa on a space-available basis. DoD beneficiaries therefore benefit from access to VA providers with specialties not present among Navy providers, including pulmonary critical care, infectious diseases, gastroenterology, nephrology, endocrinology, rheumatology, and hematology/oncology (Table 4-1). Veterans benefit from the access provided by the expanded clinical staffing. Navy inpatients and ED users also benefit from access to consultations from VA specialists (Interviews).

The pharmacy was designed to be integrated, where the DoD and the VA pharmacists could fill prescriptions for both TRICARE enrollees and veterans. This arrangement was dependent on an orders portability solution for pharmacy, which was not ready for use when the ACC opened and will not be ready until FY 2014, at the earliest. Instead, DoD pharmacists mostly serve TRICARE beneficiaries, using the DoD's AHLTA, while the VA pharmacists mostly serve veterans, using the VA's VistA.

Similarly, the efficiency of combining specialty clinics in the ACC on the west campus has been reduced by lack of interoperability between the two EHR systems. The plan was for clinical notes and information about laboratory tests, radiology, and prescriptions for recruits and other TRICARE enrollees seen in the ED and specialty clinics to be entered into VistA and for the information to be automatically populated in AHLTA. Quick, if not instant, entry into AHLTA is required because active duty servicemembers may be transferred on short notice and must take complete medical records with them. The information also might affect whether they are considered to be medically ready to be deployed. These capabilities were not ready for use when the ACC opened, necessitating the use of manual workarounds to duplicate the information entered into VistA into AHLTA, which has significantly affected productivity because of the increased paperwork load.

Conclusions Concerning Degree of Integration

The final organization of the FHCC displays various degrees of integration across services (see Table 4-2). Some services are VA only, such as long-term care and domiciliary, which only veterans can receive. Some are Navy only, such as the branch health clinics on the east campus that serve only active duty servicemembers. Inpatient mental health, medicine,

TABLE 4-2 Clinical Integration Status of the Lovell Federal Health Care Center

Directorate	Department	Division	Clinical Section
Patient Care			
	Medicine		
		Inpatient Acute/Intensive Care Unit	
		Emergency	
		Medical Specialties	
			Cardiology
			Dermatology
			Endocrinology
			Gastroenterology
			Hematology/Oncology
			Infectious Disease
			Nephrology
			Neurology
			Pulmonology
			Rheumatology
	Ambulatory Medical Care		
		Primary Care	
			Family Practice
			Internal Medicine
			Pediatrics
			Veterans' Primary Care
		Special Medical Exams	
			DoD Specialty Exams
			VA Specialty Exams
	Surgery		
		Perioperative	
			Anesthesia
			Operating Room
		Surgical Subspecialties	
			General Surgery
			Gynecology/Women's Health
			Ophthalmology
			Optometry
			Orthopedics
			Otolaryngology
			Podiatry
			Urology
	Mental Health		
		Acute Inpatient	
		Outpatient/Consultation Services	
			Consultation Liaison
			Mental Health/Life Skills

Affiliation of Head	Campus	Patients (VA, DoD, or Both)	Clinical Providers (VA, DoD, or Both)	EHR System
VA				
VA				
VA	West	Both	Both	VistA
VA	West	Both	VA	VistA
DoD				
VA	West	Both	Both	VistA
DoD	West	Both	Both	VistA
VA	West	Both	VA	VistA
VA	West	Both	VA	VistA
VA	West	Both	VA	VistA
VA	West	Both	VA	VistA
VA	West	Both	VA	VistA
VA	West	Both	VA	VistA
VA	West	Both	VA	VistA
VA	West	Both	VA	VistA
DoD				
DoD				
DoD	West	DoD	Both	AHLTA
DoD	West	DoD	Both	AHLTA
DoD	West	DoD	Both	AHLTA
VA	West	VA	VA	VistA
DoD				
DoD	West	DoD	Both	AHLTA
VA	West	Both	Both	VistA
VA				
VA				
VA	West	Both	VA	VistA
VA	West	Both	Both	VistA
DoD				
DoD	West	Both	Both	VistA
DoD	West	Both	Both	Both
VA	West	Both	Both	Both
DoD	West	Both	Both	VistA
DoD	West	Both	Both	VistA
DoD	West	Both	Both	VistA
VA	West	Both	Both	VistA
DoD	West	Both	Both	VistA
VA				
VA	West	Both	VA	VistA
DoD				
VA	West	Both	VA	VistA
DoD	Both	Both	Both	Both

continued

TABLE 4-2 Continued

Directorate	Department	Division	Clinical Section
			Mental Health Case Management
			Psychosocial Rehabilitation and Recovery Center
		Special Programs	
			Homeless
			Posttraumatic Stress Disorder
			Substance Abuse Rehabilitation Program/Addiction Treatment Program
			Vocational Rehabilitation
Patient Services			
	Ancillary Services		
		Audiology and Speech Pathology	
		Nutrition and Food Services	
		Pastoral Services	
		Pharmacy	
		Prosthetics	
	Rehabilitation		
		Kinesiotherapy	
		Occupational Therapy	
		Physiatry/Electromyography	
		Physical Therapy	
	Geriatrics and Extended Care		
		Community Living	
		Geriatric Medicine	
		Home and Community-Based Care	
	Diagnostic Services		
		Blood Donor Processing	
		Imaging and Radiation Safety	
		Pathology and Laboratory	
	Education and Training		
		Clinical Education	
		Employee/Military Education	
Dental			
	Dental Services		
		General Dentistry	
	USS Osborne		
	USS Red Rover		
	Fisher Clinic		
	Dental Prosthetic Care		

Affiliation of Head	Campus	Patients (VA, DoD, or Both)	Clinical Providers (VA, DoD, or Both)	EHR System
VA	West	VA	VA	VistA
VA	West	VA	VA	VistA
VA				
VA	West	VA	VA	VistA
VA	West	VA	VA	VistA
DoD	West	Both	Both	Both
VA	West	VA	VA	VistA
VA				
VA				
VA	West	Both	Both	VistA
VA	West	Both	VA	VistA
VA	West	Both	Both	VistA
DoD	West	Both	Both	Both
VA	West	Both	VA	VistA
VA				
VA	West	Both	VA	VistA
VA	West	Both	VA	VistA
VA	West	Both	VA	VistA
DoD	West	Both	Both	VistA
VA				
VA	West	Both	VA	VistA
VA	West	Both	VA	VistA
VA	West	VA	VA	VistA
DoD				
DoD	West	Both	DoD	DBSS
VA	Both	Both	Both	Both
VA	Both	Both	Both	VistA/CoPath
DoD				
VA	West	Both	Both	NA
DoD	West	NA	Both	NA
DoD				
DoD				
VA	West	VA	VA	VistA
DoD	East	DoD	DoD	AHLTA
DoD	East	DoD	DoD	AHLTA
DoD	East	DoD	DoD	AHLTA
DoD	East	DoD	DoD	AHLTA

continued

TABLE 4-2 Continued

Directorate	Department	Division	Clinical Section
Fleet Medicine			
	Fisher Clinic		
		Primary Care	
			Optometry
			Sick Call
		Administration	
			Active Duty Specialty Examinations/ Overseas Screening
			Medical Liaison
			Periodic Health Assessments/ Physical Examinations
			Records
	USS Tranquility		
		Primary Care	
			Recruit Primary Care
			Special Physicals
			Staff Primary Care
		Preventive Medicine	
		Recruit Evaluation Unit	
		SMART (Sports Medicine and Rehabilitation Therapy)	
	USS Red Rover		
			Audiology
			Immunizations
			Medical Assessment
			Optometry
			Women's Health
	Occupational Health and Medicine		
		Occupational Medicine	
			Hearing Conservation B237
			Immunizations 133EF
			Immunizations B237
			Occupational Health East B237
			Occupational Health West B133CA
		Preventive Medicine	
			Preventive Medicine B1007
			Preventive Medicine B237

NOTES: DBSS = Defense Blood Standard System; CoPath is an anatomic pathology system used by the Military Health System.
SOURCE: Information provided by the Lovell FHCC to the IOM committee.

Affiliation of Head	Campus	Patients (VA, DoD, or Both)	Clinical Providers (VA, DoD, or Both)	EHR System
DoD				
DoD				
DoD				
DoD	East	DoD	DoD	AHLTA
DoD	East	DoD	Both	AHLTA
DoD				
DoD	East	DoD	NA	AHLTA
DoD	East	DoD	NA	AHLTA
DoD	East	DoD	NA	AHLTA
DoD	East	DoD	NA	AHLTA
DoD				
DoD				
DoD	East	DoD	DoD	AHLTA
DoD	East	DoD	DoD	AHLTA
DoD	East	DoD	DoD	AHLTA
DoD	East	DoD	DoD	AHLTA
DoD	East	DoD	DoD	AHLTA
DoD	East	DoD	DoD	AHLTA
DoD				
DoD	East	DoD	DoD	AHLTA
DoD	East	DoD	DoD	AHLTA
DoD	East	DoD	DoD	AHLTA
DoD	East	DoD	DoD	AHLTA
DoD	East	DoD	DoD	AHLTA
VA				
DoD				
DoD	East	Both	Both	AHLTA
DoD	East	DoD	Both	AHLTA
DoD	East	DoD	Both	AHLTA
DoD	East	DoD	Both	AHLTA
DoD	West	VA	Both	VistA
DoD				
DoD	West	DoD	Both	AHLTA
DoD	East	DoD	Both	AHLTA

surgery, and emergency services are integrated, although Navy surgeons generally operate on DoD beneficiaries and VA surgeons on veterans. The main problem is the lack of EHR system interoperability, which requires manual workarounds to enter treatment information entered into VistA into AHLTA, which has reduced productivity.

For several reasons (discussed above), primary care services are separate. Specialty clinics are integrated to the extent that they have excess capacity; that is, there are not enough VA patients to fill the time of the VA providers or enough DoD patients to fill the time of the DoD providers. Only dermatology and otolaryngology routinely schedule patients regardless of the department affiliation of the beneficiary or who employs the provider.

Lack of interoperable EHR systems has significantly hindered the capacity to deliver integrated care, and the workarounds required to integrate patient information have reduced productivity. The lack of a joint or an interoperable EHR system that supports seamless clinical workflow for both VA and DoD beneficiaries is the largest contributor to the Lovell FHCC's inability to operate combined ACCs and to gain the full benefit of an integrated medical staff.

The composition and scope of outpatient clinics and provider specialties was primarily shaped by the existing staffing of the NHCGL and the NCVAMC. These were rationalized into a unified structure as much as possible, but the current organization is probably not ideally designed or sized to meet the current demand for health care services. Lovell FHCC leaders plan to integrate clinical services fully but decided to delay implementation until an interoperable EHR system is available and after completing an assessment of the changing clinical demand.

Theoretically, the merger of a VA and a military center should result in efficiencies, administrative and possibly clinical. The Lovell FHCC experience provides some insights into why the observed efficiencies will be less than expected. First, Congress placed restrictions on the degree of and legislatively mandated policies that limit efficiencies, such as the extent of staff reductions that can be achieved. Second, both departments have required the Lovell FHCC to maintain duplicative systems, business rules, standards, and reporting requirements, creating a fair degree of redundancy, administrative overhead, and duplication of effort. Third, the VA/DoD Health Resources Sharing and Emergency Operation Act of 1982 only allows the sharing of services when a facility has excess capacity, even though it may be more productive overall to combine fully utilized services.[3]

[3] According to the act, providing health care for the other department's beneficiaries may not "adversely affect the range of services, the quality of care, or the established priorities for care provided to the primary beneficiaries of the providing department."

Funding from the VA/DoD Joint Incentive Program, known as JIF awards, has played an important role in extending the range of services that could be provided by the Lovell FHCC. The JIF grants funded the start-up and initial operating costs for 2 years of services that did not exist at either the NHCGL or the NCVAMC. During the pre-2010 joint venture phase, the centers received eight grants totaling nearly $8.5 million (see Box 3-1 for brief descriptions). In addition, $111 million was provided to the VA and the DoD enterprise information technology (IT) programs to identify and fund the development of software that would enable critical information entered in one EHR system to be viewed and manipulated in the other EHR system, although, as documented in Chapter 3, most of the software was not ready for use when the FHCC began operations in late 2010 and early 2011.

The JIF program was also used to meet the emergency need for a pharmacy workaround when the interoperability capability for preventing negative drug interactions and allergic reactions was not ready for use at the time the ACC was activated. The JIF program was the only way for the DoD and the VA to jointly fund health care until the Treasury account for the Lovell FHCC was established in 2011. The award, which was supposed to be a 1-year stopgap, is being extended at $1 million a year until the joint pharmacy capability is developed as part of the VA/DoD integrated EHR initiative, currently scheduled to be ready in FY 2014.

In sum, the example of the Lovell FHCC demonstrates that it is possible to merge an MTF and a VA medical center (VAMC) into a single organization, although, as Chapter 3 documents, it was a lengthy and costly process. The start-up costs were substantial, including hundreds of meetings at all levels of the DoD (the Navy and the Office of Health Affairs) and the VA; almost $10 million in direct JIF awards; more than $100 million worth of IT software development to make the two EHR systems work together (a partial success); and $13 million to upgrade the NCVAMC's surgical facilities. Future FHCCs might be able to avoid some of these costs by adopting the solutions developed at the Lovell FHCC or, where solutions were suboptimal or failed, spend their time and resources finding other solutions.

The Lovell FHCC example also shows that there are serious limits on the extent to which such a joint health care center can be unified internally if it has to perform as an MTF for DoD purposes and as a VAMC for VA purposes. This in turn constrains the extent to which the Lovell FHCC can provide coordinated care to patients or increase efficiencies through running one instead of duplicate programs and administrative systems. To the extent that problems developing EHR interoperability software at the Lovell FHCC motivated the department secretaries of the DoD and the VA to decide to develop a single, joint EHR system, the Lovell FHCC merger experience will have eliminated a critical obstacle to VA/DoD health services integration.

PERFORMANCE MEASURES

The April 2010 EA establishing the Lovell FHCC addressed the 12 areas of agreement that the NDAA 2010 required. One of the 12 agreement areas was performance benchmarks. The DoD and the VA agreed on 15 benchmarks and how to measure their attainment in what is called the Integration Scorecard.

Integration Scorecard

The 15 benchmark measures are

1. Patient satisfaction measures meet VA and DoD benchmarks
2. Maintenance of military medical readiness
3. Stakeholders Advisory Council determination that the FHCC meets both DoD and VA missions
4. Successful annual Comptroller General review
5. Validation of fiscal reconciliation by annual independent audit
6. VA clinical and administrative performance measures exceed mean for all VA medical centers
7. Meet all access to care standards
8. Evidence-based health care measures meet or exceed the VA and DoD mean
9. Satisfactory clinical and facility inspection outcomes from external oversight/accreditation groups
10. Officer promotion/retention and enlisted advancement/retention meet or exceed Navy mean
11. Information Management/Information Technology (IM/IT) implementation timeline met and no impact on patient safety
12. Staff satisfaction and other appropriate measures identified VA and DoD as benchmarks
13. Relative value unit (or RVU)/relative weighted product (or RWP)/ dental weighted value (or DWV) production meets business plan targets
14. Maintain pre-FHCC academic and clinical research missions
15. Trainee satisfaction as measured by the Learner Perception Survey

Each of the benchmarks is based on one or more measures. For example, patient satisfaction is derived from two measures, one from a VA survey of patients, the other from a DoD survey of patients. In total, there are 37 measures for the 15 benchmarks. Each measure is reported on a 5-point scale according to a 117-page technical manual. The scale ranges from highly successful (5), to very successful (4), successful (3), unsuccessful (2), and highly unsuccessful (1).

Most of the integration benchmark results are updated monthly. Some, such as the annual audit reports and facility inspection results, are updated less often.

As of June 2012, most scores had stayed the same as they were at baseline: for example, there were 23 fives (highly successful) compared with 19 at baseline; 5 fours (very successful) compared with 7 at baseline; 6 threes (successful) compared with 6 at baseline; 1 two (unsuccessful) compared with 2 at baseline; and 1 one (highly unsuccessful) compared with a 0 at baseline (one measure, officer retention, did not have a baseline score). The scores for some measures have varied, but rarely more than one point up or down or for more than 1 or 2 months.

Two measures scored a one or a two in June 2012, which are less than successful scores: (1) the DoD component of evidence-based health care and (2) IM/IT implementation. The failure to achieve evidence-based health care goals is attributed to vacancies in the active duty provider workforce due to rotation and deployment. The delay in IM/IT has been documented in Chapter 3 of this report as well as in Government Accountability Office (GAO) reports (see below).

Most of the performance measures are specific to the VA or to the DoD rather than to the integrated performance of the FHCC, because the main purpose of the performance benchmarks was to address the concerns of the respective departments that the Lovell FHCC experiment might fail badly before the end of the 5-year demonstration period (Interviews). Also, one measure that is critical to integration—that is, the implementation of joint IM/IT capabilities—has not been successful, as noted in Chapter 3, and is unlikely to improve further until parts of the new EHR system being developed jointly by the DoD and the VA become available, beginning with a joint pharmacy program scheduled to be operational in 2014.

Integration Areas

Integration benchmarks was 1 of the 12 integration areas identified in the April 2010 EA, in accordance with the requirements of the NDAA 2011. The 12 areas that had to be addressed in the EA were

1. Governance structure
2. Patient priority system
3. Fiscal authority
4. Workforce management

5. Property
6. Contingency planning
7. Quality assurance
8. IM/IT
9. Research
10. Integration benchmarks
11. Reporting requirements
12. Contracting

The committee was not asked to report on progress in the 12 integration areas, but the NDAA 2010 directed the GAO to do so annually. In its latest report, issued in June 2012, the GAO found that 6 of the 12 were fully implemented (governance structure, patient priority system, contracting, research, quality assurance, and contingency planning), compared with 4 in 2011. Integration benchmarks was one of the 5 areas "in progress" (the others were reporting requirements, workforce management, property, and fiscal authority). The GAO found that one area—IM/IT—was delayed, requiring workarounds that were resulting in additional costs for the Lovell FHCC in terms of reduced provider productivity and increased administrative burden. The GAO found, as did this committee, that the FHCC has not quantified the extra costs, but that it has engaged the Center for Naval Analyses to assess costs and document any savings from integrated patient care (GAO, 2012).

OUTCOMES

The goals of the Lovell FHCC leadership, taken from the April 2010 EA, are to "improve access, quality, and cost effectiveness of health care delivery for the beneficiaries" of both the DoD and the VA (DoD/VA, 2010, pp. 1–2). The EA says that the FHCC should also promote "operational readiness, continued employee benefits, continued education of health care professional trainees, and approved research projects" (DoD/VA, 2010, p. 1). Patient satisfaction is another goal stated in various places. This section of the chapter analyzes the impact of the Lovell FHCC on these outcome goals to the extent they are known at the 1.5-year mark.

Some but not all of the goals of creating the Lovell FHCC are addressed by the integration benchmarks. These are access, quality of care, operational readiness, patient and provider satisfaction, and research and training opportunities. This section of the report includes summaries of what is known about outcomes in these goal areas, as well as of cost effectiveness, the goal not included in the integration benchmarks.

Access

The Integration Scorecard shows that access to VA primary care has scored a 5 on a 5-point scale every month since October 2010. Access to DoD primary care has not scored as well. It scored 5s during the early months, but has scored a mix of 2s (3 months), 3s (4 months), and 4s (4 months) since then.

TRICARE patient ratings of "getting needed care" at the FHCC increased from 64 (on a 100-point scale) in FY 2006 to 86 in FY 2010, then fell to 79 in FY 2011, the first year of the full integration (see Figure 4-9 in a later section of this chapter).

Quality of Care

Like all health care delivery systems, the Lovell FHCC reports on measures of quality, such as the Healthcare Effectiveness Data and Information Set (HEDIS) developed by the National Committee for Quality Assurance, the Surgical Care Improvement Project (SCIP), and ORYX, a set of hospital performance measures developed by the Joint Commission.

Quality of care at the FHCC as measured by HEDIS, ORYX, and SCIP scores does not indicate a significant change in either the positive or the negative direction. Generally, HEDIS scores improved for several years before the 2010 merger before declining slightly in 2011, the first full year of FHCC operation (Figures 4-1 through 4-3). Only 2 of the 18 ORYX measures reported declined from 2010 to 2011 (from 100 to 95 percent in each case) (Figures 4-4 through 4-6). Of the 9 SCIP measures, 4 were the same in 2010 and 2011, 3 were higher, and 2 were lower (from 99 to 97 percent and from 100 to 93 percent) (Figure 4-7).

In September 2011, the Lovell FHCC was 1 of 405 U.S. hospitals named a top performer on key quality measures by the Joint Commission (Joint Commission, 2011).

Quality of Inpatient Heart Attack Patient Care

The Lovell FHCC's ORYX scores for heart attack patients were 100 percent in 2008 and remained at that level in 2010 and 2011 (Figure 4-4).

Quality of Inpatient Heart Failure Patient Care

The Lovell FHCC's ORYX scores for heart failure patients were also 100 percent in all 3 years, with one exception: the percentage of heart failure patients given discharge instructions dipped to 91 percent in 2010 before returning to 100 percent in 2011 (Figure 4-5).

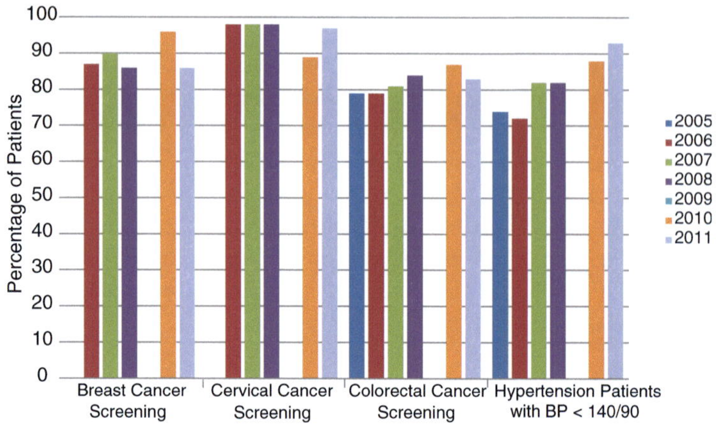

FIGURE 4-1 Selected HEDIS results for the Lovell Federal Health Care Center, 2005–2011 (percentage of patients) (Part 1).
NOTE: Results for 2009 are not included because composite measures were used that year rather than individual measures. BP = blood pressure; HEDIS = Healthcare Effectiveness Data and Information Set.
SOURCE: Provided by Lovell FHCC.

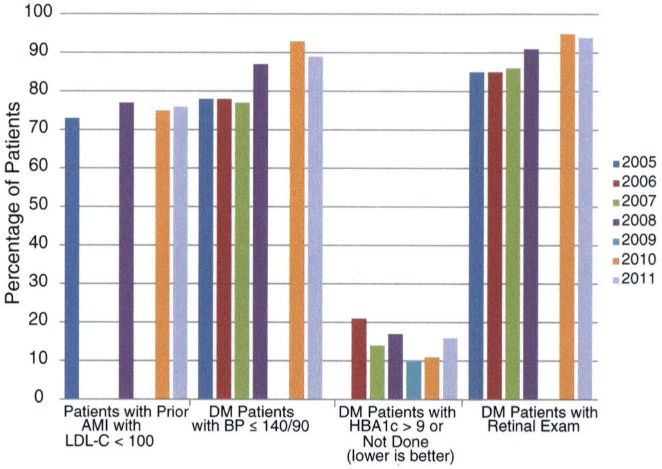

FIGURE 4-2 Selected HEDIS results for the Lovell Federal Health Care Center, 2005–2011 (percentage of patients) (Part 2).
NOTE: Results for 2009 are not included because composite measures were used that year rather than individual measures. AMI = acute myocardial infarction; BP = blood pressure; DM = diabetes mellitus; HBA1c = hemoglobin A1c (blood test for diabetes); HEDIS = Healthcare Effectiveness Data and Information Set; LDL-C = low-density lipoprotein cholesterol.
SOURCE: Provided by Lovell FHCC.

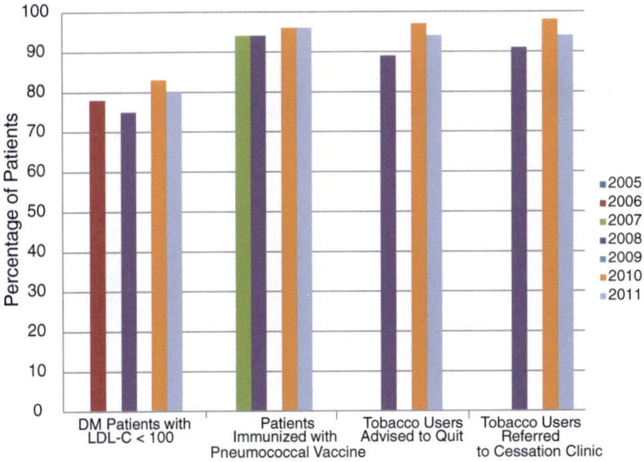

FIGURE 4-3 Selected HEDIS results for the Lovell Federal Health Care Center, 2005–2011 (percentage of patients) (Part 3).
NOTE: Results for 2009 are not included because composite measures were used that year rather than individual measures. HEDIS = Healthcare Effectiveness Data and Information Set; LDL-C = low-density lipoprotein cholesterol.
SOURCE: Lovell FHCC.

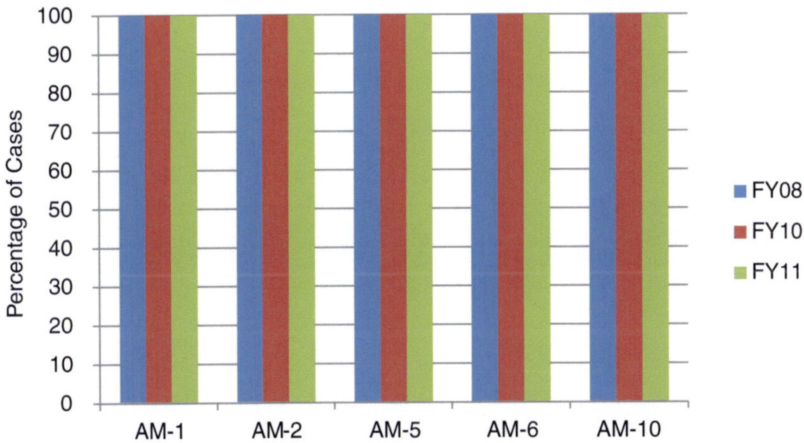

FIGURE 4-4 ORYX results for heart attack patients at the Lovell Federal Health Care Center, 2008–2011 (percentage of patients).
NOTE: Results for 2009 are not included because composite measures were used that year rather than individual measures. AM-1 = heart attack patients given aspirin at arrival; AM-2 = heart attack patients given aspirin at discharge; AM-5 = heart attack patients given beta blocker at discharge; AM-6 = heart attack patients given beta blocker at arrival; AM-10 = statin prescribed at discharge.
SOURCE: Lovell FHCC.

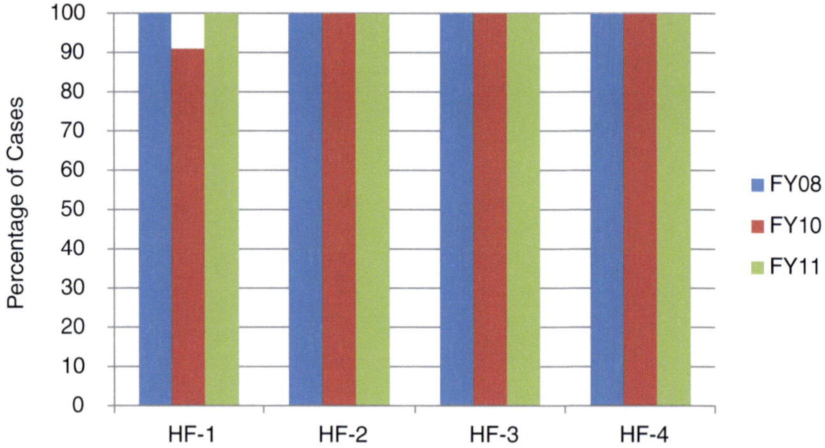

FIGURE 4-5 ORYX results for heart failure patients at the Lovell Federal Health Care Center, 2008–2011 (percentage of patients).
NOTE: Results for 2009 are not included because composite measures were used that year rather than individual measures. HF-1 = percentage of heart failure patients given discharge instructions; HF-2 = percentage of heart failure patients given an evaluation of left ventricular systolic function; HF-3 = percentage of heart failure patients given ace inhibitor or arb for left ventricular systolic dysfunction; HF-4 = percentage of heart failure patients given smoking cessation advice/counseling.
SOURCE: Lovell FHCC.

Quality of Inpatient Pneumonia Patient Care

In 2011, most of the Lovell FHCC's ORYX scores for patients with pneumonia were 100 percent, either the same or higher as they were in 2010. Two of the nine measures dipped, from 100 percent in 2010 to 95 percent in 2011 (Figure 4-6).

Quality of Inpatient Surgical Care

Five of the Lovell FHCC's seven SCIP scores in 2011 were the same or higher than in 2010, at or near 100 percent. Two measures fell: the overall rate of prophylactic antibiotic received within 1 hour prior to surgery (from 99 percent to 97 percent), and the overall rate of prophylactic antibiotic discontinuation with 24 hours after surgery (from 100 percent to 93 percent) (Figure 4-7).

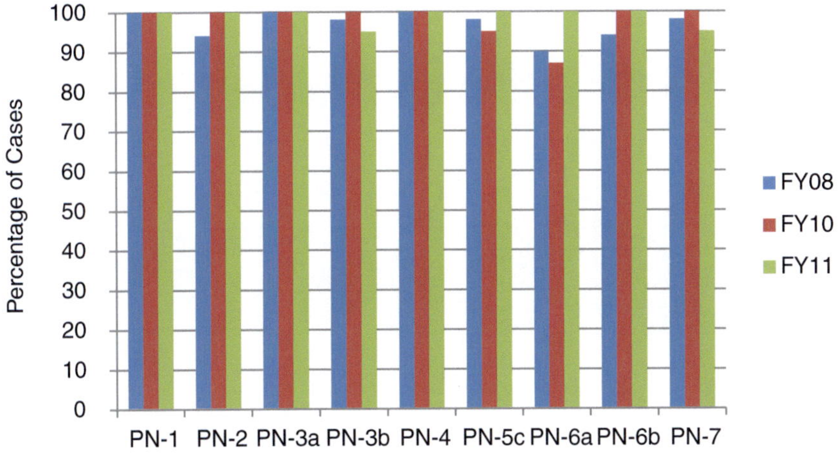

FIGURE 4-6 ORYX results for pneumonia patients at the Lovell Federal Health Care Center, 2008–2011 (percentage of patients).
NOTE: Results for 2009 are not included because composite measures were used that year rather than individual measures. PN-1 = pneumonia patient oxygenation assessed; PN-2 = pneumonia patients assessed and given pneumococcal vaccination; PN-3a = blood cultures were performed within 24 hours prior to or 24 hours after hospital arrival for patients who were transferred or admitted to the intensive care unit (ICU); PN-3b = initial emergency room blood culture was performed prior to the administration of the first hospital dose of antibiotics; PN-4 = smoking cessation advice/counseling given; PN-5c = initial antibiotic received within 6 hours of hospital arrival; PN-6a = initial antibiotic selection for community-acquired pneumonia (CAP) in immunocompetent ICU patient; PN-6b = initial antibiotic selection for CAP immunocompetent non-ICU patient; PN-7 = pneumonia patients assessed and given influenza vaccination.
SOURCE: Lovell FHCC.

Cost Effectiveness

No evidence was found regarding cost effectiveness, but some was found with regard to cost savings. The notable savings were in avoidance of construction costs and the reduction of Navy inpatient full-time equivalent (FTE) positions because the VA took over staffing of the nursing wards. There are also some operating efficiencies. However, there was no quantification of extra cost of duplicate administrative services to meet different standards and reporting requirements for similar functions.

Staff at the Lovell FHCC prepared a cost-benefit analysis of the Lovell FHCC merger in February 2009. The analysis reported that the annual savings from the Phase I move of inpatient mental health services from the

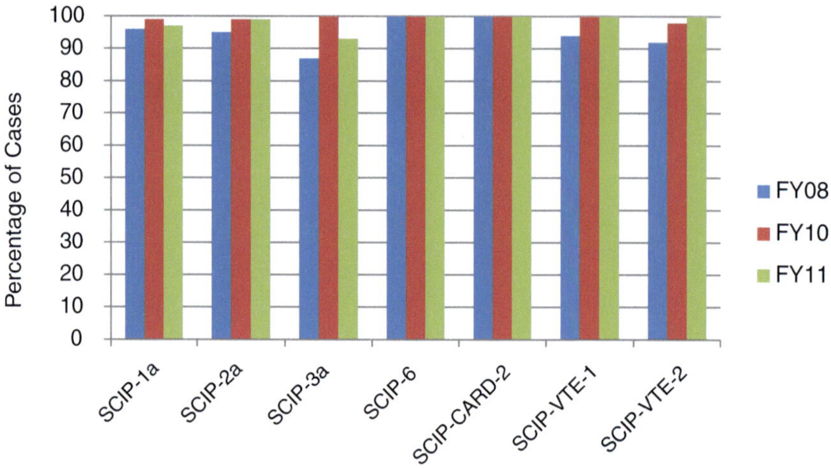

FIGURE 4-7 Selected SCIP results for the Lovell Federal Health Care Center, 2008–2011 (percentage of patients).
NOTE: Results for 2009 are not included because composite measures were used that year rather than individual measures. SCIP = Surgical Care Improvement Project; SCIP-1a = prophylactic antibiotic received within 1 hour prior to surgical incision-overall rate; SCIP-2a = prophylactic antibiotic selection for surgical patients-overall rate; SCIP-3a = prophylactic antibiotics discontinued within 24 hours after surgery end time-overall rate; SCIP-6 = surgery patients with appropriate hair removal; SCIP-CARD-2 = surgery patients on beta blocker therapy prior to admission who received a beta blocker during the perioperative period; SCIP-VTE-1 = surgery patients with recommended venous thromboembolism prophylaxis ordered; SCIP-VTE-2 = surgery patients who received appropriate venous thromboembolism prophylaxis within 24 hours prior to surgery to 24 hours after surgery.
SOURCE: Lovell FHCC.

NHGL was more than $1 million per year. The one-time cost avoidance of constructing the Navy blood processing center in the NCVAMC instead of retrofitting a building on the Navy base was $3.1 million, and the annual operating costs were $370,000 a year less. The Phase II transfer of inpatient medical, surgical, and pediatric services and the ED from the NHGL to the NCVAMC was saving more than $900,000 per year, primarily because the Navy was able to reduce staffing by more than 50 FTEs, most of them active duty servicemembers who were reassigned to other billets in North Chicago or to other Navy facilities. The analysis estimated that building the 201,000-square-foot ACC instead of the 364,000-square-foot facility the Navy had planned to build would save approximately $67 million in construction costs. Operating the combined ACC-NCVAMC facility was expected to be about $19.7 million a year less than operating both a new Navy hospital and the NCVAMC would have been.

The Lovell FHCC issued a press release when the center opened in October 2010, in which Patrick Sullivan, the director, was quoted as saying that taxpayers would be saving approximately $20 million annually from the integrated operation. He said that because of the integration, "staff members are able to care for a larger population of patients, and that by combining staffing and resources, patients are able to benefit from robust, state-of-the-art health care."[4]

Patient Satisfaction

Patient satisfaction is one of the 15 measures of the success of the integration effort agreed to by the VA and the DoD. Samples of DoD and VA beneficiaries are surveyed separately and the results are updated monthly.

The DoD conducts a quarterly survey of TRICARE beneficiaries. In 2009, the VA adopted the Consumer Assessment of Healthcare Plans and Systems survey, a nationally standardized tool. The Navy uses a survey of MTF users developed by the BUMED.

TRICARE

The TRICARE Management Activity has posted the results of its patient surveys for the years 2003–2011. In 2011, TRICARE users gave the Lovell FHCC more favorable ratings on access questions and less favorable ratings on other questions concerning physician-patient communication and quality of health care and health care providers, compared with all Navy users of TRICARE (Figure 4-8).

There was also a general drop in most ratings from 2010 to 2011, which was the first year of full integration of the Lovell FHCC. For example, the average score on a 100-point scale of patients surveyed for how well doctors communicate, which had increased from 84 in 2008 to 94 in 2010, fell to 81 in 2011 (Figure 4-9). Measures of access, such as getting care quickly and getting needed care, similarly increased until 2010, then declined from 80 to 76 and from 86 to 79, respectively (Figure 4-9). Other ratings also tended to drop in 2011, compared with 2010 (Figure 4-10). Whether these rating drops are a trend or reflect transitory effects of the first year of implementation—or are random—will not be known until several years of data are collected.

---

[4] Jonathan Friedman, Historic VA/DoD integration accomplished. http://www.lovell.fhcc.va.gov/LOVELLFHCC/features/integration.asp (accessed September 13, 2012).

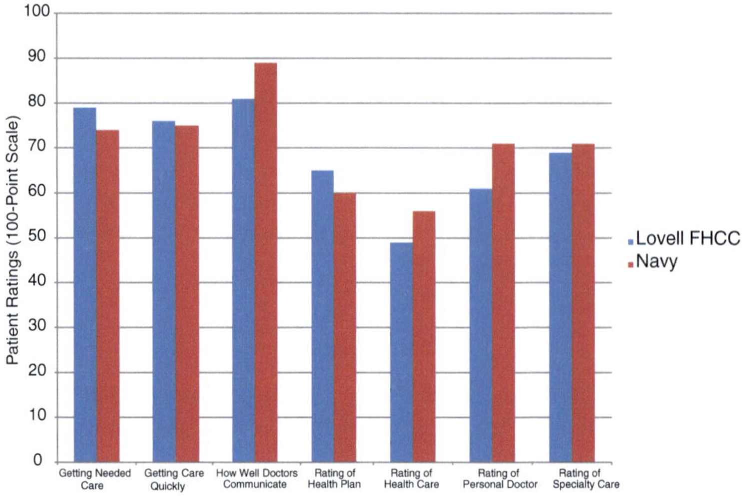

FIGURE 4-8 TRICARE patient ratings of the Lovell Federal Health Care Center, 2011 (100-point scale).
SOURCE: http://www.tricare.mil/survey/hcsurvey/annual-report.cfm (accessed September 13, 2012).

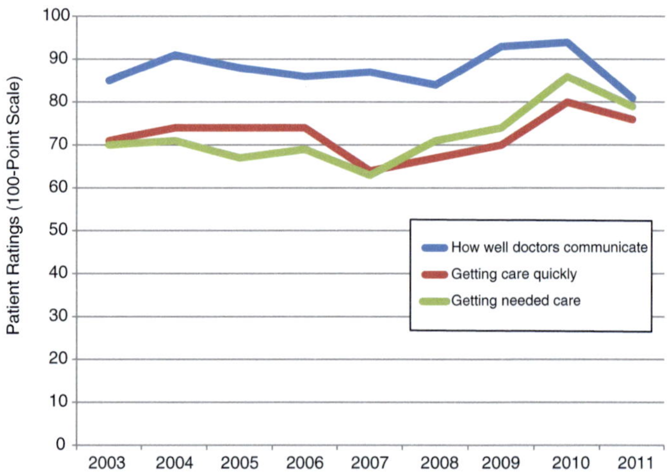

FIGURE 4-9 TRICARE patient ratings of access to care and physician-patient communication at the Lovell Federal Health Care Center, 2003–2011 (100-point scale).
SOURCE: http://www.tricare.mil/survey/hcsurvey/annual-report.cfm (accessed September 13, 2012).

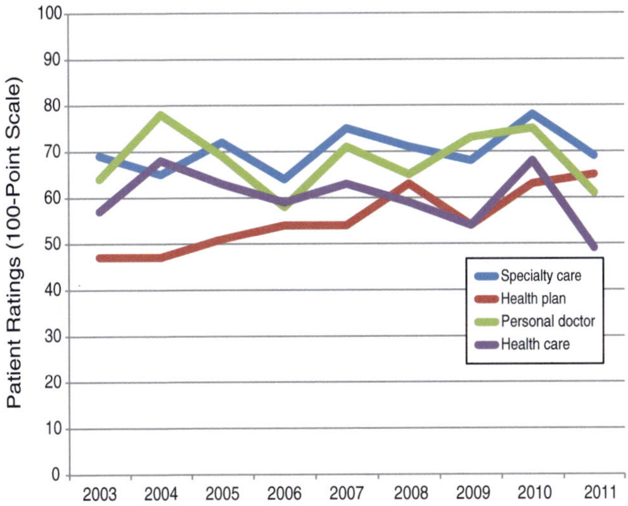

FIGURE 4-10 TRICARE patient ratings of aspects of care at the Lovell Federal Health Care Center, 2003–2011 (100-point scale).
SOURCE: http://www.tricare.mil/survey/hcsurvey/annual-report.cfm (accessed September 13, 2102).

Department of Veterans Affairs

The VA survey results show that veteran satisfaction with outpatient and inpatient care at the Lovell FHCC was higher in 2011, the first year of full integration, than in 2010. Satisfaction with outpatient care at Lovell was higher than average veteran satisfaction with VA outpatient care nationally, but the opposite was true for inpatient care (Figures 4-11 and 4-12).

Lovell Federal Health Care Center

The FHCC tracks and reports patient satisfaction by normalizing the DoD and the VA scores around the overall average score for BUMED and VISN 12, respectively, and using a 5-point scale. For example, if the DoD survey result for the FHCC deviates 16 percent or more below the overall result for BUMED as a whole, it gets 1 point. If it is between 15 and 11 percent below, it gets 2 points. If it is between 10 and 6 percent below, it gets 3 points. If it is between 5 percent above and 5 percent below the BUMED average, it gets 4 points, which is considered to be "very good." If

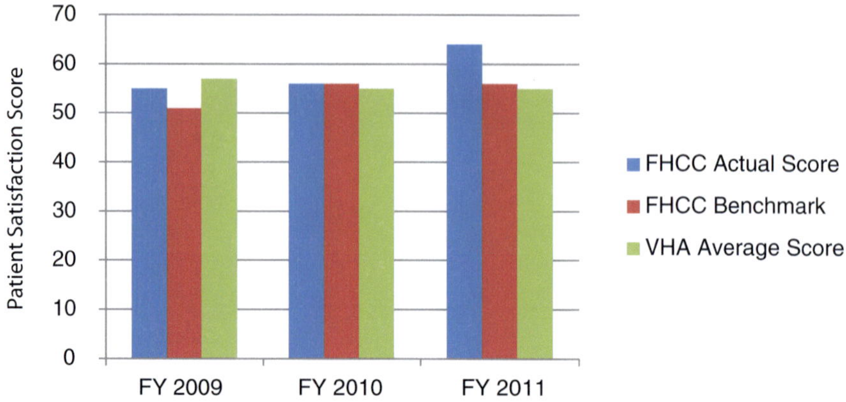

FIGURE 4-11 Department of Veterans Affairs outpatient satisfaction scores, fiscal years 2009–2011.
NOTE: The VA changed the scoring methodology in 2009, making results for 2008 and earlier noncomparable.
SOURCES: Lovell FHCC and VA, 2011.

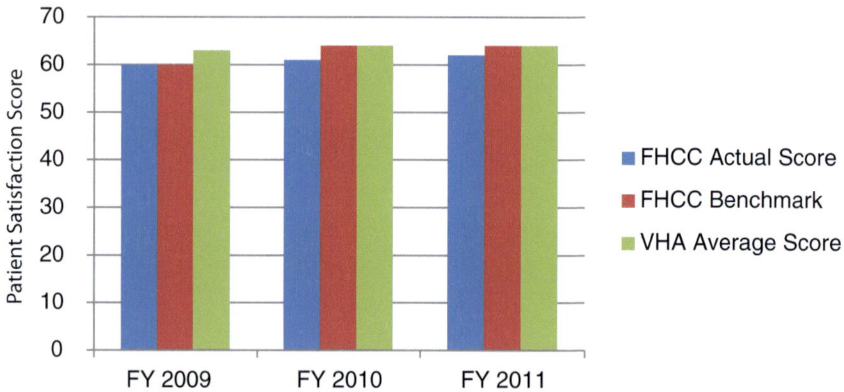

FIGURE 4-12 Department of Veterans Affairs inpatient satisfaction scores, fiscal years 2009–2011.
NOTE: The VA changed the scoring methodology in 2009, making results for 2008 and earlier noncomparable.
SOURCE: Lovell FHCC and VA, 2011.

TABLE 4-3 Department of Defense Patient Satisfaction Scale for the Lovell Federal Health Care Center

Score	Basis
5 (Excellent)	More than 5 percent above the BUMED average
4 (Very Good)	Between 5 percent above and below the BUMED average
3 (Good)	Between 5 and 10 percent below the BUMED average
2 (Fair)	Between 10 and 16 percent below the BUMED average
1 (Poor)	16 percent or more below the BUMED average

SOURCE: Lovell FHCC, 2010c.

it is more than 5 percent above the BUMED average, it gets 5 points, which is considered to be "excellent" (Table 4-3).

The similar score is derived from the VA surveys except that the comparison is the overall average for VISN 12 and the intervals are different (Table 4-4).

The benchmark considered successful is a score of 4 or higher.

Both DoD and VA patient satisfaction scores were 4s (very good) on the eve of full integration in October 2010. The measure of VA patient satisfaction was lower than the benchmark (a score of at least 4) in the early months of the integration effort and again in the summer of 2011, but the measure jumped to excellent (5) and stayed there at the beginning of the second year. The measure of DoD patient satisfaction has alternated between good (3) and very good (4) during the same initial 16-month period (Figure 4-13). These trends indicate that both sets of beneficiaries have been less satisfied than they were before the Lovell FHCC took over operations, although VA beneficiaries have been much happier recently.

TABLE 4-4 Veterans Administration Patient Satisfaction Scale for the Lovell Federal Health Care Center

Score	Basis
5 (Excellent)	More than 5 percent above the VISN average
4 (Very Good)	Between 0 and 5 percent above the VISN average
3 (Good)	Between 0 and 5 percent below the VISN average
2 (Fair)	Between 5 and 10 percent below the VISN average
1 (Poor)	10 percent or more below the VISN average

SOURCE: Lovell FHCC, 2010c.

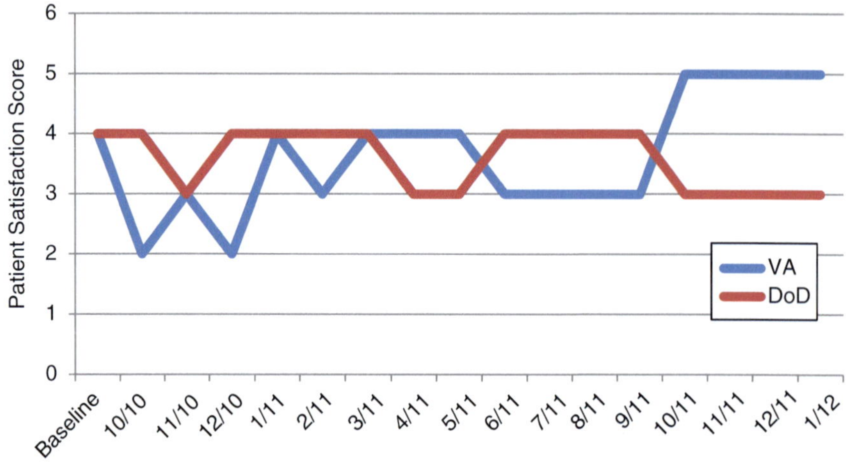

FIGURE 4-13 Lovell Federal Health Care Center patient satisfaction scores, October 2010–June 2012.
SOURCE: Lovell FHCC.

Provider Satisfaction/Morale

The FHCC is subject to an annual organizational climate survey by the Defense Equal Opportunity Management Institute which asks questions in two areas: equal employment opportunity climate and organizational effectiveness. The latest survey was conducted in January 2012. The response rate was a little more than 40 percent for both civilian and active duty responders and also proportional across pay grades/ranks.

The respondents were asked to rate their job satisfaction, their trust in the FHCC, the cohesion and the effectiveness of their work group, and their perception of the cohesion of the FHCC leadership on a 5-point scale, in which a higher number means greater satisfaction, trust, commitment, and cohesion. The results show that the ratings by FHCC personnel in January 2012 were generally comparable to those by all Navy, all DoD, and all federal civilian personnel (Figure 4-14).

The average ratings by FHCC personnel in 2012 were also comparable to the ratings done in 2011, essentially bracketing the first year of the FHCC (Figure 4-15).

Mission Readiness of Navy Staff, Recruits, and "A" School Students

The impact of the FHCC integration on the operational readiness of active duty personnel was of paramount concern to the Navy. Great Lakes is the only enlisted boot camp in the Navy and the location of many of the

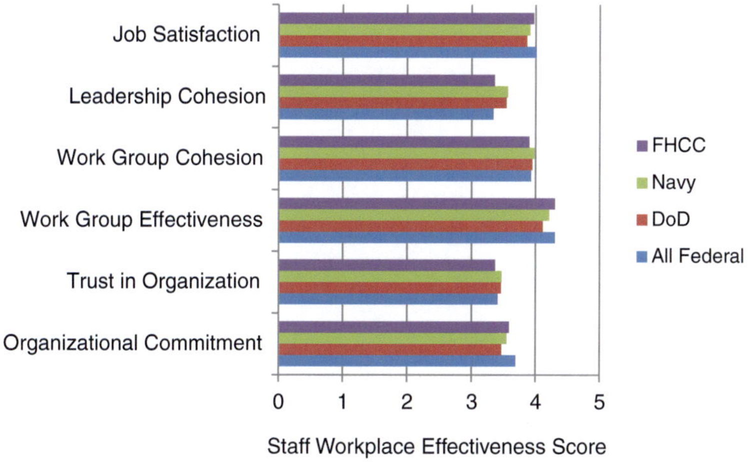

FIGURE 4-14 Average ratings of organizational effectiveness of their workplace by active duty and civilian staff at the Lovell Federal Health Care Center, all Navy facilities, all Department of Defense facilities, and all federal civilian workplaces in 2012.
NOTE: Respondents to an annual survey of the organizational climate at federal facilities administered by the Defense Equal Opportunity Management Institute were asked to give their perception of certain organizational features on a 5-point scale rate in which a higher number is better; e.g., a 4 means greater job satisfaction than a 3. DoD = Department of Defense; FHCC = Federal Health Care Center.
SOURCE: Lovell FHCC, 2012a.

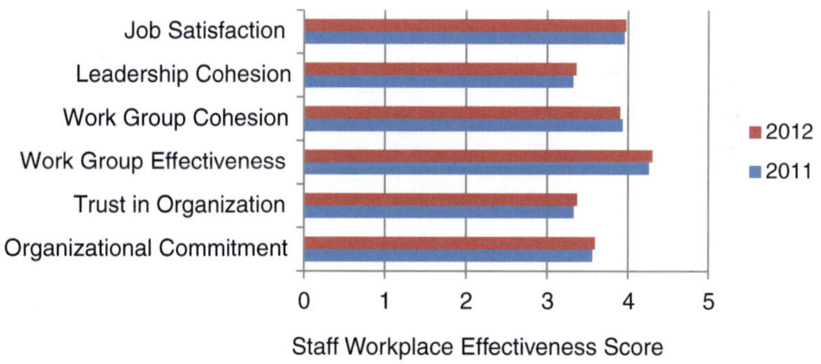

FIGURE 4-15 Average ratings of organizational effectiveness of the Lovell Federal Health Care Center by its active duty and civilian staff in 2011 and 2012.
NOTE: Respondents to an annual survey of the organizational climate at the Lovell Federal Health Care Center administered by the Defense Equal Opportunity Management Institute were asked to give their perception of certain organizational features on a 5-point scale rate in which a higher number is better; e.g., a 4 means greater job satisfaction than a 3.
SOURCE: Lovell FHCC, 2012a.

Navy's advanced training schools; therefore, a slowdown of training would negatively affect the entire Navy. On the other hand, having sailors with untreated health problems while on an extended cruise is also disruptive. This issue was mostly dealt with by keeping the recruit medical processing operation and the recruit and student health and dental clinics in place on the base, and not trying to move and integrate them with the rest of the FHCC's patient care and patient services. However, some services for Navy personnel, including recruits and students, were moved and integrated (e.g., specialty care; emergency care; acute inpatient psychiatry, surgery, and general medicine; women's health; and laboratory and pharmacy services). Administrative services such as purchasing of supplies and computer system support for the Navy branch health clinics were also centralized.

The Navy agreed on three measures of military medical readiness that collectively are being tracked as one of the 15 measures of integration success. They are the following:

- keeping recruits in temporary holding units for medical reasons after they graduate under 5 percent,
- keeping students not under instruction for medical reasons less than 2 percent, and
- keeping the medically indeterminate status of active duty staff under 5 percent.

Recruits in Temporary Holding Units for Medical Reasons After They Graduate

Enlisted recruits who graduate from boot camp but are medically unable to transfer are assigned to temporary holding units. It is the responsibility of the MTF, in this case the Lovell FHCC, to provide the care needed to keep this rate as low as possible. According to the FHCC's scorecard, Lovell has scored mostly 5s since it was launched in October 2010, meaning that the rate has been 2 percent or less (Lovell FHCC, 2010c). However, the rate jumped to more than 6 percent in January 2011 and also experienced a lesser increase (to less than 5 percent) in August and September 2011.

Enlisted Students Not Under Instruction for Medical Reasons

The percentage of enlisted students unable to attend training for medical reasons fell by half, to less than 1 percent, in September and October 2010 and, except for 1-week spikes in January 2011 and January 2012, it has trended downward to about 0.5 percent (Figure 4-16).

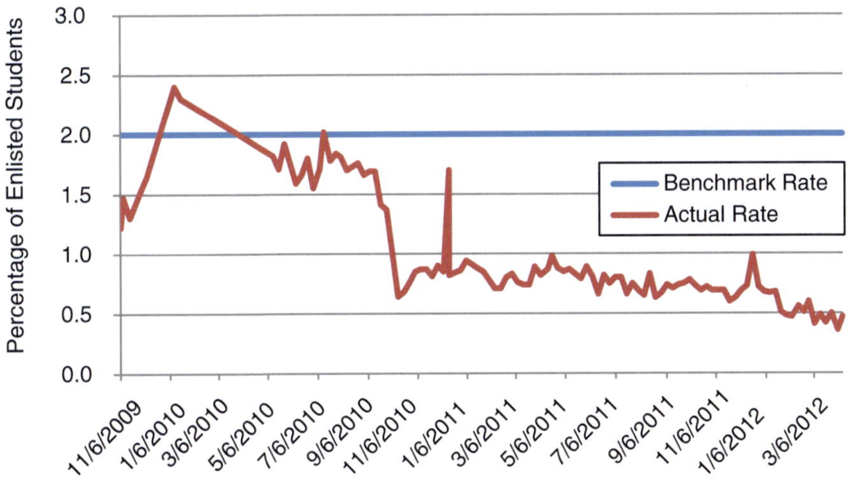

FIGURE 4-16 Percentage of enlisted students not under instruction for medical reasons, November 2009–April 2012.
NOTE: A lower score is better.
SOURCE: Lovell FHCC.

Medically Indeterminate Status

An active duty servicemember can be fully medically ready, partially medically ready, or not medically ready, or his or her medical readiness can be indeterminate. To be fully medically ready, servicemembers have to meet a list of requirements. Those who are ill or pregnant or who have acute dental problems are considered not medically ready. Those who are lacking some tests or immunizations are partially ready. Finally, those with overdue periodic health assessments, overdue periodic mental examinations, or lost medical records are classified as medically indeterminate.

In December 2010, 82 percent of active duty personnel at Great Lakes were medically ready for deployment, 4 percent were partially ready, 10 percent were not ready, and the status of 4 percent was medically indeterminate (FHCC communication). This was much better than the U.S. Armed Forces as a whole. In December 2010, the equivalent numbers were 67, 8, 13, and 12 percent, respectively (Woodson, 2011). However, Great Lakes is the Navy's major training center where most servicemembers are relatively healthy young recruits and students, and the expectations for operational medical readiness are high.

The Navy chose to track the percentage of medically indeterminate active duty servicemembers, those whose status is unknown, as its measure of active duty individual medical readiness. In addition, an MTF's percentage of personnel whose individual medical readiness status is indeterminate is a factor in the Navy's performance-based budgeting formula for MTFs.

During September 2010, the medical readiness indeterminate rate was between 4 and 5 percent. From October 2010 through January 2012, the scorecard score was 4 for most months, which means it was between 2.5 and 5 percent. It was a 5 in October 2010 and in January and June 2011, meaning it was 2.5 percent or less.

Findings and Conclusions Concerning Military Operational Readiness

The data presented on military medical readiness are consistent with the statement the RTC commander made to the committee at its third meeting. He said that the establishment of the FHCC has not had a noticeable effect on the rate of recruits who are able to graduate on time and transfer to their next assignments, some to additional training and some to immediate duty on ships. He said that when an issue does arise, it is addressed immediately and satisfactorily by the FHCC leadership. An early example was when a recruit was released from the inpatient psychiatric ward without notice to the RTC. The FHCC immediately worked out a procedure with the RTC to prevent such a reoccurrence.

Several interviewees indicated that maintaining operational readiness involved more effort than was previously necessary. They reported that it takes more time to keep medical records up to date because the DoD and the VA EHR systems do not interface and, therefore, the documentation of specialty, inpatient, and emergency services provided on the west campus must be manually entered into AHLTA. IT and laboratory services are provided centrally rather than locally, which is more cost effecive overall but can reduce responsiveness to branch health clinics' needs. Although the two campuses are only 1.5 miles apart, it takes 20–30 minutes each way to travel from one campus to the other because the roads are not direct and the naval base can be accessed only through a few secure gates. Unless the base ambulance service is used in an emergency, the transportation is often provided by hospital corpsmen, which reduces their availability in the clinic.

Training and Research

The creation of the FHCC has generated opportunities for improved training and research that are not yet exploited but are in the plans of the Lovell FHCC and its affiliated medical school, the Rosalind Franklin University of Medicine and Science. These were discussed in the presentations to the committee at its September 2011 meeting in North Chicago and in an earlier site visit to the university by the committee staff. Those discussions centered on several features of the combined FHCC, including the opportunities that the larger and more diverse patient population and the broader range of clinical services offer for both teaching and research.

Rosalind Franklin has been affiliated with the NCVAMC since 1980, when the university moved from downtown Chicago to North Chicago. The university has many doctoral and masters degree programs requiring clinical experience that is provided in part by the FHCC. There are schools of medicine, podiatry, pharmacy, and health professions, and a school of basic science that grants doctorates in the biomedical sciences. About 45 medical students a year have third-year clerkships in psychiatry, internal medicine, and neurology. There are about 40 residents a year in psychiatry and general internal medicine and 10 fellowships in endocrinology, pulmonology, infectious diseases, and cardiology. The 140 residents in podiatry do rotations at the FHCC, as well as 7 psychology students, 7 physical therapy students, 2 nurse anesthesiology students, and 18 students from other programs. The university has started a school of pharmacy, and there are plans for the 12 initial pharmacy students to rotate at the FHCC pharmacy.

The FHCC also has affiliations with Loyola University Chicago and the University of Illinois, and each year provides training for more than 400 residents, interns, and medical students, as well as students of other disciplines, including health services administration, audiology/speech pathology, biomedical engineering, dental assisting, medical technology, pharmacy, nursing, physical therapy, podiatry, psychology, and social work.

Training Opportunities

In their presentation to the committee, the director and deputy director of the FHCC said it has added new clinical disciplines for training experience, for example, family medicine, pediatrics, and hospitalist practice, as well as increased faculty and medicine. Trainees can now also be exposed to other disciplines, such as dermatology, ophthalmology, gynecology, and emergency medicine. There are more ambulatory care preceptors. The FHCC will also be able to increase the pool of speakers and the diversity of topics for grand rounds and multidisciplinary conferences.

Rosalind Franklin will be able to make greater use of the FHCC as one of its training institutions because of the expanded number of specialties and subspecialties offered there. Many VA providers have faculty appointments, and the university has now appointed Navy clinicians as faculty.

Research Opportunities

According to the integration performance benchmark, the amount of research funding at the Lovell FHCC is larger than it was leading up to

October 1, 2010. The leaderships of both Rosalind Franklin and the FHCC see the greater diversity of the patient population, now including women and children and the entire age range, as new research opportunities. The expansion of clinical staff increases the number of potential researchers.

Both institutions also mentioned having access to DoD research funding as well as to VA research funding. Although a VA clinician has had a major research program at the university on battlefield critical care, funded by the DoD, the FHCC and the university are not currently collaborating on clinical trials, although the NCVAMC and the university have in the past.

REFERENCES

DoD/VA (Department of Defense/Department of Veterans Affairs). 2008. *Good News* [newsletter]. February. http://www.tricare.mil/DVPCO/downloads/DoD-VA-Good-News-Feb-2008.pdf (accessed September 7, 2012).

DoD/VA. 2010. Executive agreement for the Department of Defense-Department of Veterans Affairs Medical Facility Demonstration Project, Federal Health Care Center. April 23. http://tricare.mil/tma/congressionalinformation/downloads/2010310/111-288%20Section%201701(d)(1)%20FHCC%20EA.pdf (accessed September 6, 2012).

Fouse, S., and B. Faber. 2011. Patient Services Directorate. Presentation to the IOM Committee on Evaluation of the Lovell Federal Health Care Center Merger by Dr. Sarah Fouse and CDR Bridgette Faber, associate director and assistant director, Patient Services Directorate, Lovell FHCC, North Chicago, IL, June 29.

GAO (U.S. Government Accountability Office). 2012. *VA/DoD health care: Costly information technology delays continue and evaluation plan lacking*. GAO-12-669. Washington, DC: GAO. http://www.gao.gov/assets/600/591895.pdf (accessed September 7, 2012).

Harnly, M. J. 2005. A qualitative analysis of resource sharing agreements between Naval Hospital Great Lakes and North Chicago Veterans Affairs Medical Center: The iron triangle theory of healthcare integration. Master's Thesis, Army-Baylor Program in Healthcare Administration, Fort Sam Houston, TX. http://www.dtic.mil/dtic/tr/fulltext/u2/a443921.pdf (accessed September 13, 2012).

Joint Commission. 2011. *Improving America's hospitals—The Joint Commission's annual report on quality and safety 2011*. http://www.jointcommission.org/2011_annual_report/ (accessed September 21, 2012).

Lovell FHCC (Captain James A. Lovell Federal Health Care Center). 2010a. *Concept of operations*. October 1. Provided by the Lovell FHCC.

Lovell FHCC. 2010b. *Interim business plan for fiscal year 2011*. Provided by the Lovell FHCC.

Lovell FHCC. 2010c. *FHCC integrated benchmarks: Tech manual*. Provided by the Lovell FHCC.

Lovell FHCC. 2012a. *Organizational climate survey synopsis*. January. Provided by the Lovell FHCC.

Lovell FHCC. 2012b. *Business plan for fiscal year 2013 through 2015*. Provided by the Lovell FHCC.

Shortell, S. M., R. R. Gillies, D. A. Anderson, K. M. Erickson, and J. B. Mitchell. 2000. *Remaking health care in America: The evolution of organized delivery systems*, 2nd Edition. San Francisco: Jossey-Bass.

VA. 2010a. Communications Department working side-by-side. *The Great Lakes News* (VISN 12 Newsletter), January. http://www.visn12.va.gov/docs/gln/Great_Lakes_News_2010_01.pdf (accessed September 7, 2012).

VA. 2010b. USS Osborne remains critical component in recruit dental readiness. *The Great Lakes News* (VISN 12 Newsletter), October. http://www.visn12.va.gov/docs/gln/Great_Lakes_News_2010_10.pdf (accessed September 7, 2012).

VA. 2011. *FY 2011 performance and accountability report*. November. http://www.va.gov/budget/report/ (accessed September 13, 2012).

VA/DoD. 2002. *The Department of Veterans Affairs and the Department of Defense report on health care resource sharing, FY 2002*. March 23. http://tricare.mil/tma/congressional information/downloads/DoD%20VA%20Sharing%20signed%20Mar%2027%202003.pdf (accessed September 16, 2012).

VA/DoD. 2007. *FY 2006 VA/DoD Joint Executive Council annual report*. February. http://www.tricare.mil/DVPCO/downloads/VADoD2006.pdf (accessed June 8, 2012).

Woodson, J. 2011. Prepared statement by Jonathan Woodson, MD, Assistant Secretary of Defense (Health Affairs), regarding the Military Health System, overview before the Senate Armed Services Committee Personnel Subcommittee, May 4. http://armed-services.senate.gov/statemnt/2011/05%20May/Woodson%2005-04-11.pdf (accessed September 7, 2012).

5

Lessons Learned from Other Federal and Private-Sector Collaborative Approaches to Health Care Services

A number of lessons emerged from the committee's examination of other collaborations in the federal and private sectors.[1] The committee confined its analysis to Department of Veterans Affairs (VA)/Department of Defense (DoD) and private-sector approaches to health care collaborations, but did not evaluate either intradepartmental health care integrations in the VA and the DoD or interdepartmental health care collaborations with other federal agencies.

DEPARTMENT OF VETERANS AFFAIRS/DEPARTMENT OF DEFENSE RESOURCE SHARING AND OTHER JOINT INITIATIVES

1978 General Accounting Office Interagency Sharing Report

In 1978, at the request of the chairman of the House Appropriations Committee, the Government Accountability Office (GAO) (at that time called the General Accounting Office) conducted a study of resource sharing among federal health care providers. The ensuing 171-page report, *Legislation Needed to Encourage Better Use of Federal Medical Resources and Remove Obstacles to Interagency Sharing* (HRD-78-54), found a very

[1] The private-sector discussion draws on a paper commissioned by the Committee on Evaluation of the Lovell Federal Health Care Center Merger on the "Collaboration Among Health Care Organizations: A Review of Outcomes and Best Practices for Effective Performance," by Thomas D'Aunno, with the assistance of Yi-Ting Chiang and Mattia Gilmartin (see Appendix D).

limited degree of sharing despite many opportunities to improve health care for beneficiaries while saving taxpayer dollars through "eliminating or consolidating underused or duplicative facilities, equipment, and staff," reducing the reliance on purchased care, and "increasing staff proficiency and improving patient care by consolidating workloads and resources" (GAO, 1978, p. 28).

The 1978 GAO report contained a number of specific recommendations for the departments, the Office of Management and Budget, and Congress, including a draft bill. In response, Congress enacted the Veterans Administration and Department of Defense Health Resources Sharing and Emergency Operations Act of 1982 (Public Law 97-174) to remove obstacles to greater sharing of health care resources between the VA and the DoD and to give military treatment facilities (MTFs) and VA medical centers (VAMCs) greater incentives to share resources. Public Law 97-174 remains the chief legislative basis for partnering between DoD's Military Health System and the Veterans Health Administration (VHA).

National Defense Authorization Act of Fiscal Year 2003

In 2002, Congress mandated initiatives intended to spur additional VA/DoD health care collaborations in the fiscal year (FY) 2003 National Defense Authorization Act (NDAA 2003).

DoD/VA Demonstration Projects

The NDAA 2003 directed the DoD and the VA to fund health care coordination demonstration projects between the two organizations' health care facilities. Seven demonstrations were implemented in 2005, "designed to improve the coordination of health care resources between VA and DoD for application elsewhere" (VA/DoD, 2006, p. 19) in the areas of budget and financial management,[2] coordinated staffing and assignment,[3] and medical information and information technology (IT)[4] (Navy Medicine, 2012).

---

[2] The sites for the budget and financial management demonstrations were the VA Pacific Islands Health Care System/Tripler Army Medical Center and the Alaska VA Health Care System/3rd Medical Group at Elmendorf Air Force Base (Navy Medicine, 2012).

[3] The coordinated staffing and assignment demonstrations were the Augusta VA Health Care System/Eisenhower Army Medical Center and the Hampton VA Medical Center/1st Medical Group at Langley Air Force Base (Navy Medicine, 2012).

[4] The medical information and information technology demonstrations were the Puget Sound VA Health Care System/Madigan Army Medical Center, the El Paso VA Health Care System/William Beaumont Army Medical Center, and the South Texas VA Health Care System/Wilford Hall Air Force Medical Center/Brooke Army Medical Center (Navy Medicine, 2012).

The demonstration sites evaluated four major IT solutions: the Laboratory Data Sharing Initiative; a DoD/VA credentials-sharing interface; the Bi-directional Health Information Exchange; and digital image sharing (DoD/VA, 2008, p. 5).

According to the final report from the DoD and the VA, there were a number of barriers to sharing. Some were amenable to policy changes, such as the different hiring authorities of the two departments, the need for procedures for paying for shared services and transferring funds, and limits on data sharing. The projects also demonstrated the importance of buy-in by all relevant local parties; the need for continuous education and training to overcome cultural differences; the problems presented by different business practices in such areas as staffing, procurement, funding, construction standards and timelines, and credentials; and the information-sharing limitations imposed by different information management (IM)/IT systems (DoD/VA, 2008, pp. 64–66).

Joint Incentive Fund

As part of the NDAA 2003, Congress also established the Joint Incentives Program to enable more collaboration between the VA and the DoD. The two secretaries were directed to contribute a minimum of $15 million per year each to a DoD-VA Health Care Sharing Incentive Fund and to use the funds to "carry out a program to identify, provide incentives to, implement, fund, and evaluate creative coordination and sharing initiatives at the facility, intraregional, and nationwide levels" (DoD/VA, 2004, p. 1). Known as the Joint Incentive Fund (JIF), the program was extended until September 30, 2015, by the NDAA 2010, the law that established the Captain James A. Lovell Federal Health Care Center (FHCC).

The JIF is administered by the VHA "under the policy guidance and direction of the HEC [Health Executive Council]," and its chief financial officer provides financial status reports to the Health HEC and to the chief financial officer of DoD's TRICARE Management Activity (AMEDD, 2012). The HEC uses the funding to promote local VA/DoD sharing by paying for initial start-up costs of a project that is expected to become self-sustaining after several years. In some cases, the projects permit existing joint venture sites to expand their collaborative activities; in other cases, the JIF projects are awarded to encourage potential joint ventures. The VA/DoD partners submit proposals each year. The Joint Facility Utilization Resource Sharing Working Group (JFURSWG) is charged by the Joint Executive Council (JEC) to review the proposed sharing activities. In its ninth year, the JIF has funded 130 projects totaling $420.6 million (Interviews).

Joint Ventures

Joint ventures are characterized by specific resource-sharing agreements encompassing multiple services resulting in joint operations. They consist of local alliances or partnerships between the DoD and the VA for the purposes of longer-term commitments of more than 5 years to facilitate comprehensive cooperation, shared risk, and mutual benefit. Joint ventures may or may not involve joint capital planning and coordinated use of existing or planned facilities. They exist along a continuum in which the medical facility missions and operations are connected, integrated, or consolidated. Joint ventures are characterized by regular and ongoing interaction in one or more of the following areas: staffing, clinical workload, business processes, management, IT, logistics, education and training, and research capabilities (VA/DoD, 2008).

Joint Market Areas

The VA and the DoD have developed criteria for identifying "joint market areas" for increased health care sharing. They are health care markets with large DoD and VA beneficiary populations where shared facilities and services would provide access to services or infrastructure not available in one or the other organization; improve efficiency through economies of scale; reduce duplication of services, infrastructure, or both; and mitigate the impact of deployment on access. The JFURSWG under the VA/DoD HEC has identified more than a dozen joint market areas and has worked with them to develop additional sharing agreements. In 2010, the selection criteria for joint market areas qualifying for focused assistance from the JFURSWG were the amount of purchased care expenditures, the degree of facility proximity, the potential enrollment population, the current working relationship, the current and planned resource sharing initiatives, and the joint construction opportunities. The 2010 sites were Phoenix, Arizona; San Diego, California; Fayetteville, North Carolina; Oklahoma City, Oklahoma; and Omaha, Nebraska (Carlisle and Henius, 2010). The sites in 2011 were St. Louis, Missouri; Columbia, South Carolina; and Temple, Texas (Cox and Ruschmeier, 2011). One of the joint market areas—Charleston, South Carolina—became a joint venture in early 2011.

The JFURSWG developed standardized reporting templates for joint ventures and joint market areas in 2010, with performance metrics. Joint ventures and joint market areas are now expected to show a reduction of at least 5 percent in overall costs or cost avoidance through use of shared initiatives (Cox and Ruschmeier, 2011).

LESSONS LEARNED FROM DEPARTMENT OF DEFENSE/ DEPARTMENT OF VETERANS AFFAIRS COLLABORATIONS

Overview

The committee reviewed the current nine formal joint ventures[5] that share resources in a variety of arrangements (see Box 5-1). To examine lessons learned from the joint ventures, related congressional testimony was examined, as well as other historical and current documentation, and personal interviews were conducted as needed for clarification. In-depth interviews with and briefings by knowledgeable DoD/VA Program Coordination Office and VHA Intergovernmental Affairs Office staff were conducted to learn the history of and ascertain the lessons learned from the creation of sharing agreements through the development phase and into the current, ongoing operations. Discussions were held at the October 2011 annual VA/DoD joint venture conference in Charleston, South Carolina, with representatives of the joint ventures, who updated attendees on their progress and described the many lessons learned from their experiences. The committee was also briefed in public session at its fourth meeting by the DoD and the VA leadership of the U.S. Air Force Medical Center, Travis Air Force Base, and the VA Northern California Health Care System joint venture. The committee arrived at its summary of lessons learned across joint ventures by considering the information collected from these sources.

Collaborations and Sharing Agreements

The VA and the DoD joint venture oversight program offices have reported on the elements of successful VA/DoD sharing and the common barriers or constraints encountered by collaborations. The following barriers and constraints are commonly cited as inhibiting successful collaboration:

- Lack of information management/information technology (IM/IT) interoperability
- Lack of joint business processes
    - o Accurate workload capture
    - o Billing processes
    - o Financial management systems that interface
- Space/new construction needs
    - o Getting facility planning and construction budget processes to align

[5] The Lovell FHCC is no longer formally classified as a joint venture because it is considered to be a unique organizational arrangement.

BOX 5-1
Currently Active Department of Veterans Affairs/ Department of Defense Joint Ventures*

Albuquerque, New Mexico (established in 1987)
377th Medical Group, Kirtland Air Force Base/New Mexico Veterans Affairs Health Care System

El Paso, Texas (established in 1987)
William Beaumont Army Medical Center/El Paso Veterans Affairs Health Care System

Honolulu, Hawaii (established in 1992)
Tripler Army Medical Center/Veterans Affairs Pacific Islands Health Care System (Spark M. Matsunaga Medical Center)

Fairfield, California (established in 1994)
60th Medical Group, David Grant Medical Center, Travis Air Force Base/Northern California Veterans Affairs Health Care System

Las Vegas, Nevada (established in 1994)
99th Medical Group, Nellis Air Force Base/Veterans Affairs Southern Nevada Health Care System (Michael O'Callaghan Federal Hospital)

Anchorage, Alaska (established in 1999)
3rd Medical Group, Elmendorf Air Force Base/Alaska Veterans Affairs Health Care System

Key West, Florida (established in 2000)
Naval Branch Health Clinic Key West/Miami Veterans Affairs Health Care System Community Based Outpatient Clinic Key West

Pensacola, Florida, and Biloxi, Mississippi (established in 2008)
Naval Hospital Pensacola/Veterans Affairs Gulf Coast Health Care Center (Biloxi)/81st Medical Group, Keesler Air Force Base/96th Medical Group, Eglin Air Force Base/325th Medical Group, Tyndall Air Force Base (5 coequal partners)

Charleston and Beaufort, South Carolina (established in 2011)
The Naval Health Clinic Charleston and the Ralph H. Johnson Veterans Affairs Medical Center jointly constructed and operate an ambulatory care clinic at the Naval Weapons Station, Charleston, South Carolina

---

* See Appendix C for brief histories of and lessons learned from these joint ventures.

- Disparity of DoD and VA rules and regulations, for example, for credentialing and for drug formularies
- Competitive health care job markets
- Leadership structures that do not align
- Restricted access to facilities on military bases (Malebranche, 2011, p. 13)

However, a number of factors common to successful joint ventures exist. They include

- Trust and integrity between VA and DoD
- A patient-centered focus
- Engaged and supportive leadership
- Regular meetings/ongoing communication
  - Monthly joint working group meetings
  - Quarterly executive management team meetings
  - Annual joint strategic planning retreats
- Addressing of issues early on
- Identifying win-win opportunities
  - It "doesn't have to be a zero sum game" (Malebranche, 2011, p. 13)

A brief history of each joint venture and a summary of self-reported lessons learned over time through trial and error is provided in Appendix C.

Summary of Lessons Learned from Department of Veterans Affairs/Department of Defense Health Care Collaborations

The committee's review of the DoD/VA collaborations highlights several aspects of the arrangements that either contributed to their success or created significant barriers. Three themes emerged consistently as contributing factors to a successful collaboration: (1) strong and committed leadership, (2) joint strategic planning and decision making, and (3) continuous and transparent communication. Four issues arose nearly as consistently as significant barriers to a combined mission: (1) separate governance structures for participating entities; (2) mixed reimbursement methodologies; (3) separate human resources policies and procedures along with high rates of turnover; and (4) the major, universally identified barrier cited by joint venture staffs, namely, the lack of a comprehensive electronic health record (EHR) system due to non-interoperable IT systems. While workarounds were devised in most sites for several of these barriers, they were uniformly labor intensive and often incomplete or inadequate to resolve the identified barriers. Finally, local context—that is, the nature of the local private health care system, the demographics of the target population, and the specific mission of the participating entities—affected the specific outcomes of the various collaborations.

Typical Factors Affecting Collaboration Success

Geographic Proximity Geographic proximity influenced the capability of the DoD and the VA to enter into collaborative efforts. A variety of terms were used to describe the new collaborative entity, the most prominent being "joint venture." Integration was commonly used to describe activities that were planned or implemented that provided a more "seamless" or less separate experience for beneficiaries utilizing each entity of the collaborative system. However, as noted previously in this report, "integration" was used to describe a wide range of sharing activities that did not always result in combining or coordinating these health care activities into a unified whole. Capability and readiness of each organization to engage in the joint ventures varied. Several of the collaborations defined operational oversight parameters through the creation of specific joint venture oversight committees. The more defined the oversight process, the more integration occurred. In addition to the three success themes outlined above, the committee identified several critical factors that strengthened collaborative services, including joint strategic planning with defined goals, objectives, and joint performance measures; membership on key operational committees; governance structures; and bilateral commitment to education and training of medical doctors and other care providers.

Strong Leadership Those joint ventures that had been in place a number of years, as well as those that were established more recently, profited from strong leadership. Commitment of senior leaders to the collaboration and operational efficacy of the enterprise was perceived as critical to success. These leaders worked together as a team to direct aspects of the joint ventures. Successful collaboration was a gradual achievement over time and persistence was found to be a critical factor. After the initial implementation of planned collaborative services, a number of different strategies, including workaround processes, were used to improve operational effectiveness as the organizational model evolved. Strong leadership that was consistent and leaders who communicated long-term organizational commitment to joint strategic goals and objectives were also critical. Where feasible, leadership transitions in demonstrations should be minimized or mitigated. Military leadership of MTFs is rotated on a predictable periodic cycle, and changes of command can disrupt developing collaborations unless a strong organizational commitment to the strategy is maintained and communicated. This was evident in the successful DoD/VA collaborations. Generally, leaders and managers of these case study models were supportive of the collaboration and committed to long-term goals to achieve better outcomes.

Open Communication Key to effective collaborations was good communication among leaders, and frequent interaction among mid-level managers, directors, and care providers. The vision for the collaboration was established and communicated by leaders. This was achieved through joint meetings and planned exchanges of information and opportunities to solve problems encountered with the system of patient care, referrals, and services. Effective collaborations for specific services occurred when DoD and VA leaders worked together early and often to establish meaningful outcome measures.

Range of Collaborative Initiatives

Collaborative initiatives included one or more of the range of services expected from large health systems. No single facility or system included a full integration or merger of all patient care services available at one or the other DoD or VA facility involved in the collaboration. Likewise, within most of the joint venture collaboration models, some of the service operations were more effective than others. Many factors influenced success of individual services or departments of the joint venture.

Specific initiatives varied across the continuum of acute care subspecialties to outpatient clinics to programs of education and training of health care professionals. Many of the collaborative organizations emphasized emergency treatment, including different strategies to improve emergency services and to decrease wait times for patients. Several joint ventures were developed because of the need to build new facilities for increased capacity. Patient care services were then developed collaboratively to promote optimal use of buildings and local area facilities and to reduce the cost of health care facility construction to the DoD or the VA system. Both acute care and outpatient care systems evolved or were actively planned, including inpatient and outpatient surgery capabilities.

Mental health services were a present and growing concern for the DoD and the VA organizations. Demand for these services increased during the time of implementation of several of the collaborations. Different strategies were identified to cope with the challenges of treating behavioral health patients of different ages and affected by military experiences or stress-related illnesses. Evaluations of these approaches on health care quality, safety, access, efficiency, and patient outcomes were not available to make generalizable conclusions.

Support services, such as pharmacy, laboratory, radiology, physical therapy, and other ancillary specialty services, were included in some measure in all of the case study collaborative organizations. Staffing for all collaborative services evaluated proved a difficult hurdle for full integration. There were instances of joint or collaborative staffing by both DoD and VA staff members. However, more often, these personnel remained separate with one or the other type of staff responsible for particular services. Personnel issues arose from differences inherent in the DoD and VA organizational cultures. These differences were difficult to surmount, often due to military readiness requirements of DoD staff members compared with civilian patient care mandates for VA staff members.

Outcomes

Intermediate outcomes and the long-term impact of these collaboration models varied with the length of time since their implementation. Financial targets were achieved by most of the joint ventures. Outcomes important to constituents were achieved at varying levels. Accountability and performance measurement were maintained through a variety of methods. In particular, many of the collaborative organizations attained better access to care for beneficiaries, reduced wait times, good patient satisfaction, improved coordination and time for referrals to subspecialties, more timely results for diagnostic tests, and better quality of care. In some cases, previously unavailable, new services were developed. In others, innovative approaches to care were initiated to address specific patient care or facility challenges. Longer-term plans were in progress for nearly all of the collaborations. As with other large-scale medical centers, leaders and members of these DoD/VA joint ventures are interested in meeting the demands of patient care that are arising from new technologies, better therapeutic interventions, and the increased need for reducing the costs of health care. To that end, many organizations are planning initiatives to address these goals, including programs for better care coordination across the joint venture and among care providers; improved processes to triage, admit, and discharge patients from the system in a more timely manner; the development of previously unavailable services; outreach to the community for better continuity of care for patients and families; and more appropriate management of medical emergencies.

Most of the DoD/VA collaborations had the goal of a "single standard of care" or improved clinical outcomes for patients as the primary focus of the joint venture. Graduate medical education, education of other licensed and unlicensed health care providers, and the best use and training of military medical personnel were important, but secondary, goals for the organizations. Educational aspects of these organizations were addressed as the situation for increased or improved opportunities for all types of students, residents, or learners arose.

Obstacles

Many obstacles were identified in achieving the vision of these joint ventures or models of DoD/VA collaboration. The obstacles were remarkably similar across the organizations. Most frequently identified were IT problems due to different and incompatible electronic data systems. Lack of shared EHR systems led to a number of cross-organizational systems problems. Efforts to address IT issues were costly and slow. Statistical data required for reporting and accreditation mandates proved more difficult to collect because of compatibility issues. Joint billing systems and procedures for sharing resources proved challenging as well. Purchasing of equipment and supplies was difficult due to different processes used by the DoD and the VA systems. Workarounds were created, but these were not always efficient.

Most of the joint ventures had issues with financing operations, financial systems, or tracking economic impacts. Efforts to address funding flow and allocation processes were an ongoing challenge. Mixed reimbursement regulations made the evaluation of revenues and expenses less accurate for the collaborative organization than for the DoD or the VA system alone. The economic impact of different staffing models using both DoD and VA personnel was difficult to measure for some of the organizations. Most included some type of joint planning or oversight as one way to improve human resource processes and financial management.

Despite systems obstacles, leaders, managers, and caregivers sought a variety of ways to address problems because of strong commitment to high-quality patient care. At the time of this evaluation, most of the organizations had in-progress plans for enhanced services going forward, for example, expanded subspecialty care, restorative medical specialties, advanced rehabilitation services, vision services, and long-term pain management plans for patients. Self-reported progress on a variety of parameters for these nine case studies of unique DoD/VA collaborative efforts was generally positive. While challenges and obstacles remain and some joint ventures have reduced their overall sharing due to changing organizational needs (e.g., Albuquerque), none reported plans for dissolution of their entire collaboration effort.

OUTCOMES AND BEST PRACTICES OF PRIVATE-SECTOR COLLABORATIVE VENTURES

The committee commissioned a review of the literature evaluating collaborative ventures among private hospitals and physician groups (see Appendix D). The review, conducted by Thomas D'Aunno, summarized the outcomes and best practices documented in the scholarly literature published in top-tier journals in the past decade (D'Aunno, 2012).

Collaboration Among Hospitals

Results from several studies show that certain initial changes in collaborative ventures among hospitals come quickly, relatively easily, and in a sequence: (1) integration of management functions (e.g., finance and accounting, human resources, managed care contracting, quality assurance and improvement programs, and strategic planning), followed by (2) integration of patient support functions (e.g., patient education), and then (3) integration of low-volume clinical services (e.g., Eberhardt, 2001).

However, integrating or consolidating larger-scale clinical services and closure of service lines typically encounters strong opposition—in many cases, clinical service integration did not occur at all. Similarly, some studies report little success at integrating the medical cultures of merged hospitals even after 3 years of effort. In short, substantial changes in core clinical services take a long time, and success is not guaranteed as conflicting interests emerge among stakeholders.

Despite these difficulties, there are examples of successful collaborations in which contextual factors and change processes made important contributions. Specifically, results from several case studies show that creating a centralized decision-making authority promotes effective collaboration, especially to the extent that this authority can develop shared values and vision with which the partner organizations must identify (Bazzoli et al., 2004). Furthermore, support from top managers is critical, but it should be complemented by buy-in from lower levels. This requires a great deal of communication within and across levels of hierarchy. Finally, at least one study identified strong and continuous external pressure on the partner organizations as a key for promoting the integration of clinical services.

Collaboration Among Physician Groups

Coddington et al. (1998) provide a useful case study of the early stages of change that focused on bringing physician partners together. They identify key phases of (1) establishing trust, (2) assessing the fit between the relative strengths of the organizations, (3) assessing the ability to deliver a high-quality product, (4) developing a business strategy, and (5) considering effects on competitive position. Similarly, Robinson (1998) emphasized the importance of fit and relative strengths of partners in bringing them together.

In general, results from studies of collaboration among physician groups emphasize the importance of managing trade-offs and tensions involved in organizational change: involving physicians versus respecting their time for patient care; slowly building trust versus frustration with slow progress; and building stakeholder buy-in versus building technical capacity (especially when buy-in and trust are enhanced by demonstrated technical capacity and improved performance).

Hospital-Physician Collaboration

Given their importance and obvious potential for problems, a relatively large number of process studies have focused on hospital-physician relationships. A major observation is the importance of developing a climate for change within the partner organizations. In turn, the role of physician leadership is universally noted as critical in developing a supportive climate for change because physician involvement is needed in both governance and management decisions. Results also highlight the importance of putting in place structures (such as incentives) and systems (especially information systems) to support changes in organizational processes and culture. As noted above, investment in management and clinical technologies and core competencies matters, as do shared vision and values.

The work of Devers and her colleagues (1994) stands out for its development of a three-part framework for assessing the extent to which consolidations achieve functional integration (business and management activities, noted above), physician-system integration (alignment of incentives and physician involvement in decision making), and clinical integration (e.g., common protocols). They find much functional integration, but little integration in the other areas—a result similar to that for collaborations among hospitals. The results are discouraging, but it appears that external context can promote change. Pressure from capitation and regulation, in particular, are related to more effective integration.

Concluding Observations from the Literature Review

Several concluding observations about the outcomes associated with collaboration among health care organizations and best practices for improving these outcomes arise from the literature review. First, there is considerable variation in the outcomes of collaborative ventures regardless of the criteria one uses to assess their performance. In fact, many, if not most, of these ventures fail to meet expectations in either the health care or the non-health fields. An exception to this result is mergers among hospitals, which seem to improve their financial performance, though not necessarily to societal advantage because available evidence indicates that improved performance comes mainly from increased market power (increased revenue) rather than efficiency gains per se.

Second, the financial performance of merged hospitals appears to be stronger than results obtained from other forms of collaboration. Mergers typically involve more centralization of authority compared with other collaborative ventures, such as alliances, and this may be an important factor in their relative success.

Third, mergers also are more costly than are alternatives for the organizations (and communities) involved, at least in terms of initial time and money needed to launch and implement them. Yet, one could argue that the risk involved in mergers seems to pay off for the hospitals themselves, though not uniformly given the variation that researchers observe in their performance.

Fourth, given substantial variation in their performance and relatively weak overall outcomes for many collaborative ventures, researchers and practitioners have begun to identify best practices for leading the *processes* involved in their implementation. Though results to date are useful, there is much more work to be done. See Box 5-2 (Box D-1 in Appendix D) for a relatively thorough checklist of best practices for implementing collaborative ventures. Few studies have examined the use of many of these practices in combination.

Fifth, the best available evidence nonetheless indicates that it is useful to conceive of these practices from the perspective of three phases or stages: (1) precollaboration activities, (2) transition work, and (3) follow-up efforts. Furthermore, these practices focus primarily on either technical tasks (e.g., due diligence with respect to antitrust issues, development of strategic plans, developing systems and incentives for change and improved performance) or people-oriented tasks (e.g., communicating effectively, involving key stakeholders, and overcoming resistance to change) (see Table 5-1 [Table D-4 in Appendix D]). Prior studies indicate that leaders need skills to focus on both technical and human tasks and, importantly, that failure to address both sets of tasks hinders implementation and performance (Battilana et al., 2010).

Sixth, the literature on collaboration and change among health care organizations in general has not given as much attention to the role of leadership as it should. To be sure, the importance of involving physicians in leadership roles is typically noted, but more fine-grained analyses are lacking (Gilmartin and D'Aunno, 2007). D'Aunno argues that effective leaders will communicate the need for change, mobilize others to accept changes, and evaluate implementation to make needed adjustments and promote optimal outcomes. Furthermore, though leaders need skills in both technical and people-oriented tasks to be effective, many individuals lack this combination of skills, which requires training or team approaches to leading change.

BOX 5-2
Checklist for Effective Implementation of Collaborative Ventures Among Health Care Organizations

I. Precollaboration Issues
   a. Cost-benefit analysis
      i. Choosing a collaboration model
      ii. Potential for reconfiguring resources through collaboration
   b. Partner selection
      i. Strategic intent
         1. Mutual and individual organizational interests
         2. Mission/vision alignment
      ii. Cultural compatibility
      iii. Context
   c. Strategic planning
      i. Planning committee
      ii. Setting priorities

II. Transition Issues
   a. Governance
      i. Monitoring and evaluation
      ii. Problem analysis and solution
   b. Decision making
   c. Conflict management
   d. Critical success and failure factors
      i. Speed of collaboration
      ii. Communication with employees

III. Follow-Up Issues
   a. Cultural integration
   b. Human resources
      i. Redeploying; managing layoffs; reducing employee resistance
   c. Operational integration
      i. Resource allocation
   d. Ongoing governance

SOURCE: D'Aunno et al., 2012.

Finally, relatively fragmented and narrow disciplinary approaches have hindered both research and practice in this area. For example, the vast majority of studies of hospital mergers focus on their financial performance (Vogt and Town, 2006), with little attention given to other key outcomes, such as access to care, and, similarly, with little attention to leadership using the concepts and principles discussed above. Promoting more effective col-

TABLE 5-1 Application of Best Practices to Collaboration Among Health Care Organizations: Technical and People-Focused Leadership Tasks

Technical Leadership Tasks	Best Practices
Plans and protocols for change are needed (see Box 5-2 [Box D-1 in Appendix D])	Blueprints are needed to manage complexity and promote due diligence and effective decision making by leaders of change (e.g., conducting thorough premerger assessment of potential partners)
Technical capacity building	Investment (time, money) is needed to build capacity for improved performance
Structures and systems to support change	Structures (especially incentives) and systems (especially information systems) are needed to promote change and to improve organizational performance
People-Focused Leadership Tasks	
External pressure	In most cases, external pressure/support for change increases both its speed and likelihood of success
Buy-in from all levels; critical role of central authority and shared vision	Support from top managers and leaders is essential, but buy-in is also needed from lower-level staff; a centralized group with authority for implementation of changes is critical, especially to develop a shared vision and goals for change
Communication	Communication is needed at all levels: What is the vision; why change is needed; what progress has been achieved
Role of physician leaders	Involvement of physician leaders, both formal and informal, in key decisions is critical to success
Managing tensions, trade-offs inherent in change	Involving physicians versus respecting their time for patient care; time needed to build trust versus frustration with slow progress; building stakeholder buy-in versus building technical capacity (especially when buy-in and trust are enhanced by demonstrated technical capacity and improved performance)
Core versus peripheral organizational features	Change in peripheral features of organizations, including management and support services, is easier to achieve than change in either core clinical services or organizational culture

SOURCE: D'Aunno et al., 2012.

laboration in health care will require a broader, interdisciplinary approach. Indeed, it is likely that current collaborative ventures among health care organizations may face greater challenges than in the past due to the increased complexity of the organizations themselves, including, for example, the difficulty of integrating their information technologies.

LESSONS LEARNED FROM OTHER FEDERAL AND PRIVATE-SECTOR COLLABORATIVE APPROACHES

The committee's review of both the DoD/VA and the private-sector collaborations suggests several lessons for the consideration of future attempts to combine federal health care facilities. First, while reduced expenditures and improved quality of care are among the top stated goals of these collaborative efforts, the published evidence does not support these expectations. Second, both public and private efforts demonstrate the importance of several key features of collaborative ventures that heavily influence their outcomes. These key features are

- strong, stable, and committed leadership;
- shared vision and values for the collaboration;
- clear and combined governance structures;
- combined, or at least compatible, policies at the department level;
- shared strategic planning and decision making;
- interoperable IT systems;
- compatible administrative processes;
- clear mechanisms to share resources, both human and financial; and
- constant and transparent communication.

These internal features then interact with pressures from and features of the external environment to determine the outcome of the collaboration.

Lessons Learned Relevant to the Lovell Federal Health Care Center

The Lovell FHCC was intended to address several lessons learned and barriers often cited by VA/DoD joint ventures seeking to improve services or reduce costs, or both. One is the need for strong leadership. Others are the problems caused by the differing accounting and billing systems of the VA and the DoD, which make it difficult to determine how much each partner should pay, and those caused by differing workforce policies, which put people with different pay levels doing the same jobs next to each other. The joint ventures are unanimous in citing the problem of incompatible IM/IT systems.

Strong Leadership

The departments chose local leaders for the Lovell FHCC merger process who were committed to its success. The Navy has consistently selected commanders of the naval hospital who strongly support the FHCC concept and even assigned a commanding officer to an unusually long tour of duty—4 instead of 2 years—for the period leading up to the launch of the FHCC in 2010. In addition, it was decided at the beginning to appoint the director of the North Chicago VAMC as director of the FHCC, who does not rotate as do military officers, which has provided important continuity in the key leadership position. Meanwhile, there have been four Navy medical leaders since 2003. There is also regular turnover in the active duty servicemembers leading the main subdivisions of the FHCC.

Differing Financial Systems

Differing financial systems have made it difficult for joint ventures to function optimally in several ways. First, they make it difficult for the partners to determine the costs of the services they provide to the other partner and to bill fairly. Second, they impose constraints on what each partner can pay for, even though it would be better overall for one partner to fund the equipment or the personnel of the other partner. The Lovell FHCC was designed to pool and spend funding in a way that does differentiate the sources. Instead, the departments are developing an innovative process for assigning responsibility for funding the FHCC in proportion to each department's patient workload, which takes place after the fact. That process for reconciliation is scheduled to be completed and automated by FY 2014 and to form the basis for each department's funding of the FHCC. The Hawaii joint venture is developing an alternative joint system, called the bi-directional enhanced document referral, or eDR, system, which has four modules: billing, third-party collections, analytics, and patient referral management.

Differing Personnel Systems

The DoD and the VA personnel systems for civilians have different statutory bases—Title 5 and Title 38 of the U.S. Code, respectively—and different job descriptions, which result in differences in pay, benefits, career ladders, and bonus systems for people who do the same work. This situation affects employee morale. The FHCC expects to solve this problem by transferring everyone into the same personnel system, the VA's in this case.

Differing Electronic Health Record Systems

Each joint venture has developed workarounds for managing patients seen by both VA and DoD providers. The most advanced is Janus, the graphical user interface developed by the Hawaii joint venture, which has been chosen to be the basis for developing a joint user interface for the VA/DoD integrated EHR system. Janus was originally developed to manage prescriptions for VA patients being admitted to the Tripler Army Hospital. The planners of the Lovell FHCC were well aware of the importance of having the capability of accessing and updating VA and DoD patient health records simultaneously, and they insisted on having some basic interoperability capabilities in place. The delays in delivering those capabilities have subjected the Lovell FHCC to the same limits on seamless patient care as the joint ventures have faced.

Conclusion

Collaborations are challenging, time-consuming, and expensive, even in the best of circumstances. A literature review focused on private-sector health care collaborative ventures (see Appendix D) leads to the conclusion that there is much we do not know about how to reduce the uncertainty and to increase the success of sharing resources. Additional interdisciplinary work in this area is critical to expanding our ability to create collaborations that achieve the desired outcomes.

REFERENCES

AMEDD (U.S. Army Medical Department). 2012. AMEDD DoD/VA Healthcare Resource Sharing Program: Joint Incentive Fund information. *DOD/VA Joint Incentive Fund guide* link. http://vadodrs.amedd.army.mil/jif.html (accessed September 6, 2012).

Battilana, J., M. J. Gilmartin, M. Sengul, A.-C. Pache, and J. Alexander. 2010. Leadership competencies for planned organizational change. *Leadership Quarterly* 21(3):422–438.

Bazzoli, G. J., L. Dynan, L. R. Burns, and C. Yap. 2004. Two decades of organizational change in health care: What have we learned? *Medical Care Research and Review* 61(3):247–331.

Carlisle, M. A., and J. Henius. 2010. VA/DoD Joint market opportunities update. Presentation at the 2010 VA/DoD Joint Venture Conference, Las Vegas, NV, October 26. http://www.tricare.mil/DVPCO/downloads/lvjvc/Day3-1045_JVConfJMOUpdateBriefv45.ppt (accessed September 21, 2012).

Coddington, D. C., K. D. Moore, and R. L. Clarke. 1998. *Capitalizing medical groups: Positioning physicians for the future*. New York: McGraw-Hill.

Cox, K., and E. Ruschmeier. 2011. Joint Facility Utilization Work Group update. Presentation at the 2011 Joint Venture Conference, Charleston, SC, October 18.

D'Aunno, T. (with the assistance of Y.-T. Chiang and M. Gilmartin). 2012. Collaboration among health care organizations: A review of outcomes and best practices for effective performance. Paper commissioned by the IOM Committee on Evaluation of the Lovell Federal Health Center Merger (see Appendix D).

Devers, K. J., S. M. Shortell, R. R. Gillies, D. A. Anderson, J. B. Mitchell, and K. L. Erickson. 1994. Implementing organized delivery systems: An integration scorecard. *Health Care Management Review* 19(3):7–20.

DoD/VA (Department of Defense/Department of Veterans Affairs). 2004. Memorandum of agreement for DoD/VA Health Care Sharing Incentive Fund. http://www.tricare.mil/DVPCO/downloads/MOAforJIF.pdf (accessed July 6, 2012).

DoD/VA. 2008. Fiscal Year 2003 National Defense Authorization Act, Department of Defense and Department of Veterans Affairs Demonstration Projects: Final report. July. http://www.tricare.mil/DVPCO/downloads/DSS%20Consolidated%20Final%20Report%20v%202.31%20formatted.doc (accessed August 7, 2012).

Eberhardt, J. L. 2001. Merger failure: A five year journey examined. *Healthcare Financial Management* 55(4):37–39.

GAO (U.S. General Accounting Office). 1978 (June 14). *Legislation needed to encourage better use of federal medical resources and remove obstacles to interagency sharing*. Report to the Congress of the United States by the comptroller general. HRD-78-54. Washington, DC: GAO. http://archive.gao.gov/f0902a/106271.pdf (accessed February 16, 2012).

Gilmartin, M. J., and T. D'Aunno. 2007. Leadership research in health care: A review and roadmap. *Academy of Management Annals* 1:387–438.

Malebranche, K. T. 2011. VA/DoD collaboration and medical sharing. Briefing by Karen T. Malebranche, Acting Chief Officer for Intergovernmental Affairs, Veterans Health Administration, Department of Veterans Affairs, for the IOM Committee on Evaluation of the Lovell Federal Health Center Merger, February 25.

Navy Medicine. 2012. Joint initiatives. http://www.med.navy.mil/BUMED/DODVA/Pages/JointInitiatives.aspx (accessed July 6, 2012).

Robinson, J. C. 1998. Consolidation of medical groups into physician practice management organizations. *Journal of the American Medical Association* 279(2):144–149.

VA/DoD. 2006. *VA/DoD Joint Executive Council FY 2005 annual report*. http://www.tricare.mil/DVPCO/downloads/VADoD2005.pdf (accessed August 7, 2012).

VA/DoD. 2008. Health care resources sharing guidelines: Memorandum of understanding between VA and DoD, October 31. AMEDD DOD/VA Healthcare Resource Sharing Program link. http://vadodrs.amedd.army.mil/Policy/MOU.html (accessed July 6, 2012).

Vogt, W. B., and R. Town. 2006. How has hospital consolidation affected the price and quality of hospital care? *Research Synthesis Report No. 9*. Princeton, NJ: Robert Wood Johnson Foundation, The Synthesis Project.

6

Findings, Conclusions, and Recommendations

The Institute of Medicine was asked to form a committee to evaluate the merger of a Navy military treatment facility (MTF) and a Department of Veterans Affairs (VA) medical center in North Chicago into a federal health care center (FHCC) in terms of its benefit to the Department of Defense (DoD) and the VA compared with maintaining separate VA and DoD facilities. Specifically, the sponsor asked the committee to undertake—but not be limited to—six tasks (Box 6-1).

In addition to addressing each of the tasks outlined by the sponsor, the committee developed six recommendations regarding the Lovell FHCC merger.

STUDY TASKS

Task 1: Assessment Criteria

The committee recommends (see Recommendation 3) that the DoD and the VA conduct a comprehensive evaluation of the Lovell FHCC demonstration designed to provide the basis for determining at the end of the 5-year demonstration period whether the FHCC model has been a success and whether it should be adopted in other locations where the VA and the DoD share health care markets. Appendix B contains the framework for such an evaluation that could be adopted by the VA and the DoD.

The purpose of the evaluation is to understand how the FHCC demonstration functioned and the factors that explain its evolution and outcomes,

BOX 6-1
Substantive Study Tasks*

1. Establish criteria for near-term and longer-term assessment of the success of facility integration that can be used in follow-on assessments. Determine if success criteria would be different if the partner DoD health care facility was supporting operational units instead of basic/advanced training units, such as the Navy Health Center Great Lakes.
2. Evaluate whether performance benchmarks that DoD and VA have established in their executive agreement have been achieved.
3. Examine the lessons learned from similar mergers elsewhere in the federal and private health sectors that may be applicable to DoD/VA mergers.
4. Evaluate the most pressing concerns of the stakeholders and recommend ways to mitigate or eliminate these concerns.
5. Evaluate the specific impact of the merger on the level and quality of training received by active duty medical personnel and VA providers.

* The sixth task was to prepare a written report with findings, conclusions, and recommendations for the DoD and the VA that will be available to the general public.

which would provide lessons for designing more effective FHCCs in the future. Thus the evaluation framework looks at a much broader range of explanatory variables than internal processes (called implementation initiatives in the evaluation framework in Appendix B) that might affect outcomes, such as a single chain of command or integrated clinics. The broader framework includes the influence of the national and local contexts and of organizational capabilities and readiness. This approach makes it possible to understand not only if it is a successful demonstration (or not) but also which factors made it successful (or not).

Task 1 asks for criteria for assessing the "success" of the FHCC demonstration in the short term and the longer term. The framework in Appendix B considers short-term outcomes to be those observed in the first year or 2 and long-term outcomes to be those that emerge after 3–5 years. The Lovell FHCC is a difficult case because the phenomenon being demonstrated—an integrated health care center—was not fully in place the day it became operational and, in terms of having an electronic health record and other information management systems in place to support integrated operations, may not be fully in place within the 5-year time frame of the demonstration. Nevertheless, there will be lessons to learn, as Chapter 3 demonstrates, and some outcomes can be measured, although it might take several years to discern effects.

The executive agreement (EA) for the Lovell FHCC identifies the desired outcomes. To recapitulate from Chapter 5, they are (compared with operating separate VA and DoD health care centers in the same health care market): more accessible health care, higher-quality health care (e.g., more preventive services and continuity and coordination of care), cost savings or cost avoidance, increased market share among eligible beneficiaries, greater patient satisfaction, greater provider satisfaction, improved clinical proficiency of active duty providers, improved training programs, and better research opportunities. Operational measures for each of these outcomes need to be identified and adopted. Chapter 4 indicates that, first, data on some but not all of these outcomes are being collected monthly as part of the 15 integration benchmarks and that, second, it is difficult to discern trends in the short term.

The outcome criteria of most importance are *financial*, such as the net reduction in costs per episode of care or procedures; *clinical*, such as the numbers of preventable drug-drug interactions and allergic reactions to drugs; *patient-focused*, such as time to third appointment and standardized patient satisfaction survey results; and, in the case of the Lovell FHCC, *military operational readiness-focused*, such as the percentage of recruits unable to graduate on time for medical reasons. The evaluation framework in Appendix B suggests some intermediate-term outcomes that correspond to some of the outcomes expected of the Lovell FHCC listed above, such as higher patient volume and quality of care measures. Other metrics take longer to collect and analyze and are listed as long-term outcomes, such as cost per patient, increased market share, and health status of patients.

As part of this task, the committee was also asked to consider the differences in assessment criteria for FHCCs serving training units (such as the Recruit Training Command [RTC] at Great Lakes) and those serving operational units. Operational units are more varied and have more complex mission-related medical issues than training units. They require medical personnel with knowledge of military medicine, which VA medical personnel do not routinely have, and who respect the unique cultural identity of servicemembers in operational units. There are also service-specific differences in medical needs and the relationship between the medical and line units (e.g., Air Force medical units report to the local operational commander, while the Army and Navy medical commands are centralized). Administrative business functions would be similar for medical units serving training and operational units. Despite these differences between training and operational units, however, the criteria for success in an operational versus a training unit will be similar, although the benchmarks might be set at different levels.

Task 2: Performance Benchmarks

The departments specified 15 "integration benchmarks" that incorporate 37 measures of the degree of integration success. Most of the integration benchmark results are updated monthly (some are updated less often, such as the annual audit reports and facility inspection results). Each measure is reported on a 5-point scale from highly unsuccessful to highly successful, according to a 117-page technical manual. The resulting Integration Scorecard is reviewed monthly by the FHCC leadership and the departments.

The committee has a mostly positive evaluation of whether performance benchmarks that the DoD and the VA have established in their EA have been achieved. As of June 2012, there were 23 fives (highly successful), 5 fours (very successful), 6 threes (successful), 1 two (unsuccessful), 1 one (highly unsuccessful), and 1 unrated measure. The scores for some measures have varied, but rarely more than one point up or down or for more than 1 or 2 months since ratings began. Further details are in Chapter 4.

One measure that is critical to integration—that is, the implementation of joint information management/information technology (IM/IT) capabilities—has not been successful, as noted in Chapter 3. It is unlikely to improve further until parts of the new electronic health record (EHR) being developed jointly by the DoD and the VA become available, beginning with a joint pharmacy program scheduled to be operational in 2014.

The committee notes that most of the performance measures are specific to the VA or to the DoD rather than to the integrated performance of the FHCC, which is why the committee concluded that these alone do not constitute the basis for an adequate evaluation of the Lovell FHCC's success at achieving integration. The main purpose of the performance benchmarks was to address the concerns of the respective departments that the Lovell FHCC experiment might fail badly before the end of the 5-year demonstration period.

The Government Accountability Office (GAO) issued reports in 2011 and 2012 on the Lovell FHCC's progress toward implementing the 12 integration areas covered in the April 2010 EA. In its June 2012 report, the GAO found that 6 of the 12 were fully implemented (governance structure, patient priority system, contracting, research, quality assurance, and contingency planning), compared with 4 in 2011. Integration benchmarks was one of the five areas "in progress" (the others were reporting requirements, workforce management, property, and fiscal authority). The GAO found that one area—IM/IT—was delayed, requiring workarounds that were resulting in additional costs for the Lovell FHCC in terms of reduced provider productivity and increased administrative burden. The GAO found, as did this committee, that the FHCC has not quantified the extra costs but indicated that the FHCC has engaged the Center for Naval Analyses to assess costs and document any savings from integrated patient care (GAO, 2012).

Task 3: Lessons Learned from Other Federal and Private-Sector Health Care Mergers

The committee addressed the third task by commissioning a comprehensive overview of the private-sector health care merger literature and analyzing the lessons learned reported by the nine VA/DoD joint venture sites. The review of the private-sector merger literature appears in Appendix D, "Collaboration Among Health Care Organizations: A Review of Outcomes and Best Practices for Effective Performance," and is summarized in Chapter 5. The lessons learned from the VA/DoD joint ventures reported at the annual joint venture conferences are also summarized in Chapter 5, and short profiles of each joint venture and the lessons learned they have reported are in Appendix C, "Department of Veterans Affairs/Department of Defense Joint Ventures: Brief Histories and Lessons Learned."

Task 4: Stakeholder Concerns

The committee was not able to conduct a statistically valid survey of the most important stakeholders, the patients. However, the committee heard from stakeholders, including several veteran and retired military enrollees, at the Lovell FHCC at its third meeting, held in North Chicago.

The commanding officer of the RTC, who receives daily reports on recruits being seen at the west campus emergency room or admitted to the hospital, said that the FHCC was performing as well as the Naval Hospital/Health Clinic Great Lakes had been, for example, in the percentage of recruits unable to go to their next assignment for medical reasons.

The president of the affiliated medical school, the Rosalind Franklin University of Medicine and Science, had a positive view of the effect of the Lovell FHCC merger on medical education and training. He and senior faculty and deans told staff who visited the university earlier that the merger created additional training and research opportunities because of the larger and more varied patient base. Additionally, the performance benchmark score for trainee satisfaction, as measured by the Lerner Perception Survey each July, was 5 in July 2011, compared with the baseline score of 4. The amount of research funding, as measured quarterly, has scored 5s, compared with the baseline score of 3.

The veterans testified that they were satisfied with the care they were receiving at the Lovell FHCC. They said initially there were concerns among the veterans enrolled at the FHCC that they would not receive the same level of attention as before when the Navy started using the center but that those fears were not realized. Veterans appreciate the new facilities and mingling with active duty servicemembers and their families. The retirees appreciated the easier access to services at the west campus than when the Navy clinic was still on the naval base.

The veterans had two major concerns, however (which were consistent with earlier interviews of several veterans and retirees by committee staff). One concern was that the time it takes to fill prescriptions was much longer than before the merger, averaging at least an hour for veterans (active duty servicemembers have first priority and go to the head of the line). Although the wait times had shortened significantly more recently, they were still unacceptable. As documented in Chapter 3, the pharmacy, which is located in the ambulatory care center (ACC), was sized with the expectation that refills would be available through the VA's Consolidated Mail Order Pharmacy (CMOP) program, but the DoD did not approve of having its beneficiaries use it. At the time this report was drafted, the FHCC was preparing another executive decision memorandum requesting the use of the CMOP program to ease congestion in the pharmacy.

The other concern was the location of the mental health clinic on the third floor of the ACC, which is accessed through a balcony over the atrium between the ACC and the hospital building. The veterans said that some patients, many of them with posttraumatic stress disorder or generalized anxiety disorder, were deterred from using the service because of a fear of heights. They also feared that someone would be able to commit suicide by jumping from that location. There was a similar fear about the new four-story parking garage. This was a concern during the building of the ACC and the garage although they were considered to exceed applicable building standards. Subsequently, a veteran did commit suicide by jumping from the third story of the atrium, although not from near the mental health clinic. Consequently, steps are being taken to retrofit the atrium and the top level of the parking garage with fall protection barriers.

Task 5: Staff Training

The committee did not find that staff training was affected by the merger except in one area, which was of special concern to the Navy in agreeing to merge clinical operations with the VA in the FHCC. The concern was whether independent duty corpsmen (IDCs) and active duty advanced practice nurses (APNs) would be able to practice their skills in the merged FHCC, especially in the inpatient setting. One issue is that the Navy privileges APNs even though they are not licensed as such, while the VA requires nurses to be licensed for independent practice. Another issue is that IDCs must be ready to be deployed to locations where they are not under the direct supervision of a physician or a nurse and, therefore, must be able to perform procedures that would not be allowed in the civilian sector, including in the VA health system. As described in Chapter 3, special training of VA staff on the duties of corpsmen was provided, and several compromises were reached to allow APNs and IDCs to maintain needed clinical proficiencies at the Lovell FHCC.

RECOMMENDATIONS

Develop Uniform Policies, Procedures, and Business Practices for Federal Health Care Centers

Findings

The Lovell FHCC model is distinguished from other VA/DoD collaborative initiatives primarily by being a single organization rather than a partnership. The concept is that a health center that is operationally unified will be more cost effective and better positioned to provide high-quality health care. The implementation of the Lovell FHCC highlights the difficulty of achieving unified policies and procedures when each parent department has its own planning, operating, and reporting procedures for the same health care center functions. Some of the differences stem from different missions (e.g., the military's need to ensure and document individual medical readiness to deploy), but many others are just two ways of accomplishing the same thing (e.g., clinical credentialing).

The dilemma is that the departments operate multiple health care delivery centers—59 DoD military treatment facilities and 153 VA medical centers—to which they each want to apply common standards, business rules, administrative systems, and reporting requirements. Health system administrators are responsible for the overall performance of their health care systems and are naturally reluctant to exempt any one facility from their system's rules. The history of the Lovell FHCC implementation is replete with instances in which the FHCC was unable to obtain consensus on using a single approach to a particular function and therefore has had to carry out both. Having to operate two EHR systems is a prime example, because it affects patient care, but there are many other examples of dual systems that reduce efficiency and inhibit integrated clinical and administrative services.

The bottom-up consensus process used in implementing the Lovell FHCC accounted in part for the outcome of incomplete integration. That approach was very useful for bringing to the surface differences in department procedures and statutory authorizations that had to be addressed in implementing the Lovell FHCC and any future FHCCs, but it also made it harder to reach agreement on a single way of doing things. The process of vetting solutions up the department administrative chains was not only time-consuming, it also provided many opportunities to agree to disagree on integrated approaches. Some issues could be appealed to the Health Executive Council (HEC) or to the Joint Executive Council (JEC), but the HEC and the JEC are interdepartmental committees, not authoritative decision-making bodies. The FHCC leadership consistently pushed for unified policies and procedures but was not always successful.

Recently, the VA and the DoD agreed to develop a unified approach at the enterprise level in some cases rather than to try to facilitate local solutions. Prime examples of joint enterprise-level solutions include the efforts to develop a joint EHR system (the integrated EHR, or iEHR) and a joint disability examination process for wounded, ill, or injured servicemembers (the Integrated Disability Evaluation System, or IDES). These agreements resulted from top-down directives from the DoD and VA secretaries, who are personally monitoring progress through regular meetings.

Conclusions

Additional opportunities remain to develop enterprise-level solutions to differing department requirements and business practices. This would enable more cost-effective joint health care delivery collaborations, whether they are DoD/VA joint ventures or FHCCs. An example of an opportunity to work out a common approach would be a unified process for credentialing health care providers. Other opportunities include uniform cost accounting, civilian workforce policies, performance and quality measures, access to care standards, drug formularies, and mail-order drug refill programs. The more that common policies and processes are adopted, the more integrated FHCCs can be, which in turn should increase opportunities to achieve more accessible and cost-effective patient care.

> **RECOMMENDATION 1. Before establishing additional federal health care centers, the Department of Veterans Affairs and the Department of Defense should agree on a governance plan and common policies and procedures for joint health care delivery functions.**

Achieving additional enterprise-level agreement on single policies and processes is a critical first step in planning additional future FHCCs and would also assist the Lovell FHCC in reaching its full potential. The VA and the DoD may also have to obtain statutory authority from Congress to integrate authority, employees, and funding, and to allow the transfer of property between the two departments.

Complete Development of a Jointly Usable Electronic Health Record System Before Establishing Additional Federal Health Care Centers

Findings

The IM/IT goal for the Lovell FHCC is to "safely interface VA and DoD legacy systems to support an integrated DoD/VA facility with multiple care locations" (Filippi, 2011). The Lovell FHCC expected the software capabilities that its clinicians and other subject matter experts had identified in early 2009 as the minimum needed for integrated use of the VA and the DoD EHR systems to be in place when the FHCC opened on October 1, 2010, but they were significantly delayed. These included single registration and single sign-on (implemented in December 2010), orders portability for radiology (implemented in June 2010), and orders portability for laboratory (implemented in March 2011). Two capabilities are still not ready for implementation, namely, orders portability for pharmacy and for consults, and are not expected to be ready for several years.

Conclusions

The lack of EHR system interoperability, despite the development of workarounds (such as hiring five pharmacists to manually check both EHR systems for possible drug allergies and interactions), significantly reduced the efficiency of health care delivery for at least the first year of Lovell FHCC operations. The lack of single-entry access to both EHR systems has hindered the ability of the Lovell FHCC to deliver higher-quality or more efficient, cost-effective health care and to provide better research opportunities. The ability to seamlessly deliver electronic health information from the veteran, military beneficiary, and health care provider perspectives should be the hallmark of an FHCC.

RECOMMENDATION 2. Additional federal health care centers should not be implemented until an interoperable or joint Department of Defense/Department of Veterans Affairs electronic health record system becomes available.

The level of interoperability should be what the Center for Information Technology Leadership calls Level 4, the highest level, which is when structured electronic data in each system can be computed by the other system. At Level 3, for example, structured data in one EHR system can be viewed but not computed by the other EHR system.

The DoD and VA secretaries have committed their departments to developing such a system together—a new joint EHR system (the iEHR)—

rather than upgrading their current (now legacy) EHR systems and trying to develop interoperability software. The iEHR will be developed in phases with some modules, such as pharmacy, scheduled to be completed in 2014; the final modules are due for completion in 2017. It would be helpful for the iEHR system to have the capabilities identified by the FHCC clinical task group as the initial set of core IT capabilities required by the Lovell FHCC earlier rather than later in the development process if establishing additional FHCCs is a priority.

Develop Criteria for Selecting Future Federal Health Care Center Sites

Findings

The VA and the DoD have developed criteria for identifying "joint market areas" for increased health care sharing. They are health care markets with large DoD and VA beneficiary populations where shared facilities and services would provide access to services or infrastructure not available in one or the other organization; improve efficiency through economies of scale; reduce duplication of services, infrastructure, or both; and mitigate the impact of deployment on access. The Joint Facility Utilization Resource Sharing Working Group under the VA/DoD HEC has identified more than a dozen joint market areas and has worked with them to develop additional sharing agreements.

The VA and the DoD have adopted a definition of joint ventures. They are local alliances or partnerships formed to facilitate comprehensive cooperation, shared risk, and mutual benefit, and they are expected to last at least 5 years. To qualify as a joint venture, the departments look for regular ongoing interactions in at least several of the following areas: staffing, clinical workload, business processes, management, information technology, logistics, education and training, and research capabilities. One of the joint market areas—Charleston, South Carolina—graduated to being a joint venture in early 2011.

The VA and the DoD have not defined FHCCs and do not have criteria for choosing their locations. The Lovell FHCC is considered to be unique and is no longer a joint venture.

Conclusions

To a large extent, the criteria should address the juncture at which FHCC lower operating costs or greater effectiveness are shown to outweigh the associated significant implementation costs (i.e., a single organizational structure and integrated administrative and clinical processes) enough for the FHCC structure to be regarded as preferable to a joint venture sharing arrangement and its comparative cost effectiveness. At the time that information gathering for this report was completed (June 2012), the costs of implementing the Lovell FHCC had been substantial, while efficiencies and cost savings that might be expected had only had a limited time to transpire.

The VA and the DoD should base a decision to establish another FHCC on evidence that it would provide higher performance in quality, access, or cost effectiveness compared with other arrangements, including a joint venture agreement. An important source of evidence on the costs and benefits will be the comprehensive evaluation of the Lovell FHCC recommended below.

RECOMMENDATION 3. The Department of Veterans Affairs and the Department of Defense should develop criteria for selecting future federal health care center (FHCC) sites. The criteria should address the costs and benefits of establishing a fully integrated organization compared with the costs and benefits of other collaborative arrangements, such as joint ventures, taking into account local health care market trends, institutional capabilities and readiness, unique local circumstances, and departmental limiting factors. Only when firm criteria based on cost savings and the expectation of enhanced health care service delivery are met should the concept of a future FHCC be considered.

Analyze and Promulgate Lessons Learned from the Lovell Federal Health Care Center Experience

Findings

The leadership of the Lovell FHCC encountered numerous issues that had to be resolved to achieve an integrated organization and uniform policies and procedures. Many of the issues resulted from conflicting policies and procedures of the VA, the DoD, and the Navy. Some were the result of statutory requirements and the lack of statutory authority.

Many of the issues have been resolved by adopting the policy or procedure of one department with the agreement of the other department. In some cases, agreement on a single policy or procedure could not be reached and workarounds had to be developed to meet the requirements of the two departments. Some issues could not be resolved because of irreconcilable policy differences, such as an integrated police force including active duty masters-at-arms on the west campus. Ultimately, four critically necessary actions had to be authorized by legislation: (1) the authority to transfer civilian employees from one department to the other; (2) the authority to transfer the ACC and other Navy-built facilities and related personal property and equipment from the DoD to the VA; (3) the authority for the DoD to transfer funds to a joint Department of the Treasury account under the VA; and (4) the authority for DoD beneficiaries to be treated by the Lovell FHCC as they would be at an MTF. However, the legislation authorized these only as part of a 5-year demonstration in North Chicago.

Every difference between VA and DoD policies and procedures had to be addressed at multiple regional- and headquarters-level decision points. This often took months, and sometimes years, to resolve through numerous drafts and meetings. The extra burden of this process was very heavy, especially at the local level where planning the integration was an extra duty for most staff members.

Conclusions

The implementation of the Lovell FHCC provides a road map to issues that will be encountered in any future attempts to establish FHCCs and offers many examples of ways to overcome or bypass those impediments. It would be extremely beneficial for planners of future FHCCs, and in many cases for existing and future joint ventures, to adopt solutions developed and already approved by the VA and the DoD without having to undertake the long negotiation process that the FHCC had to go through. An important, groundbreaking contribution would be made by the FHCC staff if they developed joint DoD/VA guidance materials, including a best-practices document or guidebook to disseminate local solutions or "fixes" arrived at to solve problems that arose in the implementation of the merger.

RECOMMENDATION 4. The Department of Veterans Affairs and the Department of Defense should systematically compile and analyze the lessons learned from the Captain James A. Lovell Federal Health Care Center merger experience, including both what and what not to do, and disseminate them through onsite consultation, webinars, technical assistance, and other means to other federal health care center sites considering joint ventures and related collaborative arrangements.

Conduct a Comprehensive Evaluation of the Lovell Federal Health Care Center Demonstration

Findings

The Lovell FHCC has been in operation for less than 2 years and is still implementing parts of the integration plan. It is too early to tell how successful the overall integration effort has been or will be when the demonstration period ends in 2015. That there have been substantial one-time costs is clear, but whether these have led or will lead to lasting efficiencies or can be adopted by future FHCCs to avoid unnecessary costs is not yet known.

The Lovell FHCC is tracking certain performance indicators designed to inform about the relative degree of success or failure, for example, if the facility is providing poor, less, or more expensive care; hurting operational readiness; reducing patient satisfaction and staff morale; or providing fewer education and research opportunities. However, the VA and the DoD have not adopted a comprehensive evaluation plan to judge objectively the success of the Lovell FHCC at the end of the 5-year demonstration period and to help them to decide whether the Lovell FHCC would be applicable in other locations.

Conclusions

Without a formal evaluation plan, the success of the integration effort will be more difficult to determine after the 5-year demonstration period than it should be because not all the data needed for such an evaluation are being collected prospectively.

> **RECOMMENDATION 5. In considering the Captain James A. Lovell Federal Health Care Center merger and future collaborative arrangements, the Department of Veterans Affairs and the Department of Defense should develop a comprehensive evaluation framework with defined and measurable criteria for assessing performance that take into account local and national contexts, organizational capabilities and readiness, implementation plans, intermediate outcomes, and likely long-term impact.**

The committee offers a comprehensive evaluation framework in Appendix B.

Expand the Knowledge Base on Federal Health Care Collaborations

Findings

The DoD and the VA have not systematically analyzed the experience of the Lovell FHCC and the lessons that may be learned from it in considering if and where to establish additional integrated VA/DoD health care centers modeled after the Lovell FHCC merger.

Conclusions

The Lovell FHCC offers a number of lessons learned about what works well—and what does not—that would be useful to future FHCC decision makers and planners. The mergers of private-sector health care organizations do not provide adequate models for integration of federal health care organizations because they are narrowly based on increasing market share and revenue and usually do not involve clinical integration, only administrative consolidation. Published studies demonstrate substantial variation in performance after private-sector collaborative ventures. Nonetheless, lessons learned from private-sector mergers and pertinent data would be useful for both the Lovell FHCC and future endeavors (Appendix D contains a paper commissioned by the committee on the experiences of joint ventures and private-scector health care mergers).

RECOMMENDATION 6. The Department of Veterans Affairs (VA) and the Department of Defense (DoD) should fund studies to address the key findings and questions raised by the experiences of the Captain James A. Lovell Federal Health Care Center merger and other VA/DoD collaborative arrangements. These studies should address the implementation issues involved in establishing collaborative arrangements, including leadership, governance, communication, organizational culture, coordination, incentives, and related factors associated with improved access, quality, slowing of the increase in the cost of care, and military readiness.

REFERENCES

Filippi, D. 2011. James A. Lovell Federal Health Care Center IT informational brief. Presentation by the director of the DoD/VA Interagency Program Office to the IOM Committee on Evaluation of the Lovell Federal Health Care Center Merger at its first meeting, Washington, DC, February 25.

GAO (Government Accountability Office). 2012. *VA/DoD Federal Health Care Center: Costly information technology delays continue and evaluation plan lacking*. GAO-12-669. Washington, DC: GAO. http://www.gao.gov/products/GAO-12-669 (accessed September 21, 2012).

Appendix A

Biographical Sketches of Committee Members and Staff

COMMITTEE MEMBERS

Michael M. E. Johns, M.D. (*Co-Chair*), is the chancellor of Emory University and executive vice president for health affairs, emeritus. Before he became chancellor in 2007, he led Emory's Robert W. Woodruff Health Sciences Center from 1996 to 2007. The center is the largest, most comprehensive health care system in Georgia, and he led its extensive facilities improvement plan, which included new biomedical research, nursing school, vaccine center, and cancer institute buildings, and the complete reconfiguration and rebuilding of Emory's midtown Crawford Long Hospital (now Emory University Hospital Midtown) campus. Dr. Johns co-chaired Emory's University-wide Strategic Planning Committee that set the strategic direction of the university for the next decade or more. From 1990 to 1996, he served as dean of the School of Medicine, vice president of the medical faculty, and head of the physician practice plan at the Johns Hopkins University. Prior to that, beginning in 1984 as a professor and chair of Otolaryngology-Head and Neck Surgery at Johns Hopkins, he also served as associate dean for clinical practice and reorganized the faculty practice plan, and planned and developed the Johns Hopkins Outpatient Center. Joining the Department of Otolaryngology and Maxillofacial Surgery at the University of Virginia Medical Center in 1977, he rose from the position of assistant professor to professor. From 1975 to 1977, he served as assistant chief of the Otolaryngology Service at the Walter Reed Army Medical Center. Dr. Johns has been a significant contributor to many of the leading organizations and policy groups in health care, including the

Association of American Medical Colleges (AAMC), the Commonwealth Fund Task Force on Academic Health Centers, and the Association of Academic Health Centers (AAHC). Dr. Johns serves on the Uniformed Services University of the Health Sciences' (USUHS's) Board of Regents, as well as on various other boards, including Johnson & Johnson, the Genuine Parts Company, AMN Healthcare, the National Health Museum, and the Satcher Health Leadership Institute. He is a past member of the National Governing Board of the Clinical Center and of the Council of the National Center for Research Resources of the National Institutes of Health (NIH). He has served as a member of the board of directors and as president of the American Board of Otolaryngology, as chair of the AAHC, and as chair of the AAMC's Council of Deans. He served as editor of the *Archives of Otolaryngology* from 1992 to 2005, and serves on the editorial board of the *Journal of the American Medical Association*. Dr. Johns received his bachelor's degree from Wayne State University and graduated with distinction from the University of Michigan Medical School, where he remained for his internship and residency. He is an Institute of Medicine (IOM) member and has served as vice chair of the IOM Council and as a member of the Governing Board of the National Research Council, as well as on many committees, including as chair of the Committee on Optimizing Graduate Medical Trainee (Resident) Hours and Work Schedules to Improve Patient Safety from 2007 to 2009.

Stephen M. Shortell, Ph.D., M.P.H., M.B.A. (*Co-Chair*), is the dean of the School of Public Health, Blue Cross of California Distinguished Professor of Health Policy & Management, and professor of organization behavior in the School of Public Health and the Haas School of Business at the University of California, Berkeley. He has affiliated appointments to the Department of Sociology and serves as a member of the Center for Health Research, the Industrial Relations Institute, and the Institute for Personality and Social Research at the University of California, Berkeley, and at the Institute for Health Policy Research at the University of California, San Francisco. His research interests include organizational correlates of quality and outcomes of care; the evaluation of total quality management and community-based health improvement initiatives; strategic change in the health care sector (i.e., evolution of integrated delivery systems); and strategic alliances between physicians and other health entities. He teaches courses in strategic management of health services and organization behavior in health. Dr. Shortell was A.C. Buehler Distinguished Professor of Health Services Management and professor of organization behavior in the J.L. Kellogg Graduate School of Management at Northwestern University from 1982 to 1998. He was assistant professor from 1974 to 1976, associate professor from 1976 to 1979, and professor from 1979 to 1982 in the

School of Public Health and Community Medicine in the Department of Health Services at the University of Washington. Dr. Shortell has published 14 books and monographs, and more than 250 reports and editorials. He received his B.B.A. in business administration from the University of Notre Dame, his M.P.H. in hospital administration/public health from the University of California, Los Angeles, and his M.B.A. in business administration and Ph.D. in behavioral science from the University of Chicago Graduate School of Business. He is an IOM member and has served as a member of the IOM Council and on its executive committee. Dr. Shortell is past chair of the Gustave Lienhard Award committee. He has also served as a member of the IOM Membership Committee and the Section 11 chair of the IOM Membership Section Leaders. In addition, he has been a member of many committees, including serving as the chair of the Subcommittee on Quality Improvement Organizations' Evaluation from 2004 to 2006.

Nancy R. Adams, R.N., M.S.N., is a senior partner with Martin, Blanck & Associates (Martin-Blanck), a federal health services consulting firm based in Falls Church, Virginia. Martin-Blanck provides critical assistance to public and private sector clients focused on federal and state health care delivery systems. Martin-Blanck has more than two dozen senior executive partners with expertise in health care policy, program development, management, informatics, and strategic planning. Ms. Adams joined Martin-Blanck in August 2005 after a distinguished career as a military officer and as a senior executive in the federal government. She is one of Martin-Blanck's leading experts on federal health acquisition policies and procedures. In addition, she brings extensive clinical, administrative, and senior management experience with large, complex government health care systems, and has demonstrated experience and competency as an organizational leader, an effective communicator, and a resource manager with results that have produced performance improvements. Ms. Adams served as the source selection authority for five major, multibillion-dollar health care procurements for the Department of Defense (DoD). All procurements were accomplished on time and two awards were sustained on appeal with the General Accounting Office. In addition to shepherding the unprecedented contracting effort to completion, she also defined the business planning process and the organizational structure for the military services and TRICARE Management Activity to administer the three regional health care support contracts. Following the procurement process, Ms. Adams was the initial regional director for the TRICARE Regional Office-North and was responsible for managing the DoD health care contract for 20 state regions, worth more than $1 billion annually. From 1998 to 2002, Ms. Adams (MG rank) served as the commanding general of the Tripler Army Medical Center in Hawaii, a 266-bed tertiary care medical center with 3,000 personnel and a $245 million annual budget. She led the organization to a perfect score on the survey by the Joint Commission. She also had responsibility for TRICARE Pacific, serving 527,960 beneficiaries in Hawaii and throughout the Pacific. Prior to this command, Ms. Adams (BG rank) commanded the William Beaumont Army Medical Center at Fort Bliss, Texas, a 200-bed tertiary care medical center with 1,800 personnel serving 400,000 beneficiaries. From 1991 to 1995, she served concurrently as the chief of the Army Nurse Corps and the assistant surgeon for personnel, and was the first commander of the newly created Center for Health Promotion and Preventive Medicine. Prior to these leadership positions, she served in a variety of clinical nursing and nursing administration positions in the U.S. Army Medical Department and the DoD. Ms. Adams holds a bachelor's degree in nursing from Cornell University and a master's degree in nursing from Catholic University. She is a fellow in the American Academy of Nursing (AAN).

George K. Anderson, M.D., M.P.H., is executive director of the Association of Military Surgeons of the United States (AMSUS). AMSUS, the nonprofit society of the federal health agencies, operates from a headquarters located in Bethesda, Maryland. He is an experienced physician executive who, prior to his current position at AMSUS, was an independent medical technology consultant. He served as chief executive officer at Oceania, Inc., a medical software company, from 1999 to 2001, and as chief executive officer of the Koop Foundation from 1997 to 1998. Dr. Anderson was in military service for 30 years and retired from active duty in the grade of major general. He served in the Air Force as a flight surgeon, an aerospace medicine staff officer, and a commander of several medical organizations in Korea, Germany, and the United States. He serves as a director of the Environmental Tectonics Corporation, in Southhampton, Pennsylvania, as well as on several advisory boards and groups. Dr. Anderson received his M.P.H. degree from Tulane University and his M.D. degree from the University of Michigan Medical School. He is a past president of the American College of Preventive Medicine, a past chairman of the American Board of Preventive Medicine, and currently serves on the IOM Board on the Health of Select Populations (BSP) and the Defense Health Board.

Peter B. Angood, M.D., is the chief executive officer of the American College of Physician Executives (ACPE). Prior to joining the ACPE, he provided senior executive health care consultant experience for small-, medium-, and large-size health care organizations across a variety of focus areas. He recently completed a 2-year engagement with the National Quality Forum (NQF) as a senior advisor on patient safety and continues with the NQF part time to help guide projects focused on improving national patient safety and health care quality. He also recently provided technical expertise on projects related to the National Priorities Partnership's goal of improving the safety of America's health care system. Prior to engaging as a health care consultant, Dr. Angood was the chief patient safety officer and a vice president for the Joint Commission, where he oversaw the annual development of the commission's national patient safety goals and several other enterprise-wide patient safety initiatives. He continues to work with the World Health Organization's Alliance for Patient Safety initiative after helping to lead early development of the organization's Collaborating Center for Patient Safety Solutions and other patient safety programs. After initially practicing with the hospitals of McGill University, Dr. Angood was subsequently recruited into surgery faculty and hospital administrative positions at the University of Pennsylvania, Yale University, and Washington University in St. Louis. Prior to joining the Joint Commission, he was a professor of surgery, anesthesia, and emergency medicine at the University of Massachusetts Medical School. Dr. Angood is a fellow of the Royal College of Surgeons (Canada), the American College of Surgeons, and the American College of Critical Care Medicine. He has a history of active committee involvement with numerous professional medical societies and recently served as president for the Society of Critical Care Medicine, a 14,000-member international organization. Dr. Angood is author of approximately 130 peer-reviewed articles, abstracts, editorials, and book chapters. His research interests have addressed leading-edge clinical care problems, patient safety, injury prevention, benchmarking, outcomes management, resource utilization, health services, medical education, advanced medical and telemedicine technologies, and the utility of simulation technology. Dr. Angood received his medical degree from the University of Manitoba in Canada and completed his training in general surgery at McGill University in Montreal, as well as fellowship training in trauma surgery and critical care medicine at the University of Miami/Jackson Memorial Hospital in Miami.

Lawton R. (Robert) Burns, Ph.D., M.B.A., is chair of the Health Care Management Department, James Joo-Jin Kim Professor, and professor of health care management in the Wharton School at the University of Pennsylvania. He is also director of the Wharton Center for Health Management & Economics. He teaches courses on health care strategy, strategic change, organization and management, managed care, and integrated delivery systems. From 1998 to 2002, he was a visiting professor in the Department of Preventive Medicine at the University of Wisconsin School of Medicine, where he taught corporate strategy to physicians. Dr. Burns taught previously in the Graduate School of Business at the University of Chicago and the College of Business Administration at the University of Arizona. He has analyzed physician-organization integration over the past 25 years. In recognition of this research, he was named the Edwin L. Crosby Memorial Fellow by the Hospital Research and Educational Trust in 1992. Dr. Burns has also published several papers on the array of vehicles for integrating physicians and hospitals, the structure and performance of physician networks, the market forces that shape the growth of group practices and investor-owned networks, and the organizational options for physicians in a consolidating industry. In addition to this research, Dr. Burns has conducted extensive analyses of the Allegheny Health Education & Research Foundation bankruptcy, and is now completing a book on the bankruptcy and the Philadelphia hospital market. He has completed a book on supply chain management in the health care industry, titled *The Health Care Value Chain* (Jossey-Bass, 2002). The study focuses on the strategic alliances and partnerships developing between pharmaceutical firms and distributors, disposable manufacturers, medical device manufacturers, group purchasing organizations, and organized delivery systems. He has also completed a companion volume, *The Business of Healthcare Innovation* (Cambridge University Press, 2005), which examines the market structure and trends in the pharmaceutical, biotechnology, medical device, and information system sectors of the global health care industry. Dr. Burns received an Investigator Award from the Robert Wood Johnson Foundation to study the reasons for failure in organizational change efforts by health care providers. Dr. Burns served on the editorial board of *Health Services Research*. He is a past member of the Grant Review Study Section for the Agency for Health Care Policy & Research. He is also a life fellow of Clare Hall at the University of Cambridge. He received his doctorate in sociology and his M.B.A. in health administration from the University of Chicago. Dr. Burns served on the IOM Board on Health Care Services from 2003 to 2006.

Emmanuel G. Cassimatis, M.D., is president and chief executive officer of the Educational Commission for Foreign Medical Graduates (ECFMG®) and chair of the board of directors of the Foundation for the Advancement of International Medical Education and Research, a separate, nonprofit foundation of the ECFMG. Prior to joining the ECFMG on July 1, 2009, he served as the vice president for affiliations and international affairs and the associate dean for clinical affairs and professor of psychiatry, F. Edward Hébert School of Medicine, USUHS. In addition to his duties at the ECFMG, Dr. Cassimatis continues to serve as professor of psychiatry at the USUHS School of Medicine. Dr. Cassimatis served on active duty with the U.S. Army for more than 25 years. His military assignments included tours as director of psychiatric residency training at the Walter Reed Army Medical Center, psychiatry consultant to the Army Surgeon General, and director of medical education for the U.S. Army Medical Department. His military awards include the Defense Superior Service Medal and the Legion of Merit (with Oak Leaf Cluster). Dr. Cassimatis is a member of the U.S. Medical License Examination Composite Committee and the World Federation for Medical Education Executive Council, and president of the Hellenic American Psychiatric Association (APA). He was a delegate to the American Medical Association (AMA) House from the AMSUS for many years, and was a member and chair of the AMA's Council on Medical Education, Section Council on Federal and Military Medicine, and Specialty and Service Society. Dr. Cassimatis also completed 4 years on the Institutional Review Committee and 7 years on the board of directors of the Accreditation Council for Graduate Medical Education (ACGME), the last 2 years as chair. He is a life fellow of AMSUS, a fellow of the American Academy of Psychoanalysis and Dynamic Psychiatry, and a distinguished life fellow of the APA. Dr. Cassimatis is a graduate of the University of Chicago, the Harvard Medical School, and the Washington Psychoanalytic Institute. He recently served on the IOM Committee on Qualifications of Professionals Providing Mental Health Counseling Services under TRICARE from 2009 to 2010.

Timothy C. Flynn, M.D., became senior associate dean for clinical affairs at the University of Florida College of Medicine and chief medical officer for Shands Hospital at the University of Florida in September 2010. In both roles, he serves as a point person for planning and implementing quality and patient safety initiatives, areas he has focused on throughout his career at the College of Medicine, and especially while serving as interim senior associate dean for clinical affairs. In his 26 years with the college, Dr. Flynn has filled a number of leadership roles, including chief of surgery at the Malcom Randall Veterans Affairs Medical Center, program director for the general surgery residency, and associate dean for graduate medical education. As a professor of surgery, he has distinguished himself nationally in graduate medical education and academic surgery. After his Navy service and his residency, he served as an assistant professor at the University of Texas Medical School for 4 years before going to the University of Florida in 1984. He has held several national appointments with the Veterans Administration. He is a member of the Alpha Omega Alpha Honor Medical Society and has served as president of the Alachua County Medical Society. In 2010, he was elected chair of the ACGME's board of directors. In addition, he is chair of the American College of Surgeons Board of Governors, a past chair of the American Board of Surgery, and former president of the Association of Program Directors in Surgery and the Association of VA Surgeons. Dr. Flynn graduated from Louisiana State University with a bachelor's degree in zoology in 1971 and earned his medical degree from the Baylor College of Medicine in 1974. He completed his surgery residency at the University of Texas Health Science Center in Houston, Texas, and is board certified in general surgery, vascular surgery, and surgical critical care.

Larry M. Manheim, Ph.D., is a research professor in the Institute for Healthcare Studies and the Department of Physical Medicine and Rehabilitation, Northwestern University Feinberg School of Medicine. His interests have involved using large datasets to (1) look at aging and individual risks of high medical costs, disability, and long-term care use; (2) analyze hospital and post-acute care organization responses to changes in Medicare payment rules using Medicare data; and (3) evaluate cost effectiveness of health care system interventions using primary interview and Medicare data. Dr. Manheim has a master's degree in statistics and a Ph.D. in economics from the University of California, Berkeley.

John E. Maupin, Jr., D.D.S., M.B.A., is president and chief executive officer of Morehouse School of Medicine (MSM) and has more than 30 years of experience in health care administration, public health, and academic medicine. Prior to joining MSM on July 1, 2006, Dr. Maupin served as president of Meharry Medical College in Nashville, Tennessee, for 12 years. His other senior administrative positions have included executive vice president and chief operating officer of MSM; executive director, Morehouse Medical Associates; chief executive officer of Southside Healthcare, Inc., Atlanta, Georgia; deputy commissioner for Medical Services, Baltimore City Health Department, Baltimore, Maryland; and dental director and chief of medical staff, West Baltimore Community Health Center. Dr. Maupin was a career dental officer in the U.S. Army Reserves, retiring in 1997 with more than 28 years of service, including 2 years of active duty at the Walter Reed Army Medical Center in Washington, DC, and 9 months of active duty service during Desert Shield/Desert Storm. He has served on numerous health-related task forces, scientific panels, and advisory councils. Most notably, he was recently appointed to the National Health Care Workforce Commission. Dr. Maupin is past president of the National Dental Association and the Association of Minority Health Profession Schools. He also currently serves on the board of directors of LifePoint Hospitals, Inc., a nonurban, acute care hospital management company; HealthSouth, Inc., a national rehabilitative health care services management company; and Regions Financial Corporation, a regional multibank holding company. Dr. Maupin attended San Jose State College and earned a D.D.S. degree in 1972 from Meharry Medical College School of Dentistry. The following year he completed a general dentistry residency at Provident Hospital in Baltimore, Maryland, and subsequently received an M.B.A. degree in 1979 from Loyola College in Baltimore.

Karen L. Miller, R.N., Ph.D., is the senior vice chancellor for academic and student affairs at the University of Kansas Medical Center. She has also served as the dean of and a professor at the University of Kansas Schools of Nursing and Health Professions since 1996. Prior to her dean's appointment, Dr. Miller was the vice president and a chief nursing officer at the Children's Hospital, Denver, and an associate professor at the University of Colorado Health Sciences Center. Dr. Miller has more than 35 years of health care executive experience. She completed her baccalaureate degree at Case Western Reserve University and received her master's and doctoral degrees from the University of Colorado. Her research has been in the areas of health systems, finance, and patient care outcomes in health care. Throughout her career, she has published and presented on organizational leadership in health care, financial management of clinical services, and nursing workforce issues. Dr. Miller is the president of KU HealthPartners, Inc., a University of Kansas faculty practice plan and direct clinical services corporation for nursing and allied health professionals. She also serves on the board of directors of the University of Kansas Hospital and the board of directors of the University of Kansas Research Institute. Among past national appointments, Dr. Miller was a member of the 2002 Commission on Workforce for Hospitals & Health Systems of the American Hospital Association. In 2004, Dr. Miller completed a 4-year term on the National Advisory Council on Nursing Education and Practice of the U.S. Department of Health and Human Services and she served from 1995 to 2000 on the National Advisory Council of the National Institute of Nursing Research (NINR) of the NIH. She served on the Workforce Advisory Council for the AAHC from 2005 to 2007 as a representative for nursing and allied health professions. In 2008, she completed a 2-year term as president of the Board of the Friends of the NINR. Dr. Miller commenced service on the board of directors of the Watson Caring Science Institute during 2011. She was named a fellow of the AAN in 1995 and a fellow of the Association of Schools of Allied Health Professions in 2010.

Frances M. Murphy, M.D., M.P.H., is president of Sigma Health Consulting, LLC, a health services consulting firm located in Silver Spring, Maryland. Dr. Murphy serves as a consultant on health care management, public health, neurosciences and mental health, health information technology, and veterans' and military health. She has focused particularly on health information technology, in addition to the transformation of health care delivery systems. Prior to establishing Sigma Health Consulting, Dr. Murphy had a distinguished federal career, including more than 25 years as a physician, educator, researcher, and health care executive. From 1999 to 2002, she served as the Department of Veterans Affairs' (VA's) deputy under secretary for health (DUSH) and chief operating officer for the VA's integrated health care system. From 2002 to 2006, she served as the DUSH for health policy coordination and worked extensively on improving mental health care services as the VA's member of the President's New Freedom Commission on Mental Health. Dr. Murphy chaired the VA secretary's Mental Health Task Force and led the Veterans Health Administration's Action Agenda: Achieving the Promise—Transforming VA Mental Healthcare. From 1983 to 1987, Dr. Murphy served in the U.S. Air Force as the staff neurologist at Andrews Air Force Base, Maryland, and on the faculty of the USUHS. She is board certified in neurology and earned her M.D. from the Georgetown University School of Medicine and her M.P.H. from the USUHS. She currently serves on the IOM's Committee on the Readjustment Needs of Military Personnel, Veterans, and Their Families: Phase 2, and has been appointed to serve as a member of the BSP and the National Academy's Institutional Review Board.

J. Marc Overhage, M.D., Ph.D., is the chief medical informatics officer for Siemens Health Services. Prior to joining Siemens, he was the founding chief executive officer of the Indiana Health Information Exchange (IHIE) and was director of medical informatics at the Regenstrief Institute, Inc., and a Sam Regenstrief Professor of Medical Informatics at the Indiana University School of Medicine. He has spent more than 25 years developing and implementing scientific and clinical systems and evaluating their value. With his colleagues from the Regenstrief Institute, he created a community-wide electronic medical record (called the Indiana Network for Patient Care) containing data from many sources, including laboratories, pharmacies, and hospitals in central Indiana. The system currently connects a majority of acute care hospitals in central Indiana and includes inpatient and outpatient encounter data, laboratory results, immunization data, and other selected data. In order to create a sustainable financial model, Dr. Overhage helped create the IHIE, a not-for-profit corporation. In addition, he has developed and evaluated clinical decision support, including inpatient and outpatient computerized physician order entry and the underlying knowledge bases to support them. He practiced general internal medicine for more than 20 years, including in the ambulatory, inpatient, and emergency care settings. Over the last decade, Dr. Overhage has played a significant regional and national leadership role in advancing the policy, standards, financing, and implementation of health information exchange. He serves on the National Committee for Vital and Health Statistics and the Health Information Technology Standards Committee, as well as serving on the board of directors of the NQF and being engaged in a number of national health care initiatives. Dr. Overhage is a member of the IOM and a fellow of the American College of Medical Informatics and the American College of Physicians. He received the Davies Recognition Award for Excellence in

Computer-Based Patient Recognition for the Regenstrief Medical Record System. Dr. Overhage received his B.A., with high honors, in physics from Wabash College and his Ph.D. in biophysics and his M.D. from the Indiana University School of Medicine. Dr. Overhage was a resident in internal medicine, a medical informatics and health services research fellow, and then chief medical resident at the Indiana University School of Medicine.

Susanne Tropez-Sims, M.D., M.P.H., is associate dean of clinical affiliations and professor of pediatrics at Meharry Medical College, and adjunct professor of pediatrics at the Vanderbilt School of Medicine in Nashville, Tennessee. She directs the Adolescent Clinic at Meharry. She specializes in general pediatric care, adolescent medicine, and child abuse. She directed an HIV/AIDS prevention program entitled MINDS (Moving in New Directions) in two public schools in Davidson County for 5 years. She joined the faculty at the Louisiana State University Medical Center in 1988 as the director of the pediatric emergency room and, in 1989, she became the division chief of the ambulatory division. During this period, Dr. Tropez-Sims was also the maternal and child health director for the New Orleans Health Department. Under her leadership, the Child Abuse Program became more organized and became an integral part of the pediatric residency and the emergency residency training. She received an award from the state of Louisiana Council for Child Abuse for her contribution in this area. Dr. Tropez-Sims was instrumental in improving and ensuring the medical services for two school-based clinics (G.W. Carver Junior/Senior High School and Booker T. Washington Junior/Senior High School) in New Orleans. In 1982, she joined the faculty at the University of North Carolina at Chapel Hill and served as director of the Outpatient Pediatric Clinic for the Wake Area Health Education Center. She was a child medical examiner for North Carolina, training physicians, police, social workers, and lawyers across the state in the evaluation of child abuse. In 1997, she received the first national American Academy of Pediatrics Martin Ushkow Community Service Award for her work in school health. Dr. Tropez-Sims is a graduate of the University of North Carolina School of Medicine, where she received her M.D. and M.P.H. in maternal and child health. She was the second minority to complete her internship and residence in pediatrics at the North Carolina Memorial Hospital in Chapel Hill, North Carolina.

Carolyn (Cindy) Watts, Ph.D., became professor and chair of the Department of Health Administration at the Virginia Commonwealth University in August 2010. Prior to this appointment, she was a professor in the Department of Health Services at the University of Washington, where she held adjunct appointments in the Department of Economics and the Evans School of Public Affairs. She served as the director of the health policy analysis and the process track of the M.P.H. program; as a director of the extended M.P.H. program in health services; and as a core faculty member of the Institute for Public Health Genetics. Her research work has focused on organizational, reimbursement, and regulatory issues in health care markets, and health care industry structure and incentives. An accomplished scholar, her work is widely published in academic literature. In addition to her academic appointments, Dr. Watts has worked extensively with numerous provider and policy organizations. She was a board member of the Virginia Mason Medical Center in Seattle, chaired the 2006 Washington State Certificate of Need Program Task Force, was director of the Washington Health Legislative Conference, and has been a consultant to the Washington State Hospital Association. Dr. Watts received her M.A. and Ph.D. degrees in political economics from the Johns Hopkins University.

CONSULTANTS

David K. Barnes is the head of Advanced Policy Solutions, Bethesda, Maryland. Mr. Barnes is the former director of the Social Security Administration's (SSA's) Office of Disability Evaluation Policy. At the SSA, he oversaw development, implementation, and analysis of disability decision-making policy for both the Social Security Disability Insurance and the Supplemental Security Income disability programs. In his 27-year career, Mr. Barnes developed a reputation not only as a preeminent authority on disability policy and decision making but also as a respected expert in research and development, personnel management, team building, procurement, rule making, and litigation.

Thomas A. D'Aunno, Ph.D., is the executive vice dean of the Mailman School of Public Health at Columbia University. His research focuses on the organization and management of health care services. He has a particular interest in leadership, organizational change, and performance improvement, and has examined these issues in a variety of national studies of health care organizations that have been funded by the National Institute on Drug Abuse, the Agency for Healthcare Research and Quality, and the Pew Memorial Trust. Dr. D'Aunno was previously a faculty member at the University of Chicago, the University of Michigan, and, most recently, at INSEAD, where he held the Novartis Chair in Healthcare Management. He has published articles in leading management and health journals, including the *Administrative Science Quarterly*, the *Academy of Management Journal*, the *Academy of Management Review*, the *Journal of the American Medical Association*, and the *Journal of Health and Social Behavior*. Dr. D'Aunno has been a member of the editorial boards of several journals, including the *Administrative Science Quarterly*, the *Journal of Health and*

Social Behavior, and the *Academy of Management Review*. In addition, he has consulted and taught executive education courses on several topics, including leadership, performance management, high-performance teams, organizational design, and organizational change. Dr. D'Aunno is a past chairman of the Academy of Management Division of Health Care Management and a recipient of that division's award for career distinguished service.

PRINCIPAL STAFF

Frederick (Rick) Erdtmann, M.D., M.P.H., is currently the director of the BSP and the Medical Follow-up Agency at the IOM. Prior to joining the IOM, he was a career military physician in the U.S. Army. While in the military, he served as chief of several large departments of preventive medicine at U.S. and overseas installations. He also was commander of the military community hospital at Ft. Carson, Colorado, and later served as hospital commander for the Walter Reed Army Medical Center. Dr. Erdtmann had several assignments at the Army Surgeon General's Office, where he worked on military health care policies. He received his undergraduate degree from Bucknell University and an M.P.H. degree from the University of California, Berkeley. He is a graduate of Temple University's Medical School and is board certified in the specialty of preventive medicine. The board that Dr. Erdtmann directs was responsible for managing a major study involving the disability decision process for the SSA and two other disability-related studies for the Veterans Administration in the recent past.

Michael McGeary is a senior program officer at the BSP, serving concurrently as the director of the Committee on Evaluation of the Lovell Federal Health Care Center Merger and the Committee of Medical Experts to Assist Social Security on Disability Issues. He recently served as the director of the Committee on Social Security Cardiovascular Disability Criteria. He is a political scientist specializing in health, science, and technology policy analysis and program evaluation. Before 2004, he was an independent consultant to government agencies, foundations, and nonprofit organizations in issues of science and technology. Between 1981 and 1995, Mr. McGeary was at the IOM and the National Academy of Sciences, where he was staff director of more than a dozen major reports on such topics as federal funding of research and development; graduate education and employment of scientists and engineers; and priority setting, funding, and management of the NIH. From 2004 to 2007, he was staff director for the IOM committees that recommended improvements in the systems for determining disability of the SSA and the VA, respectively. Mr. McGeary is a graduate of Harvard

College and completed all requirements for a doctorate in political science from the Massachusetts Institute of Technology except the dissertation.

Susan R. McCutchen is a senior program associate at the BSP supporting the work of the Committee on Evaluation of the Lovell Federal Health Care Center Merger and the Committee of Medical Experts to Assist Social Security on Disability Issues. She has been on staff at the National Academies for more than 30 years and has worked in several institutional divisions and with many different boards, committees, and panels within those units. The studies in which she has participated have addressed a broad range of subjects and focused on a variety of issues, including science and technology for international development, technology transfer, aeronautics and the U.S. space program, natural disaster mitigation, U.S. education policy and science curricula, needle exchange for the prevention of HIV transmission, the scientific merit of the polygraph, human factors/engineering, research ethics, disability compensation programs, health hazard evaluation, and medical and public health preparedness for catastrophic events, including nuclear detonations. She has assisted in the production of more than 50 publications and was an editor for *A 21st Century System for Evaluating Veterans for Disability Benefits* and *Assessing Medical Preparedness to Respond to a Terrorist Nuclear Event: Workshop Report*. Ms. McCutchen has a B.A. in French, with minors in Italian and Spanish, from Ohio's Miami University, and an M.A. in French, with a minor in English, from Kent State University.

LaVita Sullivan is a senior program assistant with the BSP supporting the work of the Committee on Evaluation of the Lovell Federal Health Care Center Merger and the Committee of Medical Experts to Assist Social Security on Disability Issues. Prior to joining the National Academies in 2008, Ms. Sullivan spent 5 progressive years with the DoD, where she served as a program analyst and contributed to the streamlining of administrative processes and procedures. She is a certified event planner and is currently pursuing her undergraduate degree in communications at the University of Maryland University College.

Appendix B

Framework for Evaluating Department of Veterans Affairs/Department of Defense Health Care Collaborations

In the process of its deliberations, the committee created a framework (Table B-1) to guide its evaluation of the Lovell Federal Health Care Center (FHCC) merger that may prove useful to assess future collaborations between the Departments of Defense (DoD) and Veterans Affairs (VA), whether these take the form of shared service arrangements, joint ventures, or partial or full mergers. The five major categories for consideration include (1) national and local contexts, (2) organizational capabilities and readiness, (3) implementation initiatives, (4) intermediate outcomes, and (5) long-term impact. Each of these is discussed in turn.

NATIONAL AND LOCAL CONTEXTS

Whether various forms of continued or expanded collaboration between DoD and VA medical facilities make sense will depend to a large degree on the national and local contexts within which such collaborations might be realized. Among the most important of these are the current DoD and VA departmental policies, goals, and objectives. The Lovell FHCC "integration," for example, was inherently constrained by the need to conform to many divergent DoD and VA policies. In some respects, the degree of success of the integration was achieved through major "work-arounds" of current national VA and DoD policies and business processes. In the extreme, one could imagine a fully merged "Federal Health Service" that would totally absorb and integrate current DoD and VA health care policies and institutions. For a variety of reasons, this may not be feasible in the near future. In the meantime, any future collaborations must recog-

TABLE B-1 Framework for Evaluating Department of Veterans Affairs and Department of Defense Health Care Collaborations*

National and Local Contexts	Organizational Capabilities and Readiness	Implementation Initiatives	Intermediate Outcomes First 2 Years	Long-Term Impact 3–5 Years
• Department of Veterans Affairs and Department of Defense (DoD) policies, goals, objectives • Number and location of facilities • Size and number of people served • Local health care market—public and private sectors • Local labor market • Other	• Shared vision • History of working together • Culture • Leadership • Information technology capabilities • Care management • Care improvement • Performance measurement • Training and human resources development • Financial reserves • Other	• Combining departments and services • Transferring personnel • Orienting employees • Communication/education • Developing policies • Developing shared electronic health records • Other	• Increased operational readiness for recruits • Expanding patient volume to critical mass to maintain competency • More in-house surgery—added posttraumatic stress disorder unit • Increased professional opportunities for staff • Residency opportunities • Healthcare Effectiveness Data and Information Set, DoD, Joint Commission benchmark measures • Employee satisfaction • Patient experience measures • Other	• Operating efficiencies • Costs per patient • Patient functional health status measures • Increased market share in local area • Other

* It is important to evaluate shared services, joint ventures, and partial and full mergers, etc., against their *own* stated goals and objectives in addition to those expected by external parties, including accreditation bodies, payers, and others.

nize the constraints imposed by the existence of separate executive branch departments with differing missions, statutory requirements, departmental policies, administrative procedures, organizational cultures, performance standards, and reporting requirements.

Other important contextual factors include the current degree of interdependence among DoD and VA facilities relative to collocation, current sharing of services, various informal arrangements, opportunities for medical and health professional education and research, and related factors. Other additional factors include the number of people served by the entities involved, their demographic characteristics and health needs, and the characteristics of the local private-sector health care marketplace. Further considerations include the strength of the local economy, the availability of workforce, and related resources. Relationships with medical and affiliated health professions schools are also an important consideration.

Despite the national policy challenges, the local context was quite favorable for the Lovell FHCC integration. For instance, the Navy and the VA facilities were located very close together, allowing the VA to accommodate Navy beneficiaries and improve the capacity of its medical facility and the Navy to save money by not having to replace its obsolete inpatient facility. In addition, the VA patient population offered a more varied and complex health care treatment mix to allow Navy clinical personnel to keep up their skills, while the overall increase in the number of patients created some economies of scale and staffing efficiencies. For the VA, in addition to increasing use, the larger and more varied patient base, including women and children, provided increased training and potential research opportunities for medical students and residents.

Into the future, changes in demand for both DoD and VA facilities will be an important consideration for the success of collaborative activities. The veteran population enrollment for VA health care services is projected to decline over the next decade, and immediate indicators suggest a reduced future demand. Another factor to be considered is the difference between the requirements of more standard health care operations as opposed to recruit training sites, such as that found in the Lovell FHCC merger.

The country's slow economic recovery, the burden of debt, and related factors may also affect how the nation chooses to provide health care to its military personnel and veterans.

ORGANIZATIONAL CAPABILITIES AND READINESS

The second key component in considering future collaborations is a rigorous realistic assessment of the capabilities and readiness of the involved parties. While there are many important factors to consider, among the most critical are the governance and the stability of leadership of the involved entities; the budget authorities and restrictions; the electronic health record (EHR) system and information technology infrastructure capabilities; the human resource systems, capabilities, and personnel resources; and the care processes and management/improvement/performance measurement systems (including outcomes that can be compared against external benchmarks).

The single biggest barrier for the more complete clinical implementation of the Lovell FHCC was the incompatibility of the DoD and the VA EHR systems and the resultant technical challenges and barriers. The time necessary to integrate various features of the two systems was seriously underestimated, resulting in delays and incremental "one-off" workarounds. The problem of having to reconcile two different human resources systems was solved by the decision to move all the Navy civilians into the VA personnel system, although the active duty servicemembers could not be moved. A great deal of time and energy had to be spent addressing cultural differences between the Navy and the VA, which would also be expected from potential mergers between the VA and other branches of the services that have their own distinct cultures. Chapter 2 of this report provides the history of the Lovell FHCC merger and Chapter 3 gives a more detailed description of the implementation process.

DoD and VA entities considering further collaborative opportunities also need to assess their current care management and quality improvement processes, and their ability to generate performance measures. To their credit, the Lovell FHCC leaders developed a set of standardized performance measures in the areas of patient access, quality of care, patient satisfaction, provider satisfaction, and mission readiness that are tracked on a regular basis.

Finally, the financial resources available to implement further collaborations must be assessed relative to the challenges of implementation. Because of its status as the first demonstration of an integrated VA/DoD health care facility, the Lovell FHCC received substantial resources from the departments that might not be available to future integration efforts and, if provided, would significantly increase the cost side of the cost-benefit equation.

IMPLEMENTATION INITIATIVES

An accurate documentation of the actual changes made at the Lovell FHCC is critical to evaluating the successes and failures in North Chicago to inform other collaborations between DoD and VA facilities. The central question involves *change*. Specifically, what changes are made by whom, with whom, and with what results? Examples include the acculturation of shared mission and vision through the establishment of joint governance and leadership structures (see Organizational Capabilities and Readiness), joint business offices and a joint strategic planning process, development of multidisciplinary teams and ongoing and continuous communication mechanisms, the combining of departments and services, the transferring of personnel, staff orientation, shared EHR system implementation, and many other such changes.

INTERMEDIATE OUTCOMES

Intermediate outcomes can be categorized in terms of cost and efficiency, clinical processes and outcomes, patient experience, and education and research. Cost and efficiency measures include various measures of productivity as well as cost per patient. Clinical process measures would include the Healthcare Effectiveness Data and Information Set, the DoD, and the Joint Commission benchmark measures. They might also include patient and staff satisfaction measures. Research and education measures could include the amount of research funding generated but also the number of articles published in peer-reviewed journals, particularly articles jointly authored by DoD and VA researchers.

Each potential collaboration should also be evaluated on intermediate outcomes based on its unique organizational mission, strategic goals, and objectives. Some examples at the Lovell FHCC included developing in-house surgical capacity, upgrading the emergency department, extending the range of specialty services provided onsite, increasing professional opportunities for staff, improving the operational readiness of the recruits and other active duty servicemembers, and increasing the clinical competence of Navy providers.

LONG-TERM IMPACT

While intermediate outcomes can usually be observed within a year or 2 of implementing an expanded collaboration, it is also important to examine the longer-term impact that emerges over a 3- to 5-year period. The impact can be measured by responses to key questions. For example, are the initial positive outcomes sustained over time (e.g., in the areas of health care value and efficiency, access, patient clinical outcomes, patient functional health status outcomes, patient experience measures, and related metrics)? Is there growth in the patient population served, admissions, and other indicators of service use? These data should be compared with comparable data available from private-sector institutions to better examine the overall nature of a DoD/VA health service impact in a given geographic area. Finally, it should be asked what additional innovations in new program development have taken place as a result of the collaborative activity established several years earlier.

While the committee's framework can be used retrospectively to assess the Lovell FHCC experience, its greater potential is as a template for evaluating and learning from future collaborations between the DoD and the VA. It can be used both by an external entity to provide an independent assessment of collaborative activity as well as by the collaborating institutions themselves to assess their ongoing progress.

Appendix C

Department of Veterans Affairs/ Department of Defense Joint Ventures[1]: Brief Histories and Lessons Learned

The committee reviewed the current nine formal joint ventures that share resources in a variety of arrangements, and arrived at its summary of lessons learned across them by considering the information collected from a number of sources (see Chapter 5).

ALBUQUERQUE, NEW MEXICO: 377TH MEDICAL GROUP, KIRTLAND AIR FORCE BASE/NEW MEXICO VETERANS AFFAIRS HEALTH CARE SYSTEM

Brief History

The first formally designated Department of Defense (DoD)/Department of Veterans Affairs (VA) joint venture was established in 1987 between the Air Force's 377th Medical Group (377th MDG) at Kirtland Air Force Base (Kirtland AFB) and the New Mexico Veterans Affairs Health Care System (NMVAHCS), located in Albuquerque, New Mexico. The Kirtland AFB Hospital and the Albuquerque VA Medical Center (VAMC), located two miles apart, had shared some services since at least the 1970s, for example, laboratory tests performed at no cost by the VA for DoD patients in the early part of that decade. With an eye toward achieving efficiency and cost savings, DoD and VA officials in Albuquerque have envisioned, created agreements for, and supported the increase of their shared services. The first

[1] The Lovell FHCC is no longer formally classified as a joint venture because it is considered to be a unique organizational arrangement.

formal sharing agreement was signed in March 1976. Under the agreement, the VA provided medical services and laboratory tests on a reimbursement basis. In the 1980s, the Air Force was faced with renovating its hospital at a cost of $26 million at the same time that the VA was planning the construction of a new Albuquerque VAMC. Rather than renovate the Air Force hospital, the VA agreed to include a 40-bed inpatient medical-surgical unit for the 377th MDG to staff and manage in the new VA facility, to be called the New Mexico Regional Federal Medical Center, which opened in 1987. The Air Force also agreed to manage the emergency room and, in 1989, constructed an ambulatory care center next to the hospital. The VA provided all ancillary services to the Air Force–staffed inpatient unit. The joint venture underwent a major change in 2002, when the Air Force, due to substantial reductions in personnel stationed at Kirtland, closed the inpatient unit and revised the interagency sharing agreement to allow the purchase of inpatient services from the VA (GAO, 1978; Simmons, 1989; VA/DoD, 2002).

In a recent development, the DoD invested $2.9 million for the renovation of its same-day-surgery unit, which was completed in 2011. As of the end of February 2012, the director of the joint venture indicated that the associated sharing agreement is pending review and approval by the Air Force Medical Support Agency, and the reopening was anticipated for March 2012.[2] The sharing agreement will be between the 377th MDG and the NMVAHCS for the VA to occupy DoD ambulatory surgery space in exchange for providing 30 free surgeries a month for DoD beneficiaries (VA/DoD, 2011b).

Lessons Learned

Lessons learned at the Albuquerque joint venture include that successful agreements are worked out over time and through extensive planning efforts. Sharing agreements or joint ventures are unique to their locations and will not work unless the arrangement is cost effective for both partners. Leadership, personalities, and communications are important, and cultural issues must be overcome. Leadership needs to make strategic plans in the anticipation of accommodating the fluctuating availability of resources in an unpredictable environment. Sharing partners and their leaders must be committed, flexible, open-minded, and patient in their planning efforts, and they must look for opportunities to expand and modify arrangements as needed (Anderson, 1995; Baine, 1995; Carlton, 2000; Rogers, 2007; Spaulding and Catton, 2008; VA/DoD, 2011b).

---

[2] Personal communication with Patricia L. Ospino, M.B.A., Joint Venture Director, February 24, 2012.

EL PASO, TEXAS: WILLIAM BEAUMONT ARMY MEDICAL CENTER, FORT BLISS/EL PASO VETERANS AFFAIRS HEALTH CARE SYSTEM

Brief History

The William Beaumont Army Medical Center (WBAMC) and the El Paso Veterans Affairs Health Care System (EPVAHCS) have shared resources since the early 1970s. At that time, the VA canceled plans to build a hospital in El Paso when the Army agreed to provide inpatient care to VA beneficiaries in the WBAMC, which was then under construction. The El Paso DoD/VA joint venture started in 1987, when the VA needed to replace its outpatient clinic. A working group between the two organizations agreed to an arrangement in which the VA built its new, larger VA Eastside El Paso Clinic (VA Clinic) adjacent to the WBAMC. The clinic opened in 1995, and each floor is physically connected and has open access to the WBAMC. The Army provides inpatient care to VA beneficiaries in El Paso, who account for 26 percent of inpatient services provided at the WBAMC. VA staff share an 8-room ambulatory surgical suite and 16-bed recovery area on the fourth floor of the WBAMC with Army staff. The VA Clinic's staff provides primary and behavioral health care, specialty services, dental services, and ambulatory surgery to veterans and has two ambulatory surgery suites available for use by the WBAMC. In 2008, the VA opened a 29,000-square-foot addition to the clinic for physical therapy, behavioral health, and podiatry programs. While the WBAMC underwent renovations to its post-anesthesia care unit (completed in 2009), the VA allowed Army staff to use the ambulatory surgery suite in the clinic. The Texas Tech University School of Medicine has a consortium agreement with the EPVAHCS and the WBAMC to train residents in internal medicine and psychiatry. The WBAMC's graduate medical education program (GME) is open to VA medical residents (AMEDD, 2012; DoD/VA, 2002, 2008b; GAO, 2007; Hite, 2011; U.S. Senate, 1980; VA, 2012b; VA/DoD, 2002, 2006).

Because of Defense Base Realignment and Closure (BRAC) actions and other shifts of personnel, Fort Bliss is expanding substantially. By 2014, it is slated to be the third largest Army installation in the United States after Fort Bragg and Fort Hood. TRICARE Prime enrollment at the WBAMC is expected to double, to more than 110,000. In anticipation of this large increase in demand for health care, the Army began to plan for a major expansion of health care facilities, including a new $966 million hospital in a new location about 10 miles away in East El Paso. The new WBAMC hospital replacement project was awarded in 2009, ground was broken in 2011, and the inpatient facility is scheduled to open in 2016 (Wirtemburg and Ancker, 2008).

The VA wanted to relocate with the new Army facility and possibly share space for outpatient services—rather than build a separate ambulatory care facility—and also possibly jointly staff ambulatory surgery services. The VA is expecting its patient load to increase by nearly 5,000, to 41,000, and also wanted its clinic to be near the new access to the emergency room and specialty consultations at the new WBAMC, and to have continuity of care, sharing of ancillary services, and better GME opportunities. There was an effort to size the new inpatient facility to provide services for both DoD and VA beneficiaries, with the VA paying a proportionate share of the construction costs (approximately 25 percent), but differing construction planning and funding cycles made this approach impossible to achieve. In August 2012, Army Major Bryan Walrath, program manager for the U.S. Army Health Facility Planning Agency, reported that what will happen to the Beaumont facility is yet to be determined, indicating that "a big part of that question will be answered when it's known if the Veterans Administration clinic, now located in a wing attached to Beaumont, will stay or eventually move to its own facility at the new hospital site" (Kolenc, 2012).

Lessons Learned

Lessons learned in El Paso include that open communication and information sharing are paramount to the success of a joint venture, and that trust and cooperation are key elements of the collaboration. There must be strong and committed leadership and a solid management structure, including middle management as well as subcommittees and work groups, sufficient to cohesively address important issues. DoD/VA team members (along with leadership as needed) should brainstorm together in a joint effort to resolve the major issues and creatively collaborate on plans and documentation. This kind of communication involves being specific about situations that arise to encourage more targeted discussions and practical solutions and to create a paper trail. By doing this, staff from both organizations will come to understand each other better and identify with the positive community effort they are undertaking. Staff should also commingle as much as possible to further their community identification. Unions should be part of the discussions from the beginning and as often as feasible (Perdue and Ancker, 2007, 2011; VA/DoD, 2006; Wirtemburg and Ancker, 2008).

HONOLULU, HAWAII: TRIPLER ARMY MEDICAL CENTER/ VETERANS AFFAIRS PACIFIC ISLANDS/HEALTH CARE SYSTEM (SPARK M. MATSUNAGA MEDICAL CENTER)

Brief History

The Tripler Army Medical Center (TAMC) and the Veterans Affairs Pacific Island Health Care System (VAPIHCS) joint venture is unusual because it was established through a 1991 memorandum signed by Hawaii Senator Daniel Inouye and by Undersecretary of the Army John W. Shannon. It became an official joint venture in 1992. Its purpose was to provide a better and broader range of health care for beneficiaries and to promote the use of a single inpatient facility that would obviate the need for the VA to build one separately, thus reducing both construction costs and the expense associated with beneficiaries going out to the community to seek medical care. In this sharing arrangement, the TAMC hosts the VA, with VA staff providing outpatient, mental health, dental health, and nursing home care. The VAPIHCS arranges and pays for the care of veterans at the TAMC, in the local community, or at VA facilities in California as needed (AMEDD, 2011; Hite, 2011; Perlin, 2006).

TAMC's E-Wing inpatient ward, staffed by VA personnel, was established in 1994, was renovated in 1999, and became the site of the VA's Regional Office Center and the VAPIHCS administrative services in 2000. In 1997, the VA Day Hospital Program was relocated to the campus adjacent to the VA-staffed psychiatric ward. A new parking facility and the Center for Aging were completed in 2000. That same year, the VAPIHCS Spark M. Matsunaga VA Ambulatory Care Center, located adjacent to the TAMC campus, opened and began to provide primary care services, including mental health, specialty services, radiology, and optometry. The VA's Post-Traumatic Stress Disorder Recovery Rehabilitation Program residential program relocated to the fifth floor of the TAMC after moving from Hilo in 2006. The first telehealth initiative began in 2009, as did the opening of the VA Dialysis Unit managed by VA staff for the use of both VA and DoD beneficiaries. A Joint Sleep Studies Unit was completed in 2010 (AMEDD, 2011; Committee on Veterans' Affairs, U.S. Senate, 2002; DoD, 2010; Hite, 2011; Pacific Region Health Systems, 2011; Perlin, 2006).

Lessons Learned

The Hawaii joint venture offers a number of lessons learned. Good leadership from both partners that creates a cooperative atmosphere based on mutual trust and from staff who address issues on an ongoing basis is needed. Sharing equally and reaching consensus despite differences between the organizations are important, with the underpinning of well-documented agreements and understandings. It is important for both organizations to be dedicated to the common joint venture mission, to work hard and envision success, and to further progress by developing new initiatives created by working groups and multidisciplinary teams. To accomplish the joint venture goals, open and honest communication is paramount, as is creative thinking to find solutions. Patients need to be the focus (patient-centered care) while saving money in the federal health care system at the same time (Horner and Holes, 2007, 2008; Horner et al., 2006).

Potential Contributions to Other Joint Ventures and Sharing Locations

The Hawaii joint venture has provided potentially useful electronic sharing technology models for other joint venture and sharing agreement arrangements. Its pilot project graphic user interface (GUI), or Janus, is a promising technological collaborative development with Pacific Telehealth & Technology Hui that was begun in 2003. In 2011, it was announced that Janus would be used as part of the VA's joint electronic health record to access records and radiological imagery, including laboratory and pharmacy, allowing clinicians to view data from the two systems, and that the single GUI for the Veterans Health Information Systems and Technology Architecture (VistA) and the Armed Forces Health Longitudinal Technology Application (AHLTA) was being tested in the Tripler Army Medical Center in Honolulu. Future capabilities for Janus II are being developed through collaboration with the same company and will include intranet capabilities and radiology imaging sharing. In 2008, document management and referral management tools with four modules—bi-directional enhanced document referral (eDR) system, Charge Master Billing System, Joint Analytic Repository, and VistA Fee/IPAC Interface (a patch that allows the VA to pay the DoD within the VistA system)—were tested and implemented. A 2010–2012 joint venture objective is to follow up on the implementation of the eDR system and make it more efficient as an evaluation tool. If this effort is successful, it will lead to national implementation of the system at all joint venture sites as part of Joint Marketing Opportunities efforts (Brewin, 2011; Horner and Holes, 2007, 2009; Kyte and Camara, 2006; Perera, 2011; VA/DoD, 2007, 2008b, 2009a).

FAIRFIELD, CALIFORNIA: 60TH MEDICAL GROUP, DAVID GRANT MEDICAL CENTER, TRAVIS AIR FORCE BASE/NORTHERN CALIFORNIA VETERANS AFFAIRS HEALTH CARE SYSTEM

Brief History

The 1988 and the 1995 BRAC actions led to changes in the Mather and the McClellan Air Force Bases, located in Sacramento and McClellan, California, respectively. Mather became the Sacramento VA Medical Center and McClellan became a VA outpatient clinic with a DoD satellite clinic. With these developments as a backdrop, the 235-bed VA hospital in Martinez, California, closed in 1991 because of concerns that it was not safe in the event of earthquakes. A replacement clinic was built and opened in November 1992. It was regarded as a desirable VA prototype because veterans were provided a number of outpatient services they had not had before, including surgery and state-of-the-art technology. In 1994, the Air Force and its David Grant Medical Center (DGMC)/60th Medical Group (60 MDG), located at Travis Air Force Base (Travis AFB), and the Northern California Veterans Affairs Health Care System (NCVAHCS) formed a joint venture that allowed the VA to provide health care services to veterans in space allocated to them at the DGMC. This sharing agreement allowed veterans to use the emergency room, receive inpatient care, access radiation therapy, and receive specified diagnostic services. The medical/surgical unit at the DGMC (No. 5150) was operated by VA staff, while there was joint staffing at the inpatient psychiatric unit. In 1996, the VA proposed the construction of a new VA hospital, a VA outpatient clinic, and renovation to its DGMC space, but Congress decided that building a smaller outpatient clinic at Travis AFB and working through contractual arrangements would be sufficient for the VA's needs. The sharing agreement between the DoD and the VA was renewed in 2008; the current joint venture services include the above, as well as dialysis, inpatient mental health, laboratory, radiology, and pharmacy (DGMC/VANCHCS, 2006; GAO, 1996a,b, 1998, 2004; Hite, 2011; Mosher et al., 2009; Scharenbrock and Carlson, 2010; Wilder and Kelly, 2011).

The key locations for the services of this joint venture are the DGMC and the VA Fairfield Outpatient Clinic, which opened in 2001, in Fairfield, California. This is a good location because it is situated at a midpoint on the I-80 corridor between East Bay and Sacramento with the VA Medical Center located in Sacramento, and the outpatient clinics in Alameda and McClellan. The VA's Sacramento site is the location of the McClellan 60 MDG satellite clinic that provides services for DoD beneficiaries. The joint venture educational partnership is with the University of California, Davis, which is located near the DGMC (Allen and Carlson, 2009;

DGMC/VANCHCS, 2006, 2011; DoD, 2001; VA/DoD, 2000; Wilder and Kelly, 2011).

Lessons Learned

The need to have strong leadership, a single joint venture business office, an "operations guide," and an organizational chart on which to base the hiring of personnel are all offered as lessons that have been learned through this joint venture experience (DGMC/VANCHCS, 2011).

In 2011, current leadership from the Air Force and the VA discussed lessons they have learned from this joint venture. They said that a major factor in determining how well a model might work in a given location should be in the assessment of the degree of mutual dependence. Before even entering into collaboration projects, it is important to research the availability of extant federal facilities (Wilder and Kelly, 2011).

With the establishment of a joint venture, they stressed the importance of the partners meeting regularly and developing a joint strategic plan, including those to address information technology issues. Joint venture management personnel also need to work closely with veterans groups to establish trust, including sharing Joint Incentive Fund proposals with them and asking for comments (Wilder and Kelly, 2011).

When it comes to operations, both partners need to "stand at orientation" to mitigate cultural issues and promote high standards. Staff who are dedicated to the joint venture will create a smoother operation, so it is important to communicate common goals effectively, from the leadership level to personnel attending to day-to-day clinical care. This can be accomplished by shared strategic planning sessions (established between the Air Force and the VA in 2006 for the Northern California joint venture) to cement the partnership. In this case, a 3- to 5-year plan has been created on the premise of mutual dependency with mutual benefits and efforts to "understand each other's culture" (Wilder and Kelly, 2011).

Effective planning for construction projects and health facilities is important. For example, Travis AFB can bring in the VA as part of the planning process, such as the joint musculoskeletal rehabilitation facility (Wilder and Kelly, 2011).

As for the potential for a merger in Northern California, the leadership indicated that they felt it would be plausible, but that there would need to be a unified operational mechanism for supervision rather than two separate entities, e.g., VA employees and the military. However, a single chain of command and one physical "pot of money" would be better than "shuffling the money back and forth" (Wilder and Kelly, 2011).

LAS VEGAS, NEVADA: 99TH MEDICAL GROUP, NELLIS AIR FORCE BASE/VETERANS AFFAIRS SOUTHERN NEVADA HEALTHCARE SYSTEM

Brief History

The joint venture between Nellis Air Force Base's 99th Medical Group (99th MDG) and the Veterans Affairs Southern Nevada Healthcare System (VASNHS) started operations in 1994 with the opening of a new hospital on the base to replace the outdated hospital constructed in 1965. Dedicated as the Mike O'Callaghan Federal Hospital (MOFH) in 1996, the new facility marked the first hospital construction project jointly funded and planned as an "operational joint venture" by the Air Force and the VA, although the two organizations had shared resources well before then. Currently, the MOFH has 114 beds (62 DoD and 52 VA). This arrangement promotes the sharing of costs between the two organizations and the opportunity for veterans to have access to services in Las Vegas, which they had not had previously. Inpatient, limited outpatient, some parts of intensive care and the step-down unit, psychiatric, and emergency room services are shared. Staffing is complex, with some degree of integration. Planning for a new, collocated Las Vegas VAMC began in 2003 and the center opened in August 2012, with the capacity of 90 inpatient beds (22 mental health unit, 48 medical/surgical, and 20 intensive care unit), and launching with an operational outpatient mental health clinic. From August through December 2012, there will be a phased opening of other services, including the provision of "23 dental exam chairs; 13 surgical, 14 radiology, and 6 audiometric sound suites," and featuring "a telehealth unit, with bidirectional just-in-time communication capability with its outlying clinics" (VA, 2012d). With the opening of the center, sharing agreements will be enhanced, allowing Air Force patient access to clinical services currently not available at the MOFH (Collins, 2011; Hite, 2011; Irwin and Drew, 2008; MOFH, 2006; Nellis Air Force Base, 2012; Nicholson, 2005a,b; Roadman, 1999; Simmons, 1989; VA, 2006, 2007b; VA/DoD, 2002).

The Mike O'Callaghan Federal Hospital

Before 1994, VA beneficiaries did not have access to VA inpatient services in Las Vegas and they had to travel to facilities in Southern California for their care. Alternatively, DoD beneficiaries had more limited access to specialized providers prior to 1994 than after the establishment of the joint venture. In fiscal year (FY) 1990, the Air Force contributed $58 million and the VA $7 million to build the MOFH. After its 1994 opening, some operational difficulties arose, one of which was not having a system to adequately address disputes. A high-level Air Force and VA team was brought in to help resolve issues. In 1999, complications came about because of cost accounting issues, bringing to light the need for joint venture partners to have interoperable information systems. In 2002, more serious concerns about inefficiency thought to be brought about by insufficient sharing efforts between the Air Force and the VA were reported. Over time, both limited space and the MOFH concerns about the availability of beneficiary services needed to be addressed. In response, a new VA medical campus complex was proposed, approved, and subsequently funded (DoD/VA, 2002; GAO, 2004; Principi, 1999; VA/DoD, 1995).

Collocated VA Medical Campus Complex

In 2003, the VA sought a permanent location for an ambulatory care center in Las Vegas, intended to meet the needs of both the VA and the DoD, and a recommendation to build a new hospital there was made in 2004. The location was within a few miles of the MOFH facility. FY 2006 Capital Asset Realignment for Enhanced Services funding supported this construction project for a total estimated cost of $600.4 million (Collins, 2011; Ensign, 2007; MOFH, 2006, 2007; Nicholson, 2005a,b; Panangala, 2005; VA, 2003, 2007a, 2008). The state-of-the-art VA medical center opened on August 6, 2012. At the dedication, Colonel John DeGoes, the 9th Medical Group commander, commented that "this is not a divorce" and that the joint venture "will continue in Las Vegas long into the future" with "two outstanding medical centers, separated by only four miles" (Sanders, 2012).

Lessons Learned

Lessons learned in Las Vegas include that it is important to establish trust between the partners, and leadership, as well as an effective executive council, sets the tone. A joint venture is a partnership in which a single set of standards should be set forth. Both partners need to maintain consistent and open dialogue to reach their common goals and successfully share resources for the benefit of each of the populations represented. Key concerns and other issues should be recorded in formal minutes, and focusing on insignificant issues should be avoided. There should be flexibility in hiring, particularly for emergency room operations, personnel should be jointly trained from the outset, and dual credential/privileging workarounds between the DoD and the VA personnel should be created. In a few specific operational areas, the reimbursement methodology needs to be sufficient; computing technology should be adequate for unique joint venture needs; and equipment such as a patient lift system can minimize patient and staff injuries. Staff should also chronicle clinical experiences so that lessons learned can be shared for the benefit of patients and staff (e.g., that fall patients need to be actively monitored and that the early detection of MRSA [methicillin-resistant Staphylococcus aureus] minimizes internal nosocomial infection and reduces the patient's stay) (Benjamin and Feistman, 2008; DoD/VA, 2008a; Mietzner and Gerrard, 2009; VA/DOD, 2011a).

ANCHORAGE, ALASKA: 3RD MEDICAL GROUP, ELMENDORF AIR FORCE BASE/ALASKA VETERANS AFFAIRS HEALTH CARE SYSTEM

Brief History

Challenges in providing health care services to VA and DoD beneficiaries in Alaska include accessibility (long distances, rugged terrain, severe weather, a limited road system, air evacuation often needed for patient transportation); transportation costs associated with the availability of medical services and clinicians (particularly specialty); the size of the populations served (e.g., sparse in some of the more remote locations); and the opportunity for military clinicians to maintain and improve their skills through the opportunity to consistently work with patients from a broad-based population (Alaska Joint Venture, 2006).

In 1986, the Alaska Veterans Affairs Health Care System and the Air Force initiated a collaborative effort to provide inpatient services to both VA and DoD beneficiaries in a jointly planned, funded, and staffed hospital located on the Elmendorf AFB near Anchorage, Alaska. (The base has been named Joint Base Elmendorf-Richardson since 2010, when Elmendorf AFB and the Army's Fort Richardson were combined under the BRAC action in 2005.) The existing Air Force hospital at Elmendorf needed to be renovated and expanded to serve DoD beneficiaries. VA patients were being treated in area private hospitals because there was no VA inpatient facility. In 1992, after review of the original concept of operations (ConOps) that had been developed 2 years earlier (and was revised in 1998), the Air Force and the VA agreed to build a new hospital together and operate it jointly through a set of sharing agreements. The purposes of the joint venture were to use federal construction dollars more cost effectively, provide inpatient services directly to VA patients at lower cost, reduce per patient operating costs, and increase access and quality of care for both sets of beneficiaries (Alaska Joint Venture, 2006; GAO, 2004).

The project became a formal VA/DoD joint venture in 1999, and additional opportunities to collaborate for the mutual benefit of agencies and their beneficiaries have been identified and pursued since that time. Most significantly, in May 2010, the VA opened a new outpatient clinic located on an 11-acre parcel of Air Force land outside the Muldoon entrance to Elmendorf AFB. It includes a connecting walkway to the Elmendorf hospital, located outside the Air Force security checkpoint, to provide easier access for VA patients. Currently, there are shared arrangements for services at the joint venture hospital on Elmendorf AFB and at the VA outpatient clinic next door, as well as purchased care (or fee-based) arrangements with community hospitals. Primary, specialty, and mental health outpatient care are offered. The Army also hosts the VA's Fairbanks community-based outpatient clinic (CBOC), located in the Bassett Army Community Hospital at Fort Wainwright, under a VA/DoD interagency sharing agreement. The University of Alaska Anchorage, the University of Washington, and the Alaska Family Practice Residency Program are academic partners (Pendergrass, 2010; VA, 2012a).

Lessons Learned

The Alaska joint venture has yielded a number of important lessons. Both partners should be able to gain from the joint venture experience and to collaborate in a positive way toward the achievement of their separate and unified goals through joint strategic planning efforts. Staff from both organizations should approach the partnership as one team that works toward providing the best care for its collective beneficiaries, and these efforts must be consistent. There must be a commitment from the senior leaders, joint venture coordinators, and other organizational staff to establish good working relationships, including maintaining ongoing and systematic organizational communication within and outside of the collaboration. In the financial area, sound business practices must be established, resources must be shared fairly, and reimbursements must be fair and equitable. A joint business office should be set up, through which processes are thoroughly tracked and audit process are implemented to verify accuracy. In addition, it is important to have a VA or a DoD counterpart communicate these processes so everyone will be informed of all key changes. The importance of having a paper trail and maintaining documentation appropriately has also been pointed out. In this joint venture, another important lesson is that the Air Force staff need to be up-to-date in their clinical education and practice (Alaska DoD/VA Joint Venture Hospital, 2011; Anderson and Kurzejeski, 2007; Blair and Cecil, 2007; Spector and Cecil, 2008).

KEY WEST, FLORIDA: NAVAL BRANCH HEALTH CLINIC KEY WEST/MIAMI VETERANS AFFAIRS HEALTH CARE SYSTEM COMMUNITY BASED OUTPATIENT CLINIC KEY WEST

Brief History

The Naval Branch Health Clinic Key West (NBHC Key West [Jacksonville Naval Hospital]) and the Miami Veterans Affairs Healthcare System Community Based Outpatient Clinic Key West (VA CBOC Key West), in Monroe County, became the first Navy-VA joint venture in January 2000. Prior to that time, however, the DoD and the VA had developed sharing agreements for mutually beneficial services and they had shared facilities. The Naval Hospital Key West (NHKW) was commissioned in 1942, and it became the Naval Regional Medical Center (NRMC) in 1979. One year earlier, the General Accounting Office (GAO; former name for the current Government Accountability Office) had reported that the inpatient and outpatient medical services at the NHKW were underutilized and, further, that VA beneficiaries did not have health care services in the local area, which led to increased medical services costs. The VA entered into a sharing agreement with the Navy in 1986 to bring a mental health clinic into the NRMC. The following year, the NRMC facility was condemned, and the care for Navy patients was transferred to the Florida Keys Memorial Hospital. The VA mental health clinic was moved into the local community, but it returned to the newly renovated Navy clinic in 1994. In 1997, the original NRMC building was demolished and a new clinic was constructed, starting from 1998–1999 until early 2000, when the 60,000-square-foot NBHC Key West opened along with the VA CBOC Key West that shared space within the facility. In 2004, the medical and dental operations of the Naval Branch Medical Clinic integrated under the NBHC Key West brand (Cleckley and Ramirez, 2009; DoD/VA, 2006; GAO, 1978, 2000, 2004; Robinson, 2011).

The NBHC Key West and the VA CBOC Key West are both outpatient clinics, and neither offers inpatient or emergency services. The VA CBOC Key West occupies 10 percent of the 57,000-square-foot NBHC Key West facility, and the Navy pharmacy is located adjacent to the NBHC Key West. The NBHC Key West serves active duty military, their families, and other eligible beneficiaries, and offers some specialty services, but refers others out of the network. The VA CBOC Key West offers primary medical and mental health, physical therapy, dermatology, social work, and psychiatry services. The Key West joint venture partners also collaborate with the Naval Air Station Key West (NAS Key West) personnel in the areas of safety and security (Hite, 2011; NBHC, 2012; VA, 2012c).

Lessons Learned

Lessons learned from Key West include that DoD and VA leadership should communicate daily, including electronically, and meet quarterly. The strategic goals of each of the organizations should be understood by the other. Therefore, deliberations that affect the success of joint venture operations and have an impact on the clinics should be open to promote a team effort to try to meet the needs of both partners and to find resolutions to both common and unique problems. Further, communication it should be promoted on all levels of the DoD/VA interdisciplinary team, and it should include holding frequent staff meetings; providing joint training in all areas of mutual concern (e.g., clinical, safety, emergency preparedness) to achieve continuity of care for patients and to create a safe environment for both staff and patients; looking at ways to share resources; and having joint staff celebrations and recognizing the achievements of employees. In the area of staffing, departments need to consult with each other in the areas of credentialing and privileging to address any issues that may arise (Cleckley and Ramirez, 2008, 2009; DoD/VA, 2006; Hardin and Ramirez, 2007; Miavez et al., 2011).

PENSACOLA, FLORIDA, AND BILOXI, MISSISSIPPI: NAVAL HOSPITAL PENSACOLA JOINT AMBULATORY CARE CENTER/VETERANS AFFAIRS GULF COAST VETERANS HEALTH CARE SYSTEM, BILOXI CAMPUS

Brief History

Keesler Air Force Base (Keesler AFB), the 81st Medical Group (81st MDG)/Veterans Affairs Gulf Coast Veterans Health Care System (VAGCVHCS; also called the Veterans Affairs Gulf Coast Health Care System) were identified in FY 2005 as potential DoD/VA sharing agreement partners after the advent of Hurricane Katrina that led to a perceived need for the sharing of services in the Biloxi area. In 2008, these organizations were identified as a center of excellence (CoE) joint sharing site by the Joint Executive Committee, and they entered into a master sharing agreement based on a two-hospital model set up to eliminate duplication of clinical subspecialties. There are five coequal partners in this joint venture: (1) the VAGCVHCS; (2) Keesler AFB's 81st MDG; (3) the Naval Hospital Pensacola (NHP), the location of the Joint Ambulatory Care Center (JACC); (4) Eglin Air Force Base's 96th Medical Group; and (5) Tyndall Air Force Base's 325th Medical Group. Collaboration has taken place since 1996, through sharing agreements between the Navy hospital and the VA-Gulf Coast, with Navy staff treating VA patients through various arrangements for inpatient, emergency, and associated outpatient and ancillary care. The VA has provided laundry services for the Navy since 2000. Since 2001, some VA patients officially had been allowed to receive inpatient and surgical care if space was available; that same year, the VA requested increased services, for example, VA-approved inpatient admissions (Cornum and Wisnieski, 2010; Duren, 2005, 2008; GAO, 2004; Johnson et al., 2009; VA, 2011b,d; VA/DoD, 2008a, 2009b; Wyman, 2010).

The management structure of CoEs differs from other joint ventures. This DoD/VA sharing agreement involves integrated services and buildings that are not located in close proximity to one another, which sets it apart from other CoEs as well. The 81st MDG medical facility is one of the largest in the Air Force (Keesler Air Force Base, 2011). The Biloxi location is the main facility for operations, with CBOCs in Mobile, Alabama; Eglin, Florida; Pensacola, Florida; and Panama City, Florida (Irwin and Drew, 2008; Keesler Air Force Base, 2011; VA, 2011a).

The JACC, a CBOC located adjacent to the NHP, opened in 2008. Double the size of the facility it replaced, the JACC was the result of a 2002 joint recommendation by the NHP and the Biloxi VAGCHCS. In 2008, renovations began to build a VA-specified inpatient ward in the hospital. The open-access Naval Branch Health Clinic (NBHC Corry Station; also referred to as the CWO3 Gary R. Schuetz Memorial Medical Clinic at Corry Station), one of the hospital's branch health clinics, is located at the JACC but serves active duty personnel only. Joint Navy and VA clinic spaces for VA and DoD inpatient, outpatient, emergency, dental, rehabilitative medicine, and physical therapy services are available for the use of beneficiaries in the coastal counties of Alabama, Mississippi, and Florida. Academic outreach includes a residency training program accredited by the GME program through the NHP (Duren, 2005, 2008; Johnson et al., 2009; NBHC Corry Station/JACC, 2011; Robinson, 2011; VA, 2011d).

Lessons Learned

Pensacola has reported that success depends on using the strengths and separate services offered by each of the partners effectively. The partners should have equal standing at the management level, and exercising independent facility management and frequent communication are important. Sharing initiatives should be mutually beneficial, with both high-quality and coordinated patient care programs and financial benefits for each of the partners, and the missions of each should be accommodated in the streamlined construction of the initiatives. Each of the partners should be comfortable with the pace of starting or expanding sharing initiatives, and neither the staff nor the patients should feel rushed into arrangements. On the other hand, however, it has been the experience of this joint venture that the implementation of initiatives can be inordinately slowed down by the contracting process (Cornum and Wisnieski, 2010; Morro et al., 2009).

Biloxi's lessons learned include that it is important for the partners to move at a pace that is comfortable for them, that operations are undertaken when it is appropriate both for their patients and their staff, and that the contracting process itself may prolong implementation of sharing initiatives. The local environment should guide the governance structure that is created, it should be included in the operations plan, and it must encompass all elements of the joint venture, including personnel management, which must comply with the rules and regulations appropriate for the individual partners. A joint market opportunities work group that meets frequently should be created to establish best practices and to identify systemic issues to be addressed by management, particularly at the outset of the joint venture. Strategic planning summits should be held annually and should include all functional experts and the senior leadership. Communication is a key element, and it should take place at all management levels and should extend to unions. The sharing initiatives should be of benefit to all partners financially and meet their unique missions, and they should provide services that are accessible to all patients. Each partner should be allowed to do what it does best, that is, take the lead in those particular areas (Cornum and Wisnieski, 2010; Irwin and Drew, 2008; Robb and Sepich, 2008; VA, 2011c).

CHARLESTON AND BEAUFORT, SOUTH CAROLINA: RALPH A. JOHNSON VETERANS AFFAIRS MEDICAL CENTER; NAVAL HEALTH CLINIC CHARLESTON; 628TH MEDICAL GROUP, JOINT BASE CHARLESTON/ NAVAL WEAPONS STATION; NAVAL HOSPITAL BEAUFORT

Brief History

A unique and robust collaboration among the VA and the Navy and the Air Force of the DoD has been established with the most recent joint venture in Charleston-Beaufort, which has developed over time based on a complex history of sharing activities among (1) the Ralph H. Johnson Veterans Affairs Medical Center (RHJVAMC) and the Naval Health Clinic Charleston (NHCC), including the new Captain John G. Feder Joint Ambulatory Care Clinic, the location of the NHCC and the RHJVAMC CBOC (VA/DoD, 2010) in Goose Creek, South Carolina, which opened in September 2010 at a site on the Naval Weapons Station Charleston (NWSC); (2) the Air Force 628th Medical Group (628th MDG), Joint Base Charleston (JBC)/NWSC (the former Air Force 437th Medical Group [437th MDG])/ Charleston Air Force Base, the host unit until its inactivation in this role in

January 2010 [Joint Base Charleston, 2010]); and (3) the Naval Hospital Beaufort (NHB) in Beaufort, South Carolina (Hite, 2011; VA/DoD, 2010).

Becoming official in October 2011, this complex joint venture is operating under a 5-year ConOps. There are sharing agreements between the VA and the DoD to provide joint care in outpatient cardiology, orthopedics, optometry, and phlebotomy, as well as shared access to a mobile magnetic resonance imaging unit. The RHJVAMC provides care at its JACC CBOC for VA beneficiaries. The naval organizations serve DoD beneficiaries (Hite, 2011; VA/DoD, 2010).

The RHJVAMC opened in 1966. In November 2010, operations moved to Goose Creek, South Carolina, to the JACC facility where the VA shares clinic space with the DoD's NHCC. This consolidation occurred after H.R. 1720 mandated a study that included considering whether a joint-care venture with the Medical University of South Carolina (MUSC) in new facilities for both organizations would be feasible. The RHJVAMC provides primary, secondary, and tertiary care for veterans in South Carolina and Georgia, and supports veteran centers in North Charleston, South Carolina, and in Savannah, Georgia. Additional CBOCs are in Beaufort, Goose Creek, and Myrtle Beach, South Carolina, and in Savannah and Hinesville, Georgia (Hite, 2011; Perlin, 2007; U.S. Congress, 2003; VA, 2002, 2012e). MUSC residents, student trainees, and trainees from several allied health positions rotate through RHJVAMC house staff positions, and this "unique partnership … maintains the nation's only mutually supported research facility, housing collaborative biomedical research with an FY 11 VA and non-VA funding level of about $18 million … and over $10 million in funding from the VA" (MUSC, 2012).

DoD TRICARE Prime and 628th MDG enrollees receive primary, outpatient, pharmacy, laboratory, and ancillary care services at the JACC. Satellite clinics include the Naval Weapons Station Branch Medical, the Naval Nuclear Power Training Command, the Dental, the Medical Readiness/Wellness, and the Optometry Clinics, located at the NWSC (Charleston Joint Venture, 2009; Joint Base Charleston, 2010; Militarynewcomers.com, 2012; VA/DoD, 2010).

The 628th MDG offers outpatient primary care that includes physical therapy and mental health at the Charleston AFB/Joint Base Charleston facility.

The NHB provides inpatient and outpatient services at two branch health clinics, the Marine Corps Air Station at Beaufort and the Marine Corps Recruit Depot at Parris Island (Beaufort SC, 2012; Hite, 2011).

Lessons Learned

In 2006, the GAO issued a report on the VA's experiences in trying to forge partnerships with medical affiliates, specifically, in Denver and Charleston. Although the VA did not support the proposal for a joint venture in Denver, the partnership between the VA and the MUSC in Charleston was still being studied at that time and no final decision had yet been made. The GAO indicated that the Charleston and the Denver experiences yielded the following lessons: "criteria at the departmental level help provide clarity and consistency in evaluation approach; a communications strategy helps avoid misinformation and confusion; leadership support facilitates negotiations; and extensive collaboration assists negotiations" (GAO, 2006, Highlights). In 2011, the following lessons learned about what is needed for or what should be considered when undertaking a joint venture included "exclusionary fiscal processes/seamless flow of money; service footprint with measurable metrics; joint basing considerations; information technology interoperability; and deployment and staffing turnover impact" (Joint Venture Review, 2011, p. 15).

REFERENCES

Alaska DoD (Department of Defense)/VA (Department of Veterans Affairs) Joint Venture Hospital. 2011. Alaska DoD/VA Joint Venture Hospital. 2011 VA/DoD Joint Venture Conference, October. http://www.tricare.mil/DVPCO/CJVC2011.cfm [Elmendorf Joint Venture] (accessed November 29, 2011).

Alaska Joint Venture. 2006. Alaska joint venture. Presentation at 2006 Joint Venture Conference, February. www.tricare.mil/DVPCO/bummed/Navy%20JV%20Conf.Feb06.ppt (accessed October 28, 2011).

Allen, M., and K. C. Carlson. 2009. David Grant USAF Medical Center, VA Northern California Health Care System. Presentation by Col. Mark Allen, David Grant USAF Medical Center, and Ms. K. C. Carlson, VA Northern California Health Care System. http://www.tricare.mil/DVPCO/SharingConf.cfm (June 4, 2009, Breakout 7B—Joint Venture Update, Northern California VAHCS/Travis AFF) (accessed December 6, 2011).

AMEDD (U.S. Army Medical Department). 2011. Current AMEDD/VA joint ventures: Tripler Army Medical Center/VA Pacific Island Health Care System (VAPIHCS). http://vadodrs.amedd.army.mil/JV/JointVentures.html (accessed November 3, 2011).

AMEDD. 2012. William Beaumont Army Medical Center. http://www.wbamc.amedd.army.mil/ (accessed February 10, 2012).

Anderson, D., and A. Kurzejeski. 2007. Alaska VA/3MDG demonstration project: Presentation by Dan Anderson, 3rd Medical Group JV Coordinator, and Adam Kurzejeski, Alaska VA JV Coordinator. 2007 Joint Venture Conference, March 6. http://www.tricare.mil/DVPCO/el-paso/Elmendorf%20Demo%20Update.ppt (accessed October 28, 2011).

Anderson, G. K. 1995. Statement of Maj. Gen. George K. Anderson, USAF, MC, Deputy Assistant Secretary of Defense, Health Services Operations and Readiness, Department of Defense. Hearing on VA/DoD Sharing before the Committee on Hospitals and Health Care, Committee on Veterans' Affairs, House of Representatives, October 18. http://democrats.veterans.house.gov/hearings/schedule104/transcript104/sn104-12.htm (accessed January 17, 2012).

Baine, D. P. 1995. Statement of David P. Baine, Director, Health Care Delivery and Quality Issues, Health, Education, and Human Services Division, GAO. Hearing on VA/DoD Sharing before the Committee on Hospitals and Health Care, Committee on Veterans' Affairs, House of Representatives, October 18. http://democrats.veterans.house.gov/hearings/schedule104/transcript104/sn104-12.htm (accessed January 17, 2012).

Beaufort, SC. 2012. Naval Hospital Beaufort. http://www.beaufortsc.org/military/naval-hospital-beaufort.stml (accessed January 26, 2012).

Benjamin, C., and A. M. Feistman. 2008. The Mike O'Callaghan Federal Hospital: 99th Medical Group and VA Southern Nevada Healthcare System. Presentation by Chris Benjamin, Col, USAF, and Ann Marie Feistman, FACHE. 2008 VA/DoD JV Conference. http://www.tricare.mil/DVPCO/Hawaii/2008%20JV%20Conf%20-%20Las%20Vegas%20JV%20MOFH%20(99MDG-VASNHCS).ppt (accessed January 5, 2012).

Blair, H., and B. Cecil. 2007. Alaska VA/3MDG joint venture. Presentation by Hal Blair, Associate Director, Alaska VA, and COL Billy Cecil, Deputy Commander, 3rd Medical Group. 2007 Joint Venture Conference, March 6. http://www.tricare.mil/DVPCO/el-paso/Elmendorf%20JV%20Update.ppt (accessed October 28, 2011).

Brewin, B. 2011. Joint health record graphical interface contest. May 26. http://whatsbrewin.nextgov.com/2011/05/joint_health_record_graphical_interface_contest.php (accessed November 8, 2011).

Carlton, P. K. 2000. Statement of Lt. Gen Paul K. Carlton, Jr., Surgeon General, United States Air Force. *VA/DoD health care sharing*. Hearing before the Subcommittee on Health of the Committee on Veterans' Affairs, House of Representatives, May 17. Serial No. 106-39. Washington, DC: U.S. Government Printing Office. http://frwebgate.access.gpo.gov/cgi-bin/getdoc.cgi?dbname=106_house_hearings&docid=f:66495.pdf (accessed January 17, 2012).

Charleston Joint Venture. 2009. Success stories on sharing: Joint clinics (Charleston, SC). Power of VHA DOD Sharing Conference, June 3. http://www.tricare.mil/DVPCO/downloads/20090625/Breakout5aSuccessStoriesJointClinicsCharleston.ppt (accessed January 26, 2012).

Cleckley, J., and H. Ramirez. 2008. Key West VA/DoD joint venture: Naval Medical Clinic Key West/Miami VA Health Care System. Lieutenant Janiese Cleckley, BHC Key West, and Dr. Hector Ramirez, VA Miami, 2008 Joint Venture Conference. http://www.tricare.mil/DVPCO/Hawaii/2008%20JV%20Conf%20-%20Key%20West%20JV%20(NBHCKW-MVAHCS).ppt (accessed February 16, 2012).

Cleckley, J., and H. Ramirez. 2009. Naval Branch Health Clinic & VA Outpatient Clinic Key West, FL. Presentation by LT Janiese Cleckley, NBHC Key West, and Dr. Hector Ramirez, VA Key West. 2009 Joint Venture Conference. http://www.tricare.mil/DVPCO/downloads/20090625/Breakout3dJVUpdateKeyWest.ppt (accessed February 16, 2012).

Collins, C. 2011. VA medical centers: Bigger and better. December 25. *Defensemedianetwork*. http://www.defensemedianetwork.com/stories/va-medical-centers-bigger-and-better/ (accessed July 5, 2012).

Committee on Veterans' Affairs, U.S. Senate. 2002. *The fiscal year 2003 budget for veterans' programs*. Hearing before the Committee on Veterans' Affairs, United States Senate, S. Hrg. 107-744, February 14. Washington, DC: U.S. Government Printing Office. http://frwebgate.access.gpo.gov/cgi-bin/getdoc.cgi?dbname=107_senate_hearings&docid=f:82502.wais.pdf (accessed November 3, 2011).

Cornum, K., and T. Wisnieski. 2010. Biloxi/Keesler joint venture site. Presentation by Brig. Gen. Kory Cornum and Mr. Thomas Wisnieski, MPA, FACHE. 2010 VA/DoD Joint Venture Conference. http://www.tricare.mil/DVPCO/lvjvc.cfm (accessed November 11, 2011).

DGMC (David Grant USAF Medical Center)/VANCHCS (Veterans Affairs Northern California Health Care System). 2006. David Grant Medical Center, VA Northern California Health Care System: Joint venture overview. Presentation at the 2006 VA/DoD Joint Venture Conference. www.tricare.mil/DVPCO/bummed/DavidGrant.ppt (accessed December 6, 2011).

DGMC/VANCHCS. 2011. David Grant USAF Medical Center, VA Northern California Health Care System: Joint venture review. Presentation at 2011 VA/DoD Joint Venture Conference. http://www.tricare.mil/DVPCO/CJVC2011.cfm (David Grant Joint Venture) (accessed December 6, 2011).

DoD. 2001. *Department of Defense appropriations for fiscal year 2002.* Hearings before the Subcommittee on Defense of the Committee on Appropriations, United States Senate, H.R. 338, S. Hrg. 107-233, February 28. Washington, DC: U.S. Government Printing Office. http://frwebgate.access.gpo.gov/cgi-bin/getdoc.cgi?dbname=2002_sapp_def_1&docid=f:70712.pdf (accessed December 5, 2011).

DoD. 2010. Department of Defense appropriations for fiscal year 2011. Hearings before the Committee on Appropriations, United States Senate, S. 3800. http://www.gpo.gov/fdsys/pkg/CHRG-111shrg54962/pdf/CHRG-111shrg54962.pdf (accessed January 5, 2012).

DoD/VA. 2002. *Department of Defense and Department of Veterans Affairs health resources sharing: Staff report to the House Committee on Veterans' Affairs*, February 25. Pp. 123–140 in Health care sharing by the Department of Defense and the Department of Veterans Affairs' hearing before the Health Subcommittee of the Committee on Veterans'Affairs and the Military Personnel Subcommittee of the Committee on Armed Services, House of Representatives, March 7. Washington, DC: U.S. Government Printing Office. http://frwebgate.access.gpo.gov/cgi-bin/getdoc.cgi?dbname=107_house_hearings&docid=f:80528.pdf (accessed February 9, 2012).

DoD/VA. 2006. Navy Branch Health Clinic & VA Outpatient Clinic, Key West, FL. Presentation. 2006 Joint Venture Conference. www.tricare.mil/DVPCO/bummed/KeyWest.ppt (accessed February 16, 2012).

DoD/VA. 2008a. Department of Defense (DoD)/Veterans Affairs (VA) Joint Market Opportunities Work Group update. C&CS Communications and Customer Service Conference. http://tricare.mil/conferences/ccs2008/breakout.cfm (accessed August 30, 2012).

DoD/VA. 2008b (July). *Fiscal year 2003 National Defense Authorization Act.* Department of Defense and Department of Veterans Affairs Demonstration Projects. Final report. Washington, DC: DoD/VA.

Duren, R. 2005. Ground broken on new day in VA/DoD 'joint' health care. Naval Hospital Pensacola Public Affairs, May 11. http://www.navy.mil/search/display.asp?story_id=18277 (accessed November 10, 2011).

Duren, R. 2008. Military Medicine teams with VA to open joint out-patient facility. Naval Hospital Pensacola Public Affairs, September 19. http://www.globalsecurity.org/military/library/news/2008/09/mil-080919-nns03.htm (accessed November 10, 2011).

Ensign, J. 2007. Prepared statement of Hon. John Ensign, U.S. Senator from Nevada. *Hearing on construction and lease authorization needs of the Department of Veterans Affairs.* Hearing Before the Committee on Veterans' Affairs, United States Senate, S. Hrg. 109-561, April 6. Washington, DC: U.S. Government Printing Office. http://frwebgate.access.gpo.gov/cgi-bin/getdoc.cgi?dbname=109_senate_hearings&docid=f:28176.pdf (accessed January 5, 2012).

GAO (U.S. General Accounting Office). 1978 (June 14). *Legislation needed to encourage better use of federal medical resources and remove obstacles to interagency sharing.* Report to the Congress of the United States by the comptroller general. HRD-78-54. Washington, DC: GAO. http://archive.gao.gov/f0902a/106271.pdf (accessed February 16, 2012).

GAO. 1996a. *VA health care: Travis Hospital construction project is not justified*. Report to the Chairman, Subcommittee on VA, HUD, and Independent Agencies, Committee on Appropriations, U.S. Senate. GAO/HEHS-9-198. Washington, DC: GAO. http://www.gao.gov/archive/1996/he96198.pdf (accessed December 5, 2011).

GAO. 1996b. *VA health care: Travis Hospital construction project is not justified. Summary and matters for congressional consideration*. Washington, DC: GAO. GAO/HEHS-9-198. http://www.gao.gov/products/157398 (accessed December 5, 2011).

GAO. 1998. *VA hospitals: Issues and challenges for the future*. GAO/HEHS-8-32. Washington, DC: GAO. http://www.gao.gov/archive/1998/he98032.pdf (accessed December 5, 2011).

GAO. 2000. *VA and Defense health care: Evolving health care systems require rethinking of resource sharing strategies*. Washington, DC: GAO. http://www.gao.gov/archive/2000/he00052.pdf (accessed February 16, 2012).

GAO (Government Accountability Office). 2004. *VA and DOD health care: Resource sharing at selected sites*. Report to the chairman, Subcommittee on Oversight and Investigations, Committee on Veterans' Affairs, House of Representatives. GAO-04-792. Washington, DC: GAO. http://www.gao.gov/new.items/d04792.pdf (accessed January 27, 2012).

GAO. 2006. *VA health care: Experiences in Denver and Charleston offer lessons for future partnerships with medical affiliates*. GAO-06-472. Washington, DC: GAO. http://www.gao.gov/new.items/d06472.pdf (accessed January 27, 2012).

GAO. 2007. *VA health care: VA should better monitor implementation and impact of capital asset alignment decisions*. Washington, DC: GAO. http://www.gao.gov/new.items/d07408.pdf (accessed February 6, 2012).

Hardin, D., and H. Ramirez. 2007. Navy Branch Health Clinic/VA Outpatient Clinic, Key West, FL. Presentation by LCDR Dawn Hardin, BHC Key West, and Dr. Hector Ramirez, VA Key West. 2007 Joint Venture Conference. http://www.tricare.mil/DVPCO/el-paso/Key%20West%20VA%20Joint%20Venture%20Conference%202007.ppt (accessed February 16, 2012).

Hite, R. 2011. Personal communication with Robert Hite, Program Manager, Policy, Reports and Analysis, DoD VA Program Coordination Office, Office of the Assistant Secretary of Defense (Health Affairs), October 25.

Horner, B., and J. Holes. 2007. Tripler joint venture update. Presentation by Ms. Brenda Horner and Mr. John Holes. 2007 Joint Venture Conference, March 6. http://www.tricare.mil/DVPCO/el-paso/Tripler%20JV%20Conference%202007%20v3.ppt (accessed November 7, 2011).

Horner, B., and J. Holes. 2008. Tripler Army Medical Center and VA Pacific Islands Health Care System. Presentation by Brenda J. Horner and John E. Holes. 2008 VA/DoD Joint Venture Conference. http://www.tricare.mil/DVPCO/Hawaii/2008%20JV%20Conf%20-%20Hawaii%20JV%20(TAMC-VAPIHCS).ppt (accessed November 7, 2011).

Horner, B., and J. Holes. 2009. Hawaii collaboration. Presentation by Ms. Brenda Horner, Tripler Army Medical Center, and Mr. John E. Holes, VA Pacific Islands Health Care System. Power of DoD/VA Sharing Conference, June 3.

Horner, B., E. Camara, and R. Girton. 2006. DoD/VA joint venture: Joint Venture Incentive Fund proposals. Presentation by project managers Brenda Horner (TAMC) and Dr. Enrico Camara and Dr. Richard Girton (VAPIHCS). 2006 Joint Venture Conference, February. www.tricare.mil/DVPCO/bummed/Tripler.ppt (accessed November 7, 2011).

Irwin, D., and K. Drew. 2008. Elements of a joint venture. Presentation by Ms. Debra Irwin, Chief, DoD/VA Resource Sharing, Air Force Surgeon General's Office, and Ms. Kendra Drew, Director, VA/DoD Medical Sharing Office, Veterans Health Administration. 2008 Joint Venture Conference. http://www.tricare.mil/DVPCO/Hawaii/2008%20JV%20Conf%20-%20Elements%20of%20a%20JV.ppt (accessed December 7, 2011).

Johnson, J. R., R. Lockhart, and D. E. Stoops. 2009. Gulf Coast Joint Ambulatory Care Clinic (JACC). Success stories on sharing: Joint clinics. Presentation by Mr. J. Ronald Johnson, FACHE, Mr. Ralph Lockart, and Mr Dennis E. Stoops. VA/DoD Sharing Conference, June 2–4. http://www.tricare.mil/DVPCO/SharingConf.cfm (accessed November 11, 2011).

Joint Base Charleston. 2010. Joint basing takes pivotal step with activation of 628 ABW. http://www.charleston.af.mil/news/story.asp?id=123184751 (accessed February 6, 2012).

Joint Venture Review. 2011. Charleston-Beaufort: Joint venture review: Naval Health Clinic Charleston; Ralph H. Johnson Veterans Affairs Medical Center; 628 Medical Group, Joint Base Charleston; Naval Hospital Beaufort. 2011 VA/DoD Joint Venture Conference. http://www.tricare.mil/DVPCO/CJVC2011.cfm [Charleston Joint Venture] (accessed January 26, 2012).

Keesler Air Force Base. 2011. 81st Medical Group. http://www.keesler.af.mil/library/factsheets/factsheet.asp?id=4972 (accessed December 14, 2011).

Kolenc, V. 2012. The new Beaumont Army Medical Center: Contractors can benefit from Fort Bliss' $1B project. *El Paso Times*, August 13. http://www.elpasotimes.com/ci_21298898/contractors-can-benefit-from-fort-bliss-1b-project (accessed September 5, 2012).

Kyte, R., and E. Camara. 2006. DoD/VA joint venture: Joint venture demonstration project. Presentation by project managers Rosemary Kyte (TAMC) and Dr. Enrico Camara (VAPIHCS). 2006 Joint Venture Conference, February. www.tricare.mil/DVPCO/bummed/Tripler.ppt (accessed November 7, 2011).

Miavez, J., H. Ramirez, and D. Eaton. 2011. Naval Branch Health Clinic Key West & VA Outpatient Clinic Key West. Presentation by CAPT Julie Miavez, OIC, NBHC Key West, Dr. Hector Ramirez, ACOS, Ambulatory Care VA Miami, and Dr. Douglas Eaton, CMO, VA Key West. 2011 VA/DoD Joint Venture Conference. http://www.tricare.mil/DVPCO/CJVC2011.cfm [Key West Joint Venture] (accessed February 16, 2012).

Mietzner, D., and D. Gerrard. 2009. The Mike O'Callaghan Federal Hospital. Presentation by Col. David Mietzner and Dan Gerrard. 2009 Joint Venture Conference. http://www.tricare.mil/DVPCO/downloads/20090625/Breakout7bJVUpdateMikeOCallaghanFedHospitalNV.ppt (accessed January 6, 2012).

Militarynewcomers.com. 2012. Naval Weapons Station Charleston. Health care. http://www.militarynewcomers.com/NWSCHARLESTON/resources/05_health.html (accessed January 26, 2012).

MOFH (Mike O'Callaghan Federal Hospital). 2006. The Mike O'Callaghan Federal Hospital. Presentation at 2006 Joint Venture Conference, February. www.tricare.mil/DVPCO/bummed/Nevada.ppt (accessed January 5, 2012).

MOFH. 2007. Presentation on Mike O'Callaghan Federal Hospital (MOFH), March 2007, Nellis AFB, NV. 2007 Joint Venture Conference, March. http://www.tricare.mil/DVPCO/el-paso/Nellis%20Joint%20Venture%20Slides%202007c.ppt (accessed January 5, 2012).

Morro, M., D. Wyman, and K. Fogarty. 2009. Gulf Coast joint VA/DoD healthcare network "center(s) of excellence." Presentation by CAPT Maryalice Morro, BG Daniel Wyman, and Ms. Kathleen Fogarty. VA/DoD Sharing Conference, June 2–4. http://www.tricare.mil/DVPCO/SharingConf.cfm (accessed November 11, 2011).

Mosher, P., J. Majerle, and L. Kelly. 2009. Success stories on sharing: Clinical applications (hemodialysis & neurosurgery). Presentation by Peter Mosher, DGMC, John Majerle, VANCHCS, and Laura Kelly, VISN 21. The Power of DoD/VA Sharing Conference, June 4. http://www.tricare.mil/DVPCO/downloads/20090625/Breakout6aSuccessStoriesClinicalApplicationsNeurosurgeryDialysisClinicsFairfieldCA.ppt (accessed December 7, 2011).

MUSC (Medical University of South Carolina). 2012. Ralph H. Johnson Veteran's Administration Medical Center. http://academicdepartments.musc.edu/research/ord/collab_proposal/institutional_boilerplate/clinical/va.html (accessed September 5, 2012).

NBHC (Naval Branch Health Clinic). 2012. Key West Branch Health Clinic. http://www.med.navy.mil/sites/NavalHospitalJAX/AboutUs/Pages/Keywest.aspx (accessed February 16, 2012).

NBHC Corry Station/JACC. 2011. Corry Station. http://www.med.navy.mil/sites/pcola/NavyBranchHealthClinics/CorryStation/Pages/default.aspx (accessed November 9, 2011).

Nellis Air Force Base. 2012. Medical services. http://www.nellis.af.mil/library/factsheets/factsheet.asp?id=4073 (accessed January 8, 2012).

Nicholson, R. J. 2005a. Prepared statement of Hon. James Nicholson, Secretary, Department of Veterans Affairs. *Proposed fiscal year 2006 budget for Department of Veterans Affairs programs*. Hearing before the Committee on Veterans' Affairs, United States Senate, S. Hrg. 109-72, February 15. Washington, DC: U.S. Government Printing Office. http://frwebgate.access.gpo.gov/cgi-bin/getdoc.cgi?dbname=109_senate_hearings&docid=f:22412.pdf (accessed January 3, 2012).

Nicholson, R. J. 2005b. Statement of the Honorable R. James Nicholson, Secretary, Department of Veterans Affairs. *Department of Veterans Affairs budget request for FY 2006*. Hearing before the Committee on Veterans' Affairs, House of Representatives, February 16. Serial No. 109-1. Washington, DC: U.S. Government Printing Office. http://frwebgate.access.gpo.gov/cgi-bin/getdoc.cgi?dbname=109_house_hearings&docid=f:20426.pdf (accessed January 5, 2012).

Pacific Region Health Systems. 2011. http://virtual.mybaseguide.com/military/army/tripler/#page68I (accessed November 3, 2011).

Panangala, S. V. 2005. *Veterans health care issues in the 109th Congress*. CRS report for Congress, June 24. Order Code RL32961. Washington, DC: Congressional Research Service. http://www.policyarchive.org/handle/10207/bitstreams/2477.pdf (accessed January 3, 2012).

Pendergrass, S. 2010. Statement of Dr. Susan Pendergrass, Director, VA Northwest Network (VISN 20), Veterans Health Administration, Department of Veterans Affairs, before the Committee on Veterans' Affairs, United States Senate, Field Hearing in Fairbanks, Alaska. http://veterans.senate.gov/hearings.cfm?action=release.display&release_id=73308297-1724-4e95-b725-84a067127c9d (accessed November 29, 2011).

Perdue, R., and M. Ancker. 2007. ELPVAHCS-WBAMC update. Presentation by Ray Perdue and Mary Ancker. 2007 VA/DoD Joint Venture Conference. http://www.tricare.mil/DVPCO/el-paso/El%20Paso%20JV%20Update%202007.ppt (accessed February 9, 2012).

Perdue, R., and M. Ancker. 2011. El Paso joint venture update. Presentation by Ray Perdue and Mary Ancker. 2011VA/DoD Joint Venture Conference. http://www.tricare.mil/DVPCO/El-Paso.cfm [El Paso Joint Venture Update] (accessed February 9, 2012).

Perlin, J. B. 2006. Testimony of Hon. Jonathan B. Perlin, MD, PhD, Under Secretary for Health, Department of Veterans Affairs. *Field hearing on the state of VA care in Hawaii: Part II*. Hearing before the Committee on Veterans' Affairs, United States Senate, S. Hrg. 109-376, January 11. Washington, DC: U.S. Government Printing Office. http://ftp.resource.org/gpo.gov/hearings/109s/27351.txt (accessed January 5, 2012).

Perlin, J. B. 2007. Statement of Jonathan B. Perlin, MD, PhD, MSHA, FACP, Under Secretary for Health, Department of Veterans Affairs. *Department of Veterans Affairs collaboration opportunities with affiliated medical institutions and the DOD*. Hearing before the Committee on Veterans' Affairs, House of Representatives, March 8, 2006. Serial No. 109-37. Washington, DC: U.S. Government Printing Office. http://frwebgate.access.gpo.gov/cgi-bin/getdoc.cgi?dbname=109_house_hearings&docid=f:26675.pdf (accessed January 27, 2012).

Perera, D. 2011. iEHR will be in place 4 to 6 years from now, says Baker. *Fierce Government*, May 31. http://www.fiercegovernmentit.com/story/iehr-will-be-place-4-6-years-now-says-baker/2011-05-31 (accessed November 8, 2011).

Principi, A. J. 1999. Verbal testimony of Anthony J. Principi. *To receive the report of the Congressional Commission on Servicemembers and Veterans Transition Assistance*. Hearing before the Committee on Veterans' Affairs, House of Representatives, February 23. Serial No. 106-2. Washington, DC: U.S. Government Printing Office. http://frwebgate.access.gpo.gov/cgi-bin/getdoc.cgi?dbname=106_house_hearings&docid=f:56375.pdf (accessed January 3, 2012).

Roadman, C., II. 1999. Statement of Lt. Gen. Charles Roadman, II, Surgeon General, United States Air Force. Department of the Air Force presentation on the Defense Health Program to the Committee on Armed Services Subcommittee on Personnel, United States Senate, March 11. http://armed-services.senate.gov/statemnt/1999/990311cr.pdf (accessed January 17, 2012).

Robb, D. J., and C. Sepich. 2008. Gulf Coast joint VA/DoD healthcare network "center(s) of excellence." Presentation by BG Douglas J. Robb, Commander, 81st Medical Group, Keesler AFB, and Mr. Charles Sepich, Director, VA Gulf Coast Veterans Healthcare System. 2008 VA/DoD Joint Venture Conference, March 4–6. http://www.tricare.mil/DVPCO/Hawaii/2008%20JV%20Conf%20-%20Gulf%20Coast%20Healthcare%20Network.ppt (accessed December 13, 2011).

Robinson, A. M., Jr. 2011. Prepared statement of Vice Admiral Adam M. Robinson, Jr. *Defense Health Program FY12 budget*. Hearing before the Subcommittee on Defense of the Senate Committee on Appropriations, April 6. Washington, DC: U.S. Government Printing Office. http://frwebgate.access.gpo.gov/cgi-bin/getdoc.cgi?dbname=2012_sapp_def_3&docid=f:99104433.pdf (accessed January 27, 2012).

Rogers, B. 2007. Albuquerque joint venture. Presentation by Ben Rogers, CHE, NMVAHCS Joint Venture Director. 2007 Joint Venture Conference, March 8. http://www.tricare.mil/DVPCO/el-paso/JV%20ConfAlbuquerque.ppt (accessed January 17, 2012).

Sanders, J. 2012. VA medical center opens, keeps strong ties to Mike O'Callaghan. 99th Air Base Wing Public Affairs, Nellis Air Force Base. http://www.nellis.af.mil/news/story.asp?id=123315628 (accessed September 5, 2012).

Scharenbrock, C., and K. C. Carlson. 2010. Joint venture partnership successes, VANCHCS & Tribal Entities, DGMC & VANCHCS. Presentation by Dr. Christopher Scharenbrock, David Grant USAF Medical Center, and K. C. Carlson, VA Northern California Health Care System, January.

Simmons, J. 1989. Integrating federal health care resources at the local level. *Hospital & Health Services Administration* 34(1):113–122.

Spaulding, S., and K. L. Catton. 2008. Albuquerque joint venture. Presentation by Scott Spaulding, 377th Medical Group, and Kara L. Catton, New Mexico VAHCS. 2008 VA/DoD Joint Venture Conference, March. http://www.tricare.mil/DVPCO/Hawaii/2008%20JV%20Conf%20-%20Albuquerque%20JV%20(377MDG-NMVAHCS).ppt (accessed January 17, 2012).

Spector, A., and B. Cecil. 2008. Alaska. Presentation by Mr. Alex Spector, VA Director, and Colonel Billy Cecil, 3MDG Deputy Commander. 2008 VA/DoD Joint Venture Conference. http://www.tricare.mil/DVPCO/Hawaii/2008%20JV%20Conf%20-%20 Alaska%20JV%20(3MDG-VAHCS).ppt (accessed October 31, 2011).

U.S. Congress. 2003. H.R. 1720, to authorize the Secretary of Veterans Affairs to carry out construction projects for the purpose of improving, renovating, establishing, and updating patient care facilities at Department of Veterans Affairs medical centers, to provide by law for the establishment and functions of the Office of Research Oversight in the Veterans Health Administration of the Department of Veterans Affairs, and for other purposes. http://www.gpo.gov/fdsys/pkg/BILLS-108hr1720rfs/pdf/BILLS-108hr1720rfs.pdf (accessed January 27, 2012).

U.S. Senate. 1980. Hearing before the Committee on Governmental Affairs, United States Senate, Ninety-sixth Congress, Second Session, on S. 2958, Federal Interagency Medical Resources Sharing and Coordination Act of 1980, July 30. http://babel.hathitrust.org/cgi/pt?id=mdp.39015083099906 (accessed February 23, 2012).

VA. 2002. *Health care sharing by the Department of Veterans Affairs and Department of Defense*. Staff report to the House Committee on Veterans' Affairs, February 25. Hearing before the Health Subcommittee of the Committee on Veterans'Affairs and the Military Personnel Subcommittee of the Committee on Armed Services, House of Representatives, March 7. Washington, DC: U.S. Government Printing Office. http://frwebgate.access.gpo.gov/cgi-bin/getdoc.cgi?dbname=107_house_hearings&docid=f:80528.pdf (accessed January 27, 2012).

VA. 2003. *Departments of Veterans Affairs and Housing and Urban Development, and independent agencies appropriations for fiscal year 2004*. Hearings before the Subcommittee of the Committee on Appropriations, March 13. Washington, DC: U.S. Government Printing Office. http://frwebgate.access.gpo.gov/cgi-bin/getdoc.cgi?dbname=2004_sapp_va_1&docid=f:1910401.pdf (accessed January 3, 2012).

VA. 2006. *Hearing on construction and lease authorization needs of the Department of Veterans Affairs*. Hearing before the Committee on Veterans' Affairs, United States Senate, S. Hrg. 109-561, April 6. Washington, DC: U.S. Government Printing Office. http://frwebgate.access.gpo.gov/cgi-bin/getdoc.cgi?dbname=109_senate_hearings&docid=f:28176.pdf (accessed January 5, 2012).

VA. 2007a. *The VA's budget request for fiscal year 2007*. Hearing before the Committee on Veterans' Affairs, House of Representatives, February 8. Serial No. 109-30. Washington, DC: U.S. Government Printing Office. http://frwebgate.access.gpo.gov/cgi-bin/getdoc.cgi?dbname=109_house_hearings&docid=f:26103.pdf (accessed January 5, 2012).

VA. 2007b. *VA handbook 0311*. Appendix C (p. C-3). November 8. http://www1.va.gov/vapubs/viewPublication.asp?Pub_ID=381&FType=2 (accessed January 5, 2012).

VA. 2008. VA FY 2008 Congressional budget submission, Vol. III, Construction. http://www.va.gov/budget/products.asp [FY 2008 Budget Submission] (accessed January 6, 2012).

VA. 2011a. VA Gulf Coast Veterans Health Care System. http://www.biloxi.va.gov/about/ (accessed December 14, 2011).

VA. 2011b. VA Gulf Coast: Joint venture review. 2011 VA/DoD Joint Venture Conference. http://www.tricare.mil/DVPCO/CJVC2011.cfm [Keesler Joint Venture] (accessed November 11, 2011).

VA. 2011c. VA Gulf Coast: Joint venture review. 2011 VA/DoD Joint Venture Conference. http://www.tricare.mil/DVPCO/CJVC2011.cfm [Keesler Joint Venture] (accessed November 11, 2011).

VA. 2011d. VA Gulf Coast Veterans Health Care System. http://www.biloxi.va.gov/visitors/Pensacola.asp (accessed November 9, 2011).

VA. 2012a. Alaska VA Healthcare System, Fairbanks, Alaska, Community-Based Outpatient Clinic. http://www.alaska.va.gov/visitors/fairbanks.asp (accessed April 27, 2012).

VA. 2012b. El Paso VA Health Care System. http://www2.va.gov/directory/guide/facility.asp?ID=46 (accessed February 10, 2012).

VA. 2012c. Miami VA Healthcare System: Locations. Key West Outpatient Clinic. http://www.miami.va.gov/locations/KeyWest.asp (accessed February 16, 2012).

VA. 2012d. New VA medical center with state-of-the-art mental unit to open in Las Vegas. http://www.va.gov/opa/pressrel/pressrelease.cfm?id=2363 (accessed September 27, 2012).

VA. 2012e. Ralph H. Johnson VA Medical Center. About this facility. http://www.charleston.va.gov/about (accessed January 26, 2012).

VA/DoD. 1995. Hearing on VA/DoD sharing before the Subcommittee on Hospitals and Health Care, Committee on Veterans' Affairs, House of Representatives, October 18. http://democrats.veterans.house.gov/hearings/schedule104/transcript104/sn104-12.htm (accessed January 3, 2012).

VA/DoD. 2000. *VA/DoD health care sharing*. Hearing before the Subcommittee on Health of the Committee on Veterans' Affairs, House of Representatives, May 17. Serial No. 106-39. Washington, DC: U.S. Government Printing Office. http://frwebgate.access.gpo.gov/cgi-bin/getdoc.cgi?dbname=106_house_hearings&docid=f:66495.pdf (accessed December 5, 2011).

VA/DoD. 2002. *Department of Veterans Affairs and Department of Defense health resources sharing: Staff report*. Committee on Veterans' Affairs, U.S. House of Representatives, February 25. Washington, DC: U.S. Government Printing Office. http://veterans.house.gov/sites/republicans.veterans.house.gov/files/documents/vadodsha.pdf (accessed February 9, 2012).

VA/DoD. 2006. VA/DoD joint venture: Wm Beaumont Army Medical Center and El Paso VA Health Care System. Presentation at 2006 Joint Venture Conference, February. www.tricare.mil/DVPCO/bummed/ElPaso.ppt (accessed February 9, 2012).

VA/DoD. 2007. VA/DoD Joint Executive Council FY 2006 annual report. February. http://www.tricare.mil/DVPCO/downloads/VADoD2006.pdf (accessed November 7, 2011).

VA/DoD. 2008a. VA/DoD Joint Executive Council fiscal year 2007 annual report. February. http://www.tricare.mil/DVPCO/downloads/VA%20DoD%202007%20Annual%20Report%20FINAL%203-14-08.pdf (accessed December 13, 2011).

VA/DoD. 2008b. VA/DoD Joint Executive Council FY 2008 annual report, including 2009–2011 joint strategic plan. http://www.tricare.mil/DVPCO/downloads/VA%20DoD%20Joint%20Executive%20Council%20Annual%20Report.pdf (accessed November 8, 2011).

VA/DoD. 2009a. VA/DoD Joint Executive Committee FY 2009 annual report: Joint strategic plan 2010–2012. http://prhome.defense.gov/docs/2009%20VA%20DoD%20Joint%20Executive%20Council%20Annual%20Report%20and%20Joint%20Strategic%20Plan.pdf (accessed November 8, 2011).

VA/DoD. 2009b. VA/DoD Joint Executive Council FY 2008 annual report, including 2009–2011 joint strategic plan.

VA/DoD. 2010. VA/DoD Joint Executive Council annual report for FY 2010. http://www.tricare.mil/DVPCO/downloads/2010%20JEC%20Annual%20Report%20to%20Congress%20(signed).pdf (accessed January 27, 2012).

VA/DoD. 2011a. Mike O'Callaghan Federal Hospital briefing. 2011 VA/DoD Joint Venture Conference. http://www.tricare.mil/DVPCO/CJVC2011.cfm [Las Vegas Joint Venture] (accessed January 3, 2012).

VA/DoD. 2011b. New Mexico VA Health Care System, 377th Medical Group, Kirtland AFB, Albuquerque, NM. 2011 VA/DoD Joint Venture Conference. http://www.tricare.mil/DVPCO/CJVC2011.cfm [Albuquerque Joint Venture] (accessed January 17, 2012).

Wilder, D., and L. Kelly. 2011. Personal communication and discussion with the IOM Committee on Evaluation of the Lovell Federal Health Care Center Merger. Conference call with Lt. Col. Doreen Wilder, David Grant USAF Medical Center, Travis Air Force Base, California, and Laura Kelly, VA Northern California Health Care System, in public session during the committee's fourth meeting. Irvine, California, November 17–18.

Wirtemburg, D., and M. Ancker. 2008. El Paso joint venture: Wm. Beaumont Army Medical Center and El Paso VA Health Care System. Presentation by Dane Wirtemburg, ELP-VAHCS, and Mary Ancker, WBAMC. Annual 2008 VA/DoD Joint Venture Conference. http://www.tricare.mil/DVPCO/Hawaii.cfm [El Paso Joint Venture] (accessed February 9, 2012).

Wyman, D. 2010. Gulf Coast sharing success. Presentation by Brig Gen Daniel Wyman, 81 Medical Group, Keesler AFB. 2010 Military Health System Conference, January 26. http://www.health.mil/Libraries/2010_MHS_Conference_Presentations_-_Jan_26/T06_D_Wyman.pdf (accessed December 13, 2011).

Appendix D

Collaboration Among Health Care Organizations: A Review of Outcomes and Best Practices for Effective Performance[1,2]

ABSTRACT

Despite the prevalence of collaborative ventures among health care organizations, including mergers, alliances, and joint ventures, the majority of these ventures fail to significantly improve the overall performance of the organizations involved. There is a great deal of variation in the outcomes of collaborative ventures, but results from several studies indicate that key practices, including effective leadership before, during, and after these ventures are implemented, may promote their effectiveness. This paper identifies these best practices for policy makers and managers concerned with improving the outcomes of collaboration among health care organizations. To this end, I (1) review evidence on the context and outcomes of collaboration among health care provider organizations and (2) examine results concerning the processes of change and implementation practices involved in efforts to collaborate (to what extent, and how, these factors affect the outcomes of collaboration). I conclude by presenting a checklist of best practices for improving the outcomes of collaboration and discuss leadership approaches for putting these practices into effect.

---

[1] Prepared by Thomas D'Aunno, Ph.D., Columbia University, Department of Health Policy and Management, Mailman School of Public Health, with the assistance of Yi-Ting Chiang, M.P.H., and Mattia Gilmartin, Ph.D.

[2] The authors are responsible for the content of this article, which does not necessarily represent the views of the Institute of Medicine.

INTRODUCTION

Hospitals and other health care organizations across the United States are engaging in collaborative ventures—including alliances, joint ventures, and mergers and acquisitions—at an increasing rate. *Modern Healthcare*'s (2012) annual mergers-and-acquisitions reports show, for example, a 3.5 and 3.4 percent increase in the number of mergers-and-acquisitions deals in 2010 and 2011, respectively, and a 73 percent increase in the number of hospitals involved in these deals from 2009 to 2010, the greatest increase in the past decade. Health care providers may be increasing their efforts to collaborate in response to the new risks and opportunities they face, stemming primarily from the Patient Protection and Affordable Care Act (ACA) and the service delivery models it promotes, as well as related pay-for-performance reforms that aim to improve quality of care.

Unfortunately, the majority of collaborative ventures among health care organizations fail to significantly improve the overall performance of participants; there is a great deal of variation in outcomes (Bazzoli et al., 2004; Cartwright and Schoenberg, 2006; King et al., 2004). However, several study results indicate that key practices, including effective leadership before, during, and after these ventures are implemented, may promote their effectiveness (Hansen, 2009; Marks et al., 2001).

The purpose of this paper is to identify these best practices for policy makers and managers concerned with improving the outcomes of collaboration among health care organizations. I organize the paper as follows. First, I briefly define and distinguish major forms of collaboration, focusing on relationships among hospitals and physicians as the key organized providers of health care; this section also presents the conceptual framework that guided my work. Second, I review evidence on the context and outcomes of collaboration among health care provider organizations. Next, I examine results concerning the processes of change and implementation practices involved in efforts to collaborate—To what extent, and how, do these factors affect the outcomes of collaboration? I present a checklist of best practices for improving the outcomes of collaboration and discuss leadership approaches that can help put these practices into effect. I conclude with a discussion of observations about best practices for effective collaboration (Hansen, 2009).

COLLABORATION AMONG HEALTH CARE ORGANIZATIONS: DEFINITIONS AND DISTINCTIONS

This paper examines key forms of collaboration among health care providers who aim to coproduce services. I focus primarily on three major forms of collaboration among health care organizations: mergers and acquisitions, alliances, and joint ventures. Further, following Bazzoli et al. (2004), I focus on these forms of collaboration among hospitals and physician groups—the two most important organized providers of health care services.

A merger is the consolidation of two or more firms, including the pooling of their assets, into a single legal entity. The terms *merger* and *acquisition* often are used interchangeably, but there is a technical difference between them: mergers are consolidations of equal partners, while in acquisitions one organization buys the assets of another.

In contrast to mergers are alliances, which are voluntary, formal arrangements among two or more organizations for the purposes of ongoing cooperation and mutual sharing of gains and risks (Zajac et al., 2010). Alliances are similar to mergers in that often they are formed for strategic purposes; that is, they aim to promote an organization's mission and enhance organizational performance. Yet, members of alliances retain their legal independence; indeed, some alliance agreements are more informal than formal, and may involve little commitment of partners' resources.

A joint venture is a formal agreement in which parties unite to develop, for a finite time, a new legal entity by contributing funds or resources of some kind (e.g., labor). The partners exercise control over the new organization and consequently share revenues, expenses, and assets. Because the cost of starting new projects is generally high, a joint venture allows both parties to share the burden of the project, as well as any resulting profits.

In sum, I focus on mergers, alliances, and joint ventures because they represent a continuum of approaches to collaboration among health care organizations, ranging from those that change the legal status of organizations (e.g., mergers and acquisitions) to those that involve the pooling of only limited resources among partners (e.g., joint ventures) to those that are less formal and involve commitments of fewer resources than either mergers or joint ventures (e.g., alliances) (Zajac et al., 2010). Figure D-1 shows the conceptual framework that guides this review and discussion.

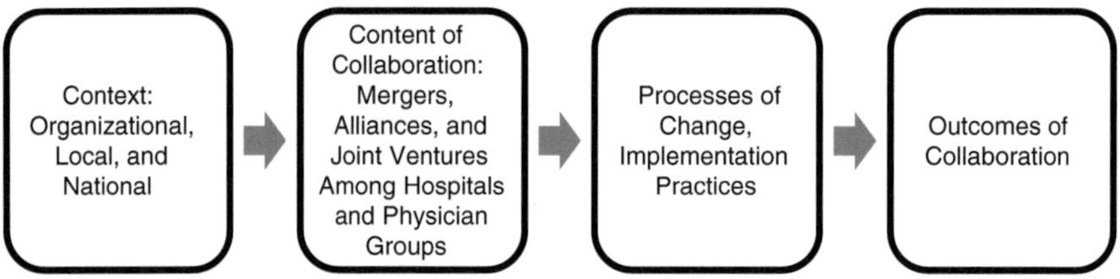

FIGURE D-1 Conceptual framework of collaboration among health care organizations.

Here, based on prior research on organizational change (Pettigrew et al., 2001; Weick and Quinn, 1999), I aim to examine factors internal to health care organizations, as well as their local and national contexts, that can promote or hinder interest in collaboration and, importantly, affect the processes and outcomes of collaboration. In response to these internal and contextual factors, organizations may seek to collaborate with other health care providers. If so, they may select among major alternative forms of collaboration (i.e., mergers, alliances, and joint ventures), which, following Bazzoli et al. (2004), I term the *content* of collaboration. Next, processes of organizational change and implementation unfold as organizations aim to achieve their desired ends. Finally, these change processes result in a variety of outcomes.

Table D-1 elaborates the framework in Figure D-1 by indicating key variables in each stage of the model. As Table D-1 shows, I define the outcomes of interest broadly to include measures of quality, cost, and access to care; financial performance; productivity; and patient and stakeholder satisfaction.

To achieve the objectives for this paper, I reviewed relevant empirical studies in both the health care and non-health care sectors. I focused heavily on studies published in top-tier journals in the past decade, in part because useful reviews of prior work were available. Though I focused primarily on studies in the health care sector, researchers have studied collaborative strategy in non-health care industries for decades, and I also draw on this work.

COLLABORATION AMONG HOSPITALS

Collaboration among hospitals, through either mergers or alliances, has been relatively substantial for many years. The Premier hospital alliance, for example, spans the nation and now includes 2,300 hospitals; Premier makes $33 billion worth of purchases per year (Zajac et al., 2010). Current interest in hospital mergers was preceded by a large national wave of mergers that occurred between 1990 and 2003, resulting in an average reduction of competitors in metropolitan areas from 6 to 4 (Vogt and Town, 2006). By the mid-2000s, at least 88 percent of metropolitan residents lived in highly concentrated hospital markets, with even greater concentration in more rural areas.

Prior work indicates that hospitals have pursued mergers and alliances primarily to maintain or improve their financial performance (Bazzoli et al., 2004). Results from studies in the 1980s (e.g., Alexander and Morrisey, 1988) show that hospitals with weak financial performance were more likely to merge or join multihospital arrangements. In contrast, studies of hospital mergers and alliances in the 1990s suggest that these efforts were

TABLE D-1 Key Variables in Collaboration Among Health Care Organizations

Organizational, Local, and National Contexts	Change Processes and Implementation Practices	Intermediate Outcomes	Long-Term Impact
• Number and location of facilities • Size and number of people served • Local health care market—public and private sectors • Community support and needs	• Early planning to manage both technical and people-focused tasks • Careful attention to roles of leadership, culture • Use of comprehensive, evidence-based checklist for implementation • Effective communications strategy—educating and orienting staff; mobilizing support • Adequate resources for transition management team	• Staff satisfaction • Meeting quality-of-care benchmark measures • Patient satisfaction • Progress toward partners' stated goals and objectives • Changes in service mix and operations: combining departments and services; transferring personnel • Developing shared information technology/electronic health records	• Operating efficiencies, productivity • Overall financial performance • Patient functional health status; patient satisfaction • Increased market share in local area • Employee and other stakeholder satisfaction • Progress on partners' stated goals and objectives for the collaboration

more a response to external market pressure than to internal weaknesses; that is, strong hospitals anticipated that managed care would have negative effects on their financial performance, and sought mergers to protect themselves (Bazzoli et al., 2003, 2004).

The potential financial benefits from hospital mergers may stem from (1) price increases facilitated by increased market power; (2) cost reduction through economies of scope, scale, and monopsony power; and (3) favorable adjustments in service and product mix (Krishnan et al., 2004). To date, Bazzoli et al. (2004) and Vogt and Town (2006) have provided the most comprehensive analyses of research that addresses these issues; their

TABLE D-2 Summary of Empirical Studies of the Effects of Hospital Mergers, Systems, and Alliances on Hospital Financial Performance and Quality of Care

	Form of Collaboration		
Outcome	Mergers	Multihospital Systems	Alliances
Hospital prices	Mergers in metropolitan areas raised hospital prices by at least 5 percent and probably significantly more; studies of mergers among geographically-proximate hospitals show price increases of 40 percent or more	Some evidence for higher prices (Dranove et al., 1996; Young et al., 2000)	Some evidence for higher prices
Cost savings	Mixed results, but balance of evidence indicates that mergers result in cost savings for participating hospitals	Little or no cost savings (Dranove and Lindrooth, 2003)	Little or no cost savings
Revenue, profit	Mergers are consistently associated with higher revenue and profits	Higher revenues and profits	Some evidence for higher revenues per patient discharge (Clement et al., 1997)
Quality of care	Results are mixed, but evidence from the best studies indicates that mergers likely decrease quality of care (Hayford, 2011)	No quality improvement, with some evidence of decreased quality (Ho and Hamilton, 2000)	No quality improvement, with some evidence of decreased quality (Ho and Hamilton, 2000)

reviews cover dozens of empirical studies. Table D-2 provides a summary of their analyses. In addition to examining the effects of hospital mergers and alliances, Bazzoli et al. (2004) reviewed studies of the effects of membership in multihospital systems; Table D-2 presents these results as a point of comparison.

Conclusions About Collaboration Among Hospitals

I draw several important conclusions from empirical studies of collaboration among hospitals. First, there is sound evidence that hospital mergers are linked to better financial performance for the participating hospitals: they have higher prices, revenues, and profits.

Second, hospital mergers lead to some cost savings, which, combined with charging higher prices, probably accounts for higher profits. Yet, the evidence on cost savings from mergers may be changing. Harrison (2011) recently reported results from a careful study of two hospital mergers that showed significant cost savings through economy of scale in the first year following a merger, but these cost savings decreased by the third year postmerger, and were no longer significant.

Third, in contrast to the results for mergers, there are fewer improvements in the financial performance of hospitals that join multihospital systems. Results from well-executed studies by Dranove and colleagues (1996; Dranove and Lindrooth, 2003) show increased prices and higher revenues for members of multihospital systems, but no cost savings.

Fourth, alliances do not seem to boost the financial performance of their member hospitals as much as mergers or multihospital systems.

Fifth, results show few quality-of-care benefits from collaboration among hospitals, and indeed there is some evidence for decreased quality of care following mergers. Some studies show no statistically significant postmerger changes in quality of care (Capps, 2005; Cuellar and Gertler, 2005), while others show a negative association. Hayford (2011), for example, analyzed 40 mergers among California hospitals from 1990 to 2006 and found that these mergers were associated with higher inpatient mortality rates among heart disease patients. Similarly, Ho and Hamilton (2000) found some evidence for decreased quality of care for heart disease patients in a study that compares hospitals' premerger to postmerger performance using measures of inpatient mortality for heart attack and stroke patients and 90-day readmission rates for heart attack patients. Discrepancies in results may be due to the difficulty in isolating the effect of mergers per se on quality of care (Gaynor, 2006).

Finally, there is some evidence that the organizational structure of hospital systems and alliances can account for variation in their financial performance (Bazzoli et al., 2004). In a national study, Bazzoli and colleagues (1999, 2000) found some systems and alliances that exercised centralized control over a variety of decisions and others in which control was decentralized. Further, Bazzoli et al. (1999, 2000) showed that members of multihospital systems generally had better financial performance than hospitals in alliances. Hospitals that belonged to highly centralized alliances had better financial performance than those belonging to more decentralized alliances. However, hospitals in moderately centralized systems performed better than those in highly centralized systems. Finally, hospitals in systems and alliances with little centralization experienced the poorest financial performance (Bazzoli et al., 2000).

In short, these results suggest that more centralized decision making in hospital systems and alliances leads to better financial performance for their members. This result may provide at least a partial explanation for the observation that "mergers among equals" seem difficult to implement (Kastor, 2001). That is, in mergers among hospitals that view themselves as equals, it may be more difficult to establish a centralized decision-making body because each party seeks to maintain its control over key decisions. Well-known examples include the failed "mergers of equals" between major teaching hospitals, in particular the Stanford University and the University of California, San Francisco, hospitals, and the Mount Sinai and the New York University hospitals (Kastor, 2001). More work is needed, however, to understand the effects of organizational characteristics, including the structure of decision making, on the financial performance of hospital systems and alliances (see Bazzoli et al., 2006; Luke, 2006; Trinh et al., 2010).

COLLABORATION AMONG PHYSICIAN GROUPS

Collaboration among physicians has occurred primarily through three types of organizations: group practices, independent practice associations (IPAs), and physician practice management companies (PPMCs) (Bazzoli et al., 2004). The number of IPAs and PPMCs has fluctuated, but the trend toward physicians working in groups has remained steady, resulting in an increased number of group practices (Boukus et al., 2009).

Studies of the relative benefits of collaboration among physician groups show results similar to those for hospitals. Identified benefits include opportunities for efficiencies in clinical care and management and greater power in negotiating contracts with insurers (Burns, 1997). Studies also show some unique benefits for physician groups: compared with the alternative of small, independent practices, mergers and alliances among physicians can increase their access to capital and management expertise (Robinson, 1998).

Most studies of collaboration among physicians have examined group practices that formed or grew through mergers or acquisitions. Summarizing results from several studies that examined the effects of collaboration among physicians, Bazzoli et al. (2004) draw three conclusions. First, there are limited cost savings; this result is similar to that reported for hospitals in multihospital systems and alliances (see Table D-2). Second, there can be important effects on physician use of resources, but these effects vary greatly and depend on the mechanisms used to monitor physician practice.

In a study of 94 physician organizations in California, for example, Kerr et al. (1995, 1996) reported the extensive use of quality assurance activities and a variety of utilization management techniques to control resource use. Yet, on balance, results from studies of physician resource use in group practices are mixed. For example, in contrast to Kerr and colleagues, Kralewski and colleagues (1996, 1998, 1999, 2000) found relatively few controls on physician resource use in the Minnesota group practices they studied. Finally, results are mixed for patient satisfaction in group medical practices.

COLLABORATION AMONG PHYSICIAN GROUPS AND HOSPITALS

Research suggests that physician groups and hospitals seek to collaborate for many reasons, only some of which overlap (Burns and Muller, 2008). Hospitals pursue closer relationships with physicians to

- capture outpatient markets;
- increase revenues and margins;
- improve care processes and outcomes;
- increase the loyalty of their physicians;
- bolster physicians' practices and incomes; and
- address weaknesses in existing hospital medical staff.

Physicians likewise enter these relationships to increase practice incomes and improve the quality of service to patients, but, otherwise, their goals diverge from those of hospitals. Physicians want to increase their access to capital and technology and increase their control in care delivery.

Although physician-hospital collaboration takes many forms, the two most prominent are physician-hospital organizations (PHOs) and integrated salary models (ISMs) (Burns and Muller, 2008). PHOs are joint ventures designed to develop new services (e.g., ambulatory care clinics) or, more commonly, to attract managed care contracts. ISMs are arrangements in which a hospital acquires a physician's practice, establishes an employment contract with the physician for a defined period, and negotiates a guaranteed base salary with a variable component based on office productivity, with some expectation that the physician will refer or admit patients to the hospital.

Within PHOs and ISMs, there are diverse relationships among physicians and hospitals that fall into three broad categories: noneconomic integration, economic integration, and clinical integration (Burns and Muller, 2008). Noneconomic integration includes hospital marketing of physicians' practices, physician use of medical office buildings, physician liaison programs, physician leadership development, and hospital support for physician technology requests. Economic integration includes the PHO and ISM models above, as well as physician recruitment, part-time compensation, leases and participating bond transactions, service-line development, and equity joint ventures. Clinical integration encompasses practice profiling, performance feedback, medical/demand/disease management programs, continuous quality-improvement programs, and linkages via clinical information systems.

If success were gauged by interest among hospitals and physicians, these collaborations are doing quite well. Other evidence, however, is mixed. On one hand, there is a wealth of evidence that suggests that physicians are satisfied with these relationships to the extent that they receive valued services (e.g., management of their practices) and are shielded from financial risk (Bazzoli et al., 2004). On the other hand, evidence is inconclusive that hospitals value these relationships. In particular, a review of the empirical literature suggests that collaboration based on economic integration yields few consistent effects on cost, quality, or clinical integration. Alliances based on noneconomic integration are widespread, but have not been subjected to rigorous academic study. Finally, alliances based on clinical integration have had positive, but weaker-than-expected, impacts on quality of care (Burns and Muller, 2008).

There may be several reasons for the varied and relatively weak performance of hospital-physician ventures. One reason is the structural form used to implement them. These ventures are typically organized, financed, and controlled by the hospital, with little physician participation. Not surprisingly, physicians balk at partnerships in which they have little power. A second, related explanation is the lack of infrastructure in many alliances. Hospitals often develop alliances as external contracting vehicles to approach the managed care market but fail to develop the internal mechanisms that will help the alliance partners to manage risk (Kale and Singh, 2009). Such mechanisms include physician compensation and productivity systems, quality monitoring and measurement, and physician selection (Burns and Thorpe, 1997). Finally, alliances often focus on taking advantage of fee-for-service reimbursement systems and seek to increase numbers of patients and procedures rather than deliver more appropriate care.

These findings suggest that careful attention to infrastructure is critical for the success of physician-hospital alliances (Zajac et al., 1991). In the absence of the mechanisms discussed above, one would expect alliances to yield little impact on quality and cost of care. In fact, two recent studies have addressed this issue directly. Cuellar and Gertler (2005) and Madison (2004) report that PHO alliances do not lower the cost of care. Indeed, they may lead to higher prices due to the combined bargaining power of the parties.

TABLE D-3 Summary of Empirical Studies of Outcomes of Collaboration Among Health Care Organizations

Outcomes	Hospital Collaboration	Physician Group Collaboration	Hospital-Physician Collaboration
Financial Performance	Higher prices; increased revenues and profit; little or no cost savings	Limited cost savings	Few consistent effects
Quality of Care	Few effects or decreased in quality	No evidence	Positive effects, but weaker than expected; inconsistent effects for clinical integration per se
Other Outcomes	The financial performance of two-hospital mergers is better than that of systems, which, in turn, have better financial performance than alliances	Mixed results for patient satisfaction; decreases in physician resource use depend on control mechanisms	Physician satisfaction increases with support services; inconclusive evidence for hospital satisfaction with hospital–physician collaboration

SUMMARY

Table D-3 summarizes the major results from studies of the outcomes associated with the three major forms of collaboration I examined. As indicated, the strongest outcome seems to be that the financial performance of hospitals benefits from collaboration with other hospitals. Results for other outcomes are mixed and, importantly, there is substantial variation in the performance of collaborative ventures.

MAKING COLLABORATION WORK: IMPLEMENTATION AND ORGANIZATIONAL CHANGE

Researchers and practitioners have proposed several explanations to account for the substantial variation observed in the performance of collaborative ventures in health care and non-health care fields. The explanations themselves vary considerably and include, for example, a focus on improving

- due diligence and partner selection prior to implementing ventures;
- leadership to implement changes more effectively once a venture begins; and
- cultural integration of the partner organizations.

Following prior work, I consider the issues that these explanations raise in a three-part sequence: precollaboration activities, transition work, and postconsolidation follow-up (Zajac et al., 2010). Perhaps most importantly, in both research and practice, we need to give greater attention to the process of organizational change and implementation practices used in collaboration efforts. Indeed, prior research indicates that some practices for implementation and leading organizational change are more effective than others (Battilana et al., 2010; Cartwright and Schoenberg, 2006; Damschroeder et al., 2009; Kale and Singh, 2009). I explore this theme in more detail below, first by proposing and discussing a checklist of best practices to overcome typical barriers to effective collaboration. Next, I discuss the role of leadership and the organizational change processes needed to put these practices into effect. I conclude this section by applying concepts, principles, and practices from the checklist and leadership and change literatures to interpret evidence from studies in health care. In doing so, I show how best practices can overcome barriers to change.

Checklist for Managing the Implementation of Collaborative Ventures

Box D-1 shows a checklist of best practices or steps that prior research indicates could prevent or mitigate typical problems that organizations and managers encounter in collaboration projects. The list draws on empirical studies from health care and non-health care fields, and is organized in chronological sequence from precollaboration to follow-up work. It is important to note, however, that prior studies have examined only a few of these practices in combination and have not examined their importance relative to each other. Thus, it is difficult to draw conclusions about the extent to which any of the practices, or combinations thereof, might be more important than others for effective collaboration among health care organizations.

Precollaboration Issues

Selecting partners effectively is critical at this stage. An important distinction is that potential partners can relate to each other symbiotically as well as competitively, or sometimes both symbiotically and competitively (Hawley, 1950; Pfeffer and Salancik, 1978). Prior work indicates that collaborative ventures may be more likely to emerge when potential partners

BOX D-1
Checklist for Effective Implementation of Collaborative Ventures Among Health Care Organizations

I. Precollaboration Issues
  a. Cost-benefit analysis
    i. Choosing a collaboration model
    ii. Potential for reconfiguring resources through collaboration
  b. Partner selection
    i. Strategic intent
      1. Mutual and individual organizational interests
      2. Mission/vision alignment
    ii. Cultural compatibility
    iii. Context
  c. Strategic planning
    i. Planning committee
    ii. Setting priorities

II. Transition Issues
  a. Governance
    i. Monitoring and evaluation
    ii. Problem analysis and solution
  b. Decision making
  c. Conflict management
  d. Critical success and failure factors
    i. Speed of collaboration
    ii. Communication with employees

III. Follow-Up Issues
  a. Cultural integration
  b. Human resources
    i. Redeploying; managing layoffs; reducing employee resistance
  c. Operational integration
    i. Resource allocation
  d. Ongoing governance

have complementary relationships such that one organization uses some services or products from the other, as opposed to a relationship in which two organizations must vie for the same resources. A common example of such complementarity or symbiosis is a rural community hospital that refers cases for tertiary care to an urban teaching hospital. A recent review of 40 studies of alliances concluded that the complementarity of partners not only promotes alliance formation, but also contributes to alliance performance (Shah and Swaminathan, 2008).

Partner selection also should take into account potential antitrust issues. Mergers, alliances, and joint ventures have often served as vehicles to leverage managed care payers, for example, and thus have run afoul of antitrust actions taken by the Federal Trade Commission and the Department of Justice (Casalino, 2006).

Considerations about the form of collaboration are also important at this stage. Each potential partner should plan carefully by constructing net present valuations of alternative relationships on a continuum ranging from maintaining the status quo (i.e., maintaining independence and arm's-length transactions with other organizations) to forming alliances or joint ventures (i.e., a formal cooperative arrangement among organizations, preserving the independent identity of each partner) to the merger of two or more organizations (Macneil, 1983). Perceptions of what each partner seeks also should be communicated clearly at this time, enabling the precise identification of similarities and differences that can form the basis for mutually beneficial exchanges.

Thus, in this early stage, there is preliminary communication and negotiation concerning mutual and individual organizational interests. As a result, the partners learn not only about each other's interests, but also about their compatibility, that is, the fit between their working styles and cultures. An organization's behavior in this stage can set a precedent for future exchanges and provides information about the expected behavior of its partner. During this phase, initial norms are being forged and commitments tested in small but important ways to determine credibility (Macneil, 1983).

Though it is important for the expectations of partners to be realistic, it turns out that many young ventures have broadly-stated goals that do not necessarily coincide with their activities. This is because goal statements reflect compromises made by partners who are, as of yet, not willing to subordinate their interests to those of the venture as a whole.

Finally, in a useful summary, Kale and Singh (2009) conclude that variation in the performance of alliances stems from variation in the management and organizational capabilities of alliance partners; Marks et al. (2001) draw a similar conclusion about mergers. In short, management literature suggests that experience in collaborative efforts (e.g., the extent to which an organization has been involved in strategic alliances previously) plays a crucial role in determining their success (Anand and Khanna, 2000; Hoang and Rothaermel, 2005).

Transition Phase

In this stage, partners should establish mechanisms for decision making and overall control of activities, or what is generally termed *governance* (Kale and Singh, 2009). Typical governance mechanisms include (1) joint ownership, in which the partners share control of some or all assets, (2) contracts that specify the rights and obligations of partners, (3) informal agreements that rely on trust and goodwill, or (4) some combination of these (Puranam and Vanneste, 2009).

Research to date does not suggest that any one of these mechanisms is superior, but rather that it is important to match a governance approach to the particular needs of a collaborative effort. Informal agreements may work effectively, for example, when the partners know each other well and activities are not complex or do not involve a high degree of risk. In any case, establishing a governance mechanism may be rocky because organizations are reluctant to grant authority to others or to sacrifice their own autonomy. It is thus critical that managers ensure that initial efforts and programs are responsive to partners' needs, in order to build their commitment to collaboration.

Collaboration projects of any form vary in the extent to which their partners are willing to commit resources to initiate and sustain programs and activities. An important weakness of many projects is their inability to gain adequate commitment of partners' resources (D'Aunno and Zuckerman, 1987). For example, there may be "free-rider" problems, in which some members of collaborations make little commitment, yet benefit from the investments of others. It is likely that such problems are directly proportional to the value that members perceive in committing resources to a project. The more value that members perceive in active participation, the more resources (including relinquishing autonomy) they are willing to commit to a project.

Of course, this leads to a challenging "chicken and egg" dilemma. On one hand, partners increase their commitment in proportion to threats from their environment and a particular partnership's ability to reduce those threats and uncertainty. On the other hand, to be effective in meeting members' needs, a partnership requires the investment of valued resources from members as well as members' willingness to coordinate efforts with each other. At some point, collaboration requires an investment of resources by partners who have no certainty of return equal to their investment. At this point, trust becomes particularly important (D'Aunno and Zuckerman, 1987).

Recent studies suggest that alliance capabilities are also important antecedents for success, mediating the effects of experience (Heimeriks and Duysters, 2007; Schilke and Goerzen, 2010). These capabilities include the ability to manage

- contract design (Argyres and Mayer, 2007; Reuer and Arino, 2007);
- interorganizational coordination (Schreiner et al., 2009);
- coordination of several alliances simultaneously (Hoffmann, 2007);

- interorganizational learning (Kale and Singh, 2007); and
- change processes (Schilke and Goerzen, 2010).

Follow-Up Issues

Many challenges in this phase result from ineffective management of key issues early in the life of a partnership. One important example comes from a study by Judge and Dooley (2006), who analyzed factors associated with both opportunistic behavior and alliance performance in the U.S. health care industry. Opportunistic behavior consists of actions primarily driven by one's own interest without regard for the interest of one's partners. These researchers found that partner trustworthiness and contractual safeguards were negatively related to opportunistic behavior, which was negatively related to alliance performance. In other words, alliances where sufficient contractual safeguards are in place, and where trust exists between partners, see less opportunistic behavior from individual partners and stronger alliance performance. Trust was found to have a stronger impact on opportunistic behavior than contractual safeguards.

LEADERSHIP COMPETENCIES FOR IMPLEMENTING ORGANIZATIONAL CHANGE[3]

I argue that using the techniques outlined in the above checklist (Box D-1) and overcoming barriers to effective collaboration is one of the defining challenges for leaders. The critical role of leadership has been largely neglected in prior work, which has focused mainly on the technical aspects of launching and managing mergers, alliances, and joint ventures, or, more often, their outcomes.

Though formal strategic assessment and planning are important elements of effective collaboration (see Box D-1), a far more challenging task is implementing change in organizations once a direction has been selected. Over the past two decades, research has explored the relationship between leadership characteristics or behaviors and organizational change (for reviews, see Bass, 1999; Conger and Kanungo, 1998; House and Aditya, 1997; Yukl, 1999, 2006). There is growing evidence that individuals' leadership characteristics and behaviors influence the success or failure of organizational change initiatives (see, e.g., Berson and Avolio, 2004; Bommer et al., 2005; Eisenbach et al., 1999; Fiol et al., 1999; Gentry and Leslie,

[3] This section of the paper, which examines leadership competencies for organizational change, draws heavily from a useful article by Battilana and colleagues (2010), which reports results from a study of leadership and organizational change in the English National Health Service (which I directed from 2002 to 2006).

2007; Higgs and Rowland, 2000, 2005; House et al., 1991; Howell and Higgins, 1990; Nadler and Tushman, 1990; Struckman and Yammarino, 2003; Waldman et al., 2004).

Most of the leadership studies that examine the relationship between leadership and change do not, however, account for the complexity of intraorganizational processes (Yukl, 1999), including the complexity of the organizational change implementation process. The fact that planned organizational change implementation involves different activities in which leadership competencies might play different roles has largely been ignored by the leadership literature (Higgs and Rowland, 2005).

In contrast, the literature on organizational change addresses the complexity of the change process (for a review, see Armenakis and Bedeian, 1999; Van de Ven and Poole, 1995) as well as the role of managers in various change implementation activities (e.g., Galpin, 1996; Judson, 1991; Kotter, 1995; Lewin, 1947; Rogers, 1962). Yet, an implicit common assumption of most of these studies is that leaders already possess the requisite competencies, skills, and abilities to engage in the different change implementation activities.

Effective Leadership for Planned Organizational Change

Notwithstanding a multitude of concepts that leadership researchers have advanced (for a review, see House and Aditya, 1997), there is general agreement that the task-oriented and person-oriented behaviors model (Bass, 1990; House and Baetz, 1979; Stodgill and Coons, 1957) remains an important foundation for managerial leadership (Judge et al., 2004). Of all the leadership competencies that are likely to influence organizational change, the ability to (1) provide effective direction for tasks (i.e., effectiveness at task-oriented behaviors), and (2) effectively engage followers (i.e., effectiveness at person-oriented behaviors) are among the most important (Nadler and Tushman, 1999).

Task-oriented skills are those related to organizational structure, design, and control, and to establishing routines to attain organizational goals and objectives (Bass, 1990). These functions are important not only for achieving organizational goals, but also for developing change initiatives (House and Aditya, 1997; Huy, 1999; Nadler and Tushman, 1990; Yukl, 2006).

Person-oriented skills include behaviors that promote collaborative interaction among organization members, establish a supportive social climate, and promote management practices that ensure equitable treatment of organization members (Bass, 1990). These interpersonal skills are critical to planned organizational change implementation because they enable

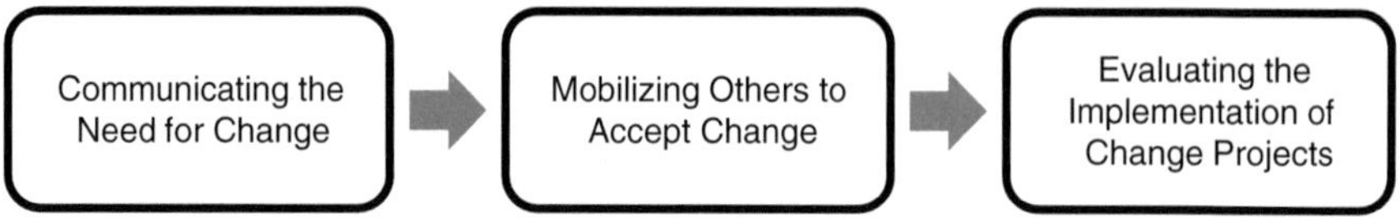

FIGURE D-2 Three key activities for effective organizational change.

leaders to motivate and direct followers (Chemers, 2001; van Knippenberg and Hogg, 2003; Yukl, 2006).

Effectiveness at task- and person-oriented behaviors requires different, but related, sets of competencies. Effectiveness at task-oriented behaviors hinges on the ability to clarify task requirements and structure tasks around an organization's mission and objectives (Bass, 1990). Effectiveness at person-oriented behaviors, on the other hand, relies on the ability to show consideration for others as well as to take into account one's own and others' emotions (Gerstner and Day, 1997; Graen and Uhl-Bien, 1995; Seltzer and Bass, 1990). Managers might be effective at both task- and person-oriented leadership behaviors, or they might be effective at only one or the other, or perhaps at neither. Managers need a mix of leadership competencies for effectively leading planned organizational change.

Leaders undertake specific activities to implement planned organizational change projects (Galpin, 1996; Judson, 1991; Kotter, 1995; Lewin, 1947; Rogers, 1962); mistakes in the execution of any of these activities or efforts to bypass some of them are detrimental to the progress of change (Armenakis and Bedeian, 1999). Prior conceptual and empirical work (Armenakis et al., 1999; Burke and Litwin, 1992; Ford and Greer, 2005; Galpin, 1996; Judson, 1991; Kotter, 1995; Lewin, 1947; Steers and Black, 1994) recurrently emphasizes three key activities associated with successful implementations of planned organizational change: communicating, mobilizing, and evaluating (see Figure D-2). *Communicating* refers to activities leaders undertake to make the case for change and to share their vision of the need for change with followers. *Mobilizing* refers to actions leaders undertake to gain coworkers' support for and acceptance of the enactment of new work routines. *Evaluating* refers to measures leaders employ to monitor and assess the impact of implementation efforts and to institutionalize changes.

Communicating the Need for Organizational Change

To destabilize the status quo and paint a picture of the desired new state for followers, leaders must communicate the need for change. Organization members need to understand why behaviors and routines must change (Fiol et al., 1999; Kotter, 1995). Resistance to change initiatives is partly attributable to organization members' emotional reactions, stemming, for example, from threats to self-esteem (Nadler, 1982), confusion and anxiety (Kanter, 1983), or stress related to uncertainty (Olson and Tetrick, 1988).

Leaders skilled at interpersonal interaction are able to monitor and discriminate among their own and others' emotions, and to use this information to guide thinking and action (Goleman, 1998; Salovey and Mayer, 1990). They are able to recognize and leverage their own and others' emotional states to solve problems and regulate behaviors (Huy, 1999). In the context of planned organizational change, consideration for others makes them likely to anticipate the emotional reactions of those involved in the change process and to take the required steps to attend to those reactions (Huy, 2002; Oreg, 2003). They are likely to emphasize communication of why the change is needed and to discuss the nature of the change and thereby reduce organization members' confusion and uncertainty.

In contrast, leaders who are effective at task-oriented behaviors are organizational architects (Bass, 1985, 1990). Rather than communicating the need for change, task-oriented leaders are likely to concentrate their energies on developing the procedures, processes, and systems required to implement planned organizational change. Because they are also more likely to keep psychological distance from their followers, task-oriented leaders may be less inclined to put emphasis on communicating activities (Blau and Scott, 1962).

Mobilizing Others to Accept Change

During implementation, leaders must mobilize organization members to accept and adopt proposed initiatives into their daily routines (Higgs and Rowland, 2005; Kotter, 1995; Oreg, 2003). Mobilizing is made difficult by participants' different personal and professional objectives and thus different outlooks on the initiative. Organization members who have something to gain will usually rally around a new initiative; those who have something to lose resist it (Bourne and Walker, 2005; Greenwood and Hinings, 1996).

The objective of mobilizing is to develop the capacity of organization members to commit to, and cooperate with, the planned course of action (Huy, 1999). To do this, leaders must create a coalition to support the change project (Kotter, 1985, 1995). Creating such a coalition is a political process that entails both appealing to organization members' cooperation and initiating organizational processes and systems that enable that cooperation (Nadler and Tushman, 1990; Tushman and O'Reilly, 1997). Mobilizing thus entails both person- and task-oriented skills.

Securing buy-in and support from the various organization members can be an emotionally-charged process (Huy, 1999). Person-oriented leaders show consideration for others and are good at managing others' feelings and emotions (Bass, 1990). They value communication as a means of fostering individual and group participation, and explicitly request contributions from members at different management levels (Vera and Crossan, 2004). Effective communicators and managers of emotions can marshal commitment to an organization's vision and inspire organization members to work toward its realization (Egri and Herman, 2000). Their inclination to take others into account makes them more likely to pay attention to individuals' attitudes toward change and to anticipate the need to involve others in the change process.

Mobilizing also implies redesigning existing organizational processes and systems in order to push all organization members to adopt the change (Kotter, 1995; Tushman and O'Reilly, 1997). For example, if a leader wants to implement a new system of quality improvement but does not change the reward system accordingly, organization members will have little incentive to adopt the new system. Redesigning existing organizational processes and systems to facilitate coalition building requires task-oriented skills.

Leaders who are effective at task-oriented behaviors are skilled in designing organizational processes and systems that induce people to adopt new work patterns (Bass, 1990). Their focus on completing tasks leads them to identify the different stakeholders involved in the change effort and to build systems that facilitate their involvement. Because they focus on structure, systems, and procedures, task-oriented leaders are more likely to be aware of the need to put in place systems that facilitate people's rallying behind new objectives. As skilled architects, they are also more likely to know how to redesign existing organizational processes and systems in order to facilitate coalition building.

Evaluating the Implementation of Change Projects

Finally, leaders need to evaluate the extent to which organization members are performing the routines, practices, or behaviors targeted in the planned change initiative. As champions of the organization's mission and goals, leaders have a role in evaluating the content of change initiatives and ensuring that organization members comply with new work routines (Yukl, 2006). Before the change becomes institutionalized, leaders need to step back to assess both the new processes and procedures that have been put in place and their impact on the organization's performance.

Leaders who are highly skilled at social interaction might be more likely to have a positive attitude toward change projects and to view change as a positive challenge (Vakola et al., 2004). Their own positive feelings and attitudes toward change might lead these leaders to overestimate the success and impact of the planned change project and thus fail to invest the required time and resources in objectively assessing the process, progress, and outcomes. To avoid dissonance, they might be reluctant to engage in a process of evaluation that could contradict their positive perception of the change (Bacharach et al., 1996).

Task-oriented leaders naturally tend to focus on the tasks that must be performed to achieve the targeted performance improvements (Bass, 1990). Their attention to structure and performance objectives attunes them to the attainment of these objectives. They are both aware of the need to analyze goals and achievements and comfortable with the need to refine processes following evaluation.

APPLICATION TO HEALTH CARE STUDIES ON THE PROCESSES AND PRACTICES OF COLLABORATION

In this section, I apply the concepts, principles, and practices summarized above to interpret the results of studies of the processes of change in collaborative ventures in health care (see Table D-4). I examine results from studies of hospital and physician collaboration, using the three major categories of these projects discussed above.

Lessons from Collaboration Among Hospitals

Results from several studies show that certain initial changes in collaborative ventures among hospitals come quickly, relatively easily, and in sequence: (1) integration of management functions (e.g., finance and accounting, human resources, managed care contracting, quality assurance and improvement programs, and strategic planning), followed by (2) integration of patient support functions (e.g., patient education), and then (3) integration of low-volume clinical services (e.g., Eberhardt, 2001).

Integrating or consolidating larger-scale clinical services and closure of service lines typically encounters strong opposition—in many cases studied, clinical service integration did not occur at all. Similarly, some studies report little success at integrating the medical cultures of merged hospitals even after 3 years of effort. In short, substantial changes in core clinical services take a long time and success is not guaranteed, as conflicting interests often emerge among stakeholders.

Despite these difficulties, however, there are examples of successful collaboration in which contextual factors and change processes made important contributions. Specifically, results from several case studies show that creating a centralized decision-making authority promotes effective collaboration, especially to the extent that this authority can develop shared

TABLE D-4 Application of Best Practices to Collaboration Among Health Care Organizations: Technical and People-Focused Leadership Tasks

Technical Leadership Tasks	Best Practices
Plans and protocols for change are needed (see Box 5-2 in Chapter 5)	Blueprints are needed to manage complexity and promote due diligence and effective decision making by leaders of change (e.g., conducting thorough premerger assessment of potential partners)
Technical capacity building	Investment (time, money) is needed to build capacity for improved performance
Structures and systems to support change	Structures (especially incentives) and systems (especially information systems) are needed to promote change and to improve organizational performance
People-Focused Leadership Tasks	
External pressure	In most cases, external pressure/support for change increases both its speed and likelihood of success
Buy-in from all levels; critical role of central authority and shared vision	Support from top managers and leaders is essential, but buy-in is also needed from lower-level staff; a centralized group with authority for implementation of changes is critical, especially to develop a shared vision and goals for change
Communication	Communication is needed at all levels: What is the vision; why change is needed; what progress has been achieved
Role of physician leaders	Involvement of physician leaders, both formal and informal, in key decisions is critical to success
Managing tensions, trade-offs inherent in change	Involving physicians versus respecting their time for patient care; time needed to build trust versus frustration with slow progress; building stakeholder buy-in versus building technical capacity (especially when buy-in and trust are enhanced by demonstrated technical capacity and improved performance)
Core versus peripheral organizational features	Change in peripheral features of organizations, including management and support services, is easier to achieve than change in either core clinical services or organizational culture

values and vision with which the partner organizations learn to identify (Bazzoli et al., 2004). Further, support from top managers is critical, but should be complemented by buy-in from lower levels. This requires a great deal of communication within and across levels of hierarchy. Finally, at least one study identified strong and continuous external pressure on the partner organizations as a key to promoting the integration of clinical services.

Lessons from Collaboration Among Physician Groups

Coddington et al. (1998) provide a useful case study of the early stages of change that focus on bringing physician partners together. The key phases are (1) establishing trust, (2) assessing the fit between the relative strengths of the organizations, (3) assessing the ability to deliver a high-quality product, (4) developing a business strategy, and (5) considering effects on competitive position. Similarly, Robinson (1998) emphasized the importance of fit and relative strengths of partners in bringing them together.

In general, results from studies of collaboration among physician groups emphasize the importance of managing trade-offs and tensions involved in organizational change, for example,

- involving physicians versus respecting their time for patient care;
- slowly building trust versus frustration with slow progress; and
- building stakeholder buy-in versus building technical capacity (especially when buy-in and trust are enhanced by demonstrated technical capacity and improved performance).

Lessons from Hospital-Physician Collaboration

Given the importance of hospital-physician collaboration and the obvious potential for complications, a relatively large number of process studies have focused on these relationships. A major observation is the importance of developing a climate for change within the partner organizations. In turn, the role of physician leadership is universally noted as critical in developing a supportive climate for change; physician involvement is needed in both governance and management decisions. Results also highlight the importance of putting in place structures (such as incentives) and systems (especially information systems) to support changes in organizational processes and culture. As noted above, investment in management, clinical technologies, and core competencies matters, as do shared vision and values.

The work of Devers and colleagues (1994) stands out for its development of a three-part framework for assessing the extent to which consolidations achieve (1) functional integration (business and management activities, noted above), (2) physician-system integration (alignment of incentives and physician involvement in decision making), and (3) clinical integration (e.g., common protocols). They find much functional integration but little integration in the other areas—a result similar to that for collaboration among hospitals. The results are discouraging, but it appears that external context can promote change—pressure from capitation and regulation, in particular, are related to more effective integration.

CONCLUDING OBSERVATIONS

I have several concluding observations about the outcomes associated with collaboration among health care organizations and best practices for improving these outcomes. First, there is considerable variation in the outcomes of collaborative ventures, regardless of the criteria one uses to assess their performance. Many, if not most, of these ventures fail to meet expectations in either the health care or the non–health care fields. An exception to this result is hospital mergers, which seem to improve members' financial performance, though not necessarily to societal advantage; available evidence indicates that improved performance comes mainly from increased market power rather than efficiency from gains.

Second, the financial performance of hospital mergers appears to be stronger than results obtained from other forms of collaboration. Mergers typically involve more centralization of authority compared with other collaborative ventures, such as alliances, and this may be an important factor in their relative success.

Third, mergers are more costly than alternatives for the organizations (and communities) involved, at least in terms of initial time and money needed to launch and implement them. Yet, one could argue that the risk involved in mergers seems to pay off for the hospitals themselves, though not uniformly, given the variation that researchers observe in their performance.

Fourth, given substantial variation in their performance and relatively weak overall outcomes for many collaborative ventures, researchers and practitioners have begun to identify best practices for leading the processes involved in their implementation. Though results to date are useful, there is much more work to be done; for example, though I presented a relatively thorough checklist of best practices for implementing collaborative ventures (see Box D-1), few studies have examined the use of many of these practices in combination.

Fifth, the best available evidence indicates that it is useful to conceive of these practices from the perspective of three phases or stages: (1) precollaboration activities, (2) transition work, and (3) follow-up efforts. Further, these practices focus primarily on either technical tasks (e.g., due diligence with respect to antitrust issues, development of strategic plans, and development of systems and incentives for change and improved performance) or people-oriented tasks (e.g., communicating effectively, involving key stakeholders, overcoming resistance to change) (see Box D-1). Prior studies indicate that leaders need skills for both technical and people-oriented tasks and, importantly, that failure to address both sets of tasks hinders implementation and performance (Battilana et al., 2010).

Sixth, in general, the literature on collaboration and change among health care organizations has not given as much attention to the role of leadership as it should. To be sure, the importance of involving physicians in leadership roles is typically noted, but more fine-grained analyses are lacking (Gilmartin and D'Aunno, 2007). I argue that effective leaders will communicate the need for change, mobilize others to accept changes, and evaluate implementation to make needed adjustments and promote optimal outcomes. Further, though leaders need skills in both technical and people-oriented tasks to be effective, many individuals lack this combination of skills, requiring the need for training or team approaches to leading change.

Finally, relatively fragmented and narrow disciplinary approaches have hindered both research and practice in this area. For example, the vast majority of studies of hospital mergers focus on financial performance (Vogt and Town, 2006), with little attention given to other key outcomes, such as access to care, and, similarly, with little attention to leadership using the concepts and principles discussed above. Promoting more effective collaboration in health care will require a broader, interdisciplinary approach. Indeed, it is likely that current collaborative ventures among health care organizations may face greater challenges than in the past due to the increased complexity of the organizations themselves, including, for example, the difficulty of integrating their information technologies. The current state of practice does not augur well for implementation of the ACA in general or accountable care organizations in particular—a type of organization that depends heavily on collaboration across organizational boundaries.

REFERENCES

Alexander, J. A., and M. A. Morrisey. 1988. Hospital-physician integration and hospital costs. *Inquiry* 25(3):388–401.

Anand, B. N., and T. Khanna. 2000. Do firms learn to create value? The case of alliances. *Strategic Management Journal* 21(3):295–315.

Argyres, N. S., and K. J. Mayer. 2007. Contract design as a firm capability: An integration of learning and transaction cost perspectives. *Academy of Management Review* 32(4):1060–1077.

Armenakis, A. A., and A. G. Bedeian. 1999. Organizational change: A review of theory and research in the 1990s. *Journal of Management* 25(3):293–315.

Armenakis, A., S. Harris, and H. Field. 1999. Paradigms in organizational change: Change agent and change target perspectives. In *Handbook of organizational behavior*, edited by R. Golembiewski. New York: Marcel Dekker. Pp. 631–658.

Bacharach, S., P. Bamberger, and W. Sonnenstuhl. 1996. The organizational transformation process: The micropolitics of dissonance reduction and the alignment of logics of action. *Administrative Science Quarterly* 41(3):477–506.

Bass, B. M. 1985. *Leadership and performance beyond expectations*. New York: Free Press.

Bass, B. M. 1990. *Bass and Stogdill's handbook of leadership*. New York: Free Press.

Bass, B. M. 1999. Two decades of research and development in transformational leadership. *European Journal of Work and Organizational Psychology* 8(1):9–32.

Battilana, J., M. J. Gilmartin, M. Sengul, A.-C. Pache, and J. Alexander. 2010. Leadership competencies for planned organizational change. *Leadership Quarterly* 21(3):422–438.

Bazzoli, G. J., S. M. Shortell, N. Dubbs, C. Chan, and P. Kralovec. 1999. A taxonomy of health networks and systems: Bringing order out of chaos. *Health Services Research* 33(6):1683–1717.

Bazzoli, G. J., C. Chan, S. M. Shortell, and T. D'Aunno. 2000. The financial performance of hospitals belonging to health networks and systems. *Inquiry* 37(3):234–252.

Bazzoli, G. J., L. M. Manheim, and T. M. Waters. 2003. U.S. hospital industry restructuring and the hospital safety net. *Inquiry* 40(1):6–24.

Bazzoli, G. J., L. Dynan, L. R. Burns, and C. Yap. 2004. Two decades of organizational change in health care: What have we learned? *Medical Care Research and Review* 61(3):247–331.

Bazzoli, G. J., S. M. Shortell, and N. L. Dubbs. 2006. Rejoinder to taxonomy of health networks and systems: A reassessment. *Health Services Research* 41(3 Pt 1):629–639.

Berson, Y., and B. J. Avolio. 2004. Transformational leadership and the dissemination of organizational goals: A case study of a telecommunication firm. *Leadership Quarterly* 15(5):625–646.

Blau, P. M., and W. R. Scott. 1962. *Formal organizations*. San Francisco: Chandler.

Bommer, W. H., G. A. Rich, and R. S. Rubin. 2005. Changing attitudes about change: Longitudinal effects of transformational leader behavior on employee cynicism about organizational change. *Journal of Organizational Behavior* 26(7):733–753.

Boukus, E., A. Cassil, and A. S. O'Malley. 2009. *A snapshot of U.S. physicians: Key findings from the 2008 Health Tracking Physician Survey*. Data Bulletin No. 35, Center for Studying Health System Change, Washington, DC.

Bourne, L., and D. Walker. 2005. Visualizing and mapping stakeholder influence. *Management Decision* 43(5):649–660.

Burke, W., and G. Litwin. 1992. A causal model of organizational performance and change. *Journal of Management* 18:523–545.

Burns, L. R. 1997. Physician practice management companies. *Health Care Management Review* 22(4):32–46.

Burns, L. R., and R. W. Muller. 2008. Hospital-physician collaboration: Landscape of economic integration and impact on clinical integration. *Milbank Quarterly* 86(3):375–434.

Burns, L., and D. Thorpe. 1997. Physician-hospital organizations: Strategy, structure and conduct. In *The organization and management of physician services: Evolving trends*, edited by R. Conners. Chicago, IL: American Hospital Publishing.

Capps, C. 2005. *The quality effects of hospital mergers*. Unpublished manuscript.

Cartwright, S., and R. Schoenberg. 2006. Thirty years of mergers and acquisition research: Recent advances and future opportunities. *British Journal of Management* 17(S1):S1–S5.

Casalino, L. P. 2006. The Federal Trade Commission, clinical integration, and the organization of physician practice. *Journal of Health Politics, Policy and Law* 31(3):569–585.

Chemers, M. M. 2001. Leadership effectiveness: An integrative review. In *Blackwell handbook of social psychology: Group processes*, edited by M. A. Hogg and R. S. Tindale. Oxford, UK: Blackwell.

Clement, J. P., M. J. McCue, R. D. Luke, J. D. Bramble, L. F. Rossiter, Y. A. Ozcan, and C. W. Pai. 1997. Strategic hospital alliances: Impact on financial performance. *Health Affairs* 16(6):193–203.

Coddington, D. C., K. D. Moore, and R. L. Clarke. 1998. *Capitalizing medical groups: Positioning physicians for the future*. New York: McGraw-Hill.

Conger, J. A., and R. N. Kanungo. 1998. *Charismatic leadership in organizations*. Thousand Oaks, CA: Sage.

Cuellar, A. E., and P. J. Gertler. 2005. How the expansion of hospital systems has affected consumers. *Health Affairs* 24(1):213–219.

Damschroder, L. J., D. C. Aron, R. E. Keith, S. R. Kirsh, J. A. Alexander, and J. C. Lowery. 2009. Fostering implementation of health services research findings into practice: A consolidated framework for advancing implementation science. *Implementation Science* 4:50.

D'Aunno, T., and H. S. Zuckerman. 1987. A life cycle model of organizational federations: The case of hospitals. *Academy of Management Review* 12(3):534–545.

Devers, K. J., S. M. Shortell, R. R. Gillies, D. A. Anderson, J. B. Mitchell, and K. L. Erickson. 1994. Implementing organized delivery systems: An integration scorecard. *Health Care Management Review* 19(3):7–20.

Dranove, D., and R. Lindrooth. 2003. Hospital consolidation and costs: Another look at the evidence. *Journal of Health Economics* 22(6):983–997.

Dranove, D., A. Durkac, and M. Shanley. 1996. Are multihospital systems more efficient? *Health Affairs* 15(Spring):100–103.

Eberhardt, J. L. 2001. Merger failure: A five year journey examined. *Healthcare Financial Management* 55(4):37–39.

Egri, C. P., and S. Herman. 2000. Leadership in the North American environmental sector: Values, leadership styles and contexts of environmental leaders and their organizations. *Academy of Management Journal* 43:571–604.

Eisenbach, R., K. Watson, and R. Pillai. 1999. Transformational leadership in the context of organizational change. *Journal of Organizational Change Management* 12(2):80–89.

Fiol, C. M., D. Harris, and R. House. 1999. Charismatic leadership: Strategies for effecting social change. *Leadership Quarterly* 10(3):449–482.

Ford, M., and B. Greer. 2005. The relationship between management control system usage and planned change achievement: An exploratory study. *Journal of Change Management* 5(1):29–46.

Galpin, T. 1996. *The human side of change: A practical guide to organization redesign*. San Francisco: Jossey-Bass.

Gaynor, M. 2006. What do we know about competition and quality in health care markets? *Foundations and Trends in Microeconomics* 2(6):441–508.

Gentry, W. A., and J. B. Leslie. 2007. Competencies for leadership development: What's hot and what's not when assessing leadership-implications for organizational development. *Organizational Development Journal* 25(1):37–46.

Gerstner, C., and D. Day. 1997. Meta-analytic review of leader member exchange theory: Correlates and construct issues. *Journal of Applied Psychology* 82(6):827–844.

Gilmartin, M. J., and T. D'Aunno. 2007. Leadership research in health care: A review and roadmap. *Academy of Management Annals* 1:387–438.

Goleman, D. 1998. *Working with emotional intelligence*. London: Bloomsbury.

Graen, G., and M. Uhl-Bien. 1995. Relationship-based approach to leadership: Development of leader-member exchange (LMX) theory of leadership over 25 years: Applying a multi-level multi-domain perspective. *Leadership Quarterly* 6(2):219–247.

Greenwood, R., and C. R. Hinings. 1996. Understanding radical organizational change: Bringing together the old and the new institutionalism. *Academy of Management Review* 21(4):1022–1054.

Hansen, M. T. 2009. *Collaboration: How leaders avoid the traps, create unity, and reap big results.* Boston: Harvard Business School Publishing.

Harrison, T. D. 2011. Do mergers really reduce costs? Evidence from hospitals. *Economic Inquiry* 49(4):1054–1069.

Hawley, A. H. 1950. *Human ecology.* New York: Ronald Press.

Hayford, T. B. 2011. The impact of hospital mergers on treatment intensity and health outcomes. *Health Services Research* 47(3 Pt 1):1008–1029.

Heimeriks, K. H., and G. Duysters. 2007. Alliance capabilities as a mediator between experience and alliance performance: An empirical investigation into the alliance capability development process. *Journal of Management Studies* 44(1):25–49.

Higgs, M., and D. Rowland. 2000. Building change leadership capability: The quest for change competence. *Journal of Change Management* 1(2):116–130.

Higgs, M., and D. Rowland. 2005. All changes great and small: Exploring approaches to change and its leadership. *Journal of Change Management* 5(2):121–151.

Ho, V., and B. H. Hamilton. 2000. Hospital mergers and acquisitions: Does market consolidation harm patients? *Journal of Health Economics* 19(5):767–791.

Hoang, H., and F. T. Rothaermel. 2005. The effect of general and partner-specific alliance experience on joint R&D project performance. *Academy of Management Journal* 48(2):332–345.

Hoffmann, W. H. 2007. Strategies for managing a portfolio of alliances. *Strategic Management Journal* 28(8):827–856.

House, R. J., and R. N. Aditya. 1997. The social scientific study of leadership: Quo vadis? *Journal of Management* 23(3):409–473.

House, R., and M. L. Baetz. 1979. Leadership: Some empirical generalizations and new research directions. *Research in Organizational Behavior* 1:341–423.

House, R. J., W. D. Spangler, and J. Woycke. 1991. Personality and charisma in the U.S. presidency: A psychological theory of leader effectiveness. *Administrative Science Quarterly* 36(3):364–396.

Howell, J. M., and C. A. Higgins. 1990. Champions of technological innovation. *Administrative Science Quarterly* 35(2):317–341.

Huy, Q. 1999. Emotional capability, emotional intelligence and radical change. *Academy of Management Review* 24(2):325–345.

Huy, Q. 2002. Emotional balancing of organizational continuity and change: The contribution of middle managers. *Administrative Science Quarterly* 47:31–69.

Judge, T. A., R. F. Piccolo, and R. Ilies. 2004. The forgotten ones? The validity of consideration and initiating structure in leadership research. *Journal of Applied Psychology* 89:36–51.

Judge, W. Q., and R. Dooley. 2006. Strategic alliance outcomes: A transaction-cost economics perspective. *British Journal of Management* 17(1):23–37.

Judson, A. 1991. *Changing behavior in organization: Minimizing resistance to change.* Cambridge, MA: Basil Blackwell.

Kale, P., and H. Singh. 2007. Building firm capabilities through learning: The role of the alliance learning process in alliance capability and firm-level alliance success. *Strategic Management Journal* 28(10):981–1000.

Kale, P., and H. Singh. 2009. Management strategic alliances: What do we know now, and where do we go from here? *Academy of Management Perspectives* 23(3):45–62.

Kanter, R. M. 1983. *The change masters.* New York: Simon & Schuster.

Kastor, J. A. 2001. *Mergers of teaching hospitals in Boston, New York, and Northern California.* Ann Arbor: University of Michigan Press.

Kerr, E. A., B. S. Mittman, R. D. Hays, A. L. Siu, B. Leake, and R. H. Brook. 1995. Managed care and capitation in California: How do physicians at financial risk control their own utilization? *Annals of Internal Medicine* 123(7):500–504.

Kerr, E. A., B. S. Mittman, R. D. Hays, B. Leake, and R. H. Brook. 1996. Quality assurance in capitated physician groups. *Journal of the American Medical Association* 276(15):1236–1239.

King, D., D. Dalton, C. Daily, and J. Covin. 2004. Meta-analyses of post acquisition performance indications of unidentified moderators. *Strategic Management Journal* 25:187–200.

Kotter, J. 1985. *Power and influence.* New York: Free Press.

Kotter, J. 1995. Leading change: Why transformation efforts fail. *Harvard Business Review* 73(2):59–67.

Kralewski, J. E., T. D. Wingert, and M. H. Barbouche. 1996. Assessing the culture of medical group practices. *Medical Care* 34(5):377–388.

Kralewski, J. E., E. C. Rich, T. Bernhardt, B. Dowd, R. Feldman, and C. Johnson. 1998. The organizational structure of medical group practices in a managed care environment. *Health Care Management Review* 23(2):76–96.

Kralewski, J. E., W. Wallace, T. D. Wingert, D. J. Knutson, and C. E. Johnson. 1999. The effects of medical group practice organizational factors on physicians' use of resources. *Journal of Healthcare Management* 44(3):167–183.

Kralewski, J. E., E. C. Rich, R. Feldman, B. E. Dowd, T. Bernhardt, C. Johnson, and W. Gold. 2000. The effects of medical group practice and physician payment methods on costs of care. *Health Services Research* 35(3):591–613.

Krishnan, R. A., S. Joshi, and H. Krishnan. 2004. The influence of mergers on firms' product-mix strategies. *Strategic Management Journal* 25(6):587–611.

Lewin, K. 1947. Frontiers in group dynamics. *Human Relations* 1:5–41.

Luke, R. D. 2006. Taxonomy of health networks and systems: A reassessment. *Health Services Research* 41(3 Pt 1):618–628.

Macneil, I. R. 1983. Values in contract: Internal and external. *Northwestern University Law Review* 78(2):340–418.

Madison, K. 2004. Hospital-physician affiliations and patient treatments, expenditures, and outcomes. *Health Services Research* 39(2):257–278.

Marks, M. L., P. H. Mirvis, and L. F. Brajkovich. 2001. Making mergers and acquisitions work: Strategic and psychological preparation. *Academy of Management Executive* 15(2):80–94.

Modern Healthcare. 2012. *18th annual hospital mergers and acquisitions report.* January 28. http://www.modernhealthcare.com/article/20120128/DATA/120129989# (accessed April 2, 2012).

Nadler, D. A. 1982. Managing transitions to uncertain future states. *Organizational Dynamics* 11:37–45.

Nadler, D. A., and M. L. Tushman. 1990. Beyond the charismatic leader: Leadership and organizational change. *California Management Review* 32(2):77–97.

Nadler, D. A., and M. L. Tushman. 1999. The organization of the future: Strategic imperatives and core competencies for the 21st century. *Organizational Dynamics* 28(1):45–60.

Olson, D. A., and L. E. Tetrick. 1988. Organizational restructuring: The impact of role perceptions, work relationships and satisfaction. *Group and Organization Studies* 13(3): 374–389.

Oreg, S. 2003. Resistance to change: Developing an individual differences measure. *Journal of Applied Psychology* 88(4):680–693.

Pettigrew, A. M., R. Woodman, and K. Cameron. 2001. Studying organizational change and development: Challenges for future research. *Academy of Management Journal* 44(4):697–713.

Pfeffer, J., and G. R. Salancik. 1978. *The external control of organizations.* New York: Harper and Row.

Puranam, P., and B. S. Vanneste. 2009. Trust and governance: Untangling a tangled web. *Academy of Management Review* 34(1):11–31.

Reuer, J. J., and A. Arino. 2007. Strategic alliance contracts: Dimensions and determinants of contractual complexity. *Strategic Management Journal* 28(3):313–330.

Robinson, J. C. 1998. Consolidation of medical groups into physician practice management organizations. *Journal of the American Medical Association* 279(2):144–149.

Rogers, E. M. 1962. *Diffusion of innovations.* New York: Free Press.

Salovey, P., and J. D. Mayer. 1990. Emotional intelligence. *Imagination, Cognition and Personality* 9:185–211.

Schilke, O., and A. Goerzen. 2010. Alliance management capability: An investigation of the construct and its measurement. *Journal of Management* 36(5):1192–1219.

Schreiner, M., P. Kale, and D. Corsten. 2009. What really is alliance management capability and how does it impact alliance outcomes and success? *Strategic Management Journal* 30(13):1395–1419.

Seltzer, J., and B. M. Bass. 1990. Transformational leadership: Beyond initiation and consideration. *Journal of Management* 16(4):693–704.

Shah, R. H., and V. Swaminathan. 2008. Factors influencing partner selection in strategic alliances: The moderating role of alliance context. *Strategic Management Journal* 29(5):471–494.

Steers, R. M., and J. S. Black. 1994. *Organizational behavior*. New York: Harper Collins.

Stodgill, R., and A. E. Coons. 1957. *Leader behavior: Its description and measurement.* Columbus: Ohio University, Bureau of Business Research.

Struckman, C. H., and F. J. Yammarino. 2003. Organizational change: A categorization scheme and response model with readiness factors. In *Research in Organizational Change and Development*, edited by R. W. Woodman and W. A. Pasmore. Greenwich, CT: JAI Press.

Trinh, H. Q., J. W. Begun, and R. D. Luke. 2010. Better to receive than to give? Interorganizational service arrangements and hospital performance. *Health Care Management Review* 35(1):88–97.

Tushman, M. L., and C. O'Reilly. 1997. *Winning through innovation: A practical guide to leading organizational change and renewal.* Cambridge, MA: Harvard Business School Press.

Vakola, M., I. Tsaousis, and I. Nikolaou. 2004. The role of emotional intelligence and personality variables on attitudes towards organizational change. *Journal of Managerial Psychology* 19(2):88–110.

Van de Ven, A. H., and M. S. Poole. 1995. Explaining development and change in organizations. *Academy of Management Review* 20(3):510–540.

van Knippenberg, D., and M. A. Hogg. 2003. A social identity model of leadership effectiveness in organizations. *Research in Organizational Behavior* 25:243–295.

Vera, D., and M. Crossan. 2004. Strategic leadership and organizational learning. *Academy of Management Review* 29(2):222–240.

Vogt, W. B., and R. Town. 2006. *How has hospital consolidation affected the price and quality of hospital care?* Research Synthesis Report No. 9. Princeton, NJ: Robert Wood Johnson Foundation, The Synthesis Project.

Waldman, D. A., M. Javidan, and P. Varella. 2004. Charismatic leadership at the strategic level: A new application of upper echelons theory. *Leadership Quarterly* 15(3):355–380.

Weick, K. E., and R. E. Quinn. 1999. Organizational change and development. *Annual Review of Psychology* 50:361–386.

Young, G. J., K. R. Desai, and F. J. Hellinger. 2000. Community control and pricing patterns of nonprofit hospitals: An antitrust analysis. *Journal of Health Politics, Policy and Law* 25(6):1051–1081.

Yukl, G. A. 1999. An evaluation of conceptual weaknesses in transformational and charismatic leadership theories. *Leadership Quarterly* 10(2):285–305.

Yukl, G. A. 2006. *Leadership in organizations*. 6th ed. Upper Saddle River, NJ: Prentice-Hall.

Zajac, E., B. R. Golden, and S. M. Shortell. 1991. New organizational forms for enhancing innovation: The case of internal corporate joint ventures. *Management Science* 37(2):170–184.

Zajac, E., T. D'Aunno, and L. R. Burns. 2010. Managing strategic alliances. In *Health care management: Organization design and behavior*. 6th ed. Albany, NY: Delmar.